Health Education in the Elementary School

Health Education in the Elementary School

Teaching for Relevance

WALTER H. GREENE **FRANK H. JENNE**
PATRICIA M. LEGOS Temple University

Macmillan Publishing Co., Inc.
New York

Collier Macmillan Publishers
London

Macmillan Publishing Co., Inc.
866 Third Avenue, New York, New York 10022

Collier Macmillan Canada, Ltd.

Library of Congress Cataloging in Publication Data

Greene, Walter H
  Health education in the elementary school.

  Includes bibliographies and index.
  1. Health education (Elementary)   I. Jenne,
Frank H., (date) joint author. II. Legos,
Patricia M., joint author. III. Title.
LB1587.A3G73   372.3'7   77–5911
ISBN 0–02–346590–5

Printing: 1 2 3 4 5 6 7 8   Year: 8 9 0 1 2 3 4

Preface

The past decade has been remarkable in terms of educational change. We have seen the advent of open schools, schools without walls, schools without failure, and storefront schools, to name a few. Much of this change seems motivated by a significant shift in our society's priorities away from spectacular space programs, military overkill, and rapid industrial expansion toward the basic human needs of the individual citizen. The battle against discrimination of all types continues unabated, medical care is rapidly coming to be regarded as a basic right, and job or career training is now directed toward the individual's economic welfare rather than toward any broad national goals.

The changes within the schools also are designed to place emphasis on the individual pupil as a human being. Teachers are becoming less directive and more facilitative; in this role they stress a need for greater freedom and decision making within (and outside) the classroom. Renewed emphasis is being placed on the teacher's task of providing a healthy emotional climate in the classroom as a stimulus to wholesome personality growth, and continued stress is placed not only on the identification of health problems of all types but also on aggressively finding help for or answers to these problems. In short, the elementary school is viewed as an organization of concerned adults interacting with children rather than one of taskmasters tutoring pupils.

The curriculum itself has been subject to the full effect of this general effort to humanize the school. Most significant here has been the shift from content to process, specifically to the skills and decision-making ability children will need in order to guide their lives and successfully deal with issues of concern to them now and in the future. This requires concern with helping students develop an awareness of their own feelings and emotions and providing them with more positive and viable alternatives for their health decisions.

v

Somewhat paradoxically, our quest for a point of departure for innovation and reform must begin with two very traditional questions: "What content is most meaningful to youngsters in health?" and "How can we teach it most effectively?" The pressures of the "space race," which peaked in the 1960s, caused the pendulum of educational philosophy to swing from an earlier preoccupation with teaching methods centered on Dewey's learning by doing to an intense interest in content. The chief result was the "new math," the "new biology," and other such projects that made up the curriculum reform movement of that era. The excessive emphasis of this movement on so-called hard subject matter for the better students prompted a counterreaction in favor of content focused on the personal needs of all students, including those who for various reasons are not so well adapted to conventional educational approaches. Efforts to reach this latter group demonstrated the need for new methods and techniques and thus brought the issue of content versus technique into better balance as applied to all students, not merely the "special" ones. Increasingly, educators are now rediscovering that how one goes about teaching is very closely related to what one tries to teach and that effective teaching depends to a great extent on the learner's interest in the subject. It is to be hoped that, this time around, educators are better prepared to realize the promise of this humanistic emphasis.

It is therefore our intent that this book have as its one central focus that of relevant human concerns. This means that within the school environment we will often be less concerned with the ambient temperature of the classroom than with the presence of security, openness, acceptance, and other factors affecting the emotional climate. Within the realm of school services we may be less concerned with height and weight records than we are with personality growth. And, most important, we may be less concerned with how comprehensive and scientifically demanding the health curriculum is than with what actually comes through to the pupils, how it is presented, and how the pupils feel about the material.

It is our feeling that effective teaching utilizes all levels of relevance. It is our general hypothesis that relevance is that which connects the affective or feeling aspects of learning and the cognitive or conceptualizing aspects. We believe, further, that a better linkage between the affective domain —the learner's concerns—and the practices of the school would reduce the discrepancy between knowledge and practices.

Although the focus of this text has been placed on the educational needs of children with respect to their lifelong health status, we recognize that the teacher and the school in general must often provide more direct assistance. The most cleverly devised learning experiences will go for naught if a child is too ill or too hungry to participate; it is fruitless to speak of love and trust within the context of a health lesson if an inept administration has allowed the school to become an armed camp with an incessantly bickering and backbiting staff. Therefore, we have challenged teachers to accept the larger role of child advocates with responsibilities far broader than mere intellectual growth. School health services and considerations for the overall school environment have thus been approached in a forthright manner designed to cut through the traditional maze of sterile policy statements, complex record systems, and legalistic referral forms. These items, although important to school nurses and physicians, often tend to obscure the classroom teacher's basic responsibility as a mature adult to help a child in need. It is the underlying elements of this very natural process that merit our intense concern.

Helping a child to grow and develop in a healthy fashion while acquiring values and insights that promise to support favorable health behavior for his or her future development is a long and arduous process that seldom appears urgent or glamorous. It is difficult and complex and the benefits are seldom immediately visible. However, we hope this text will prove useful in this endeavor, for few things in life are more important.

The task of identifying and giving proper credit to those who made it possible for the authors to write this text is difficult because of the large number of people involved. All three authors were privileged to teach at both the public school and university levels, with teaching responsibilities that ranged, collectively, from kindergarten through graduate school and included a variety of supervisory and administrative roles. Our own schooling brought us in contact with many fine teachers, but some of our best teachers were those we later sought to serve. We always found teaching and supervision to be two-way streets. More direct assistance was provided by our loyal typists, Frances Greene and Alan Older, whose work extended well beyond their clerical tasks. Our sincerest thanks go to Carol Ashton, who, as photographer and illustrator, brought an outstanding degree of personal commitment and professional expertise to her work that graces the pages of this text. Her efforts received valuable support from Dr. Donald Fork of the Department of Educational Media of Temple University, who also provided expert assistance in the preparation of our many lists of teaching materials. Finally, we are very grateful to the personnel of the Philadelphia School District, who gave Carol and her camera free access to their classrooms.

W. H. G.
F. H. J.
P. M. L.

Contents

part 1

The Goal

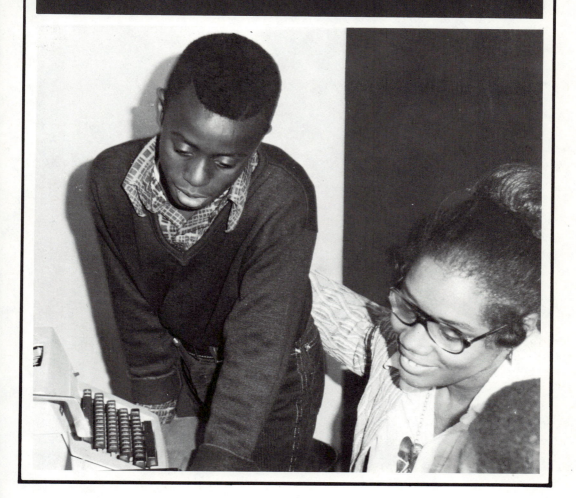

Health

One of the real advantages of entering either the general field of education or one of the health professions is the opportunity these fields provide for association with pleasant, intelligent coworkers. Genuine altruism has always been a scarce commodity, but it exists in significant quantities within these callings. One widespread shortcoming within these groups, however, is their tendency to hide simple human relationships behind clouds of complicated jargon, formalized policies, and inscrutable forms and record systems. Although technical nomenclature has its place when used properly, the really important things about health in the elementary school are much simpler and require more in the way of human sensitivity and commitment than they do technical knowledge.

YOUTHFUL POTENTIAL

Health is one of childhood's most precious resources: It means that arms and legs are intact and working properly, that children can see, hear, taste, and feel, that they can experience love, fear, pride, and other human emotions in appropriate ways, and that they have the strength and energy to carry out their plans. In short, healthy children are free of any internal restrictions that might place limits on the development of their potential. Of course, they still must learn to set their own goals, whatever these may be; it is their responsibility to use and develop their abilities. They may encounter unfair or indifferent people or simply experience bad luck; success is not guaranteed. But healthy children do not have to do battle with their own bodies and personalities; they have a running start at life that greatly shades the odds in their favor.

Unfortunately, many children fall far short of this ideal. Some have uncorrected vision problems that cause them to squint at the words before them and guess at the meaning; some come to school hungry for lack of breakfast and find themselves tired and irritable during the morning hours.

A few cannot climb a flight of stairs without experiencing breathing distress because their heart valves have been damaged by rheumatic fever. Others with very minor problems such as benign heart murmurs or mild asthma attacks have been crippled by the actions of overconcerned parents who have told them to avoid vigorous play and, in effect, consider themselves invalids. Within the emotional realm some children have been "taught" that they are not very bright or capable, that they usually do things poorly; others are "taught" that they are immoral and, when given a chance, will surely do something evil or sinful. Few children are entirely free of such impairments and a great many are severely handicapped by them.

CHILD ADVOCATES

The large majority of these restrictive health problems are either totally unnecessary or much more severe than they would be given the application of proper corrective or preventive action. As a nation we are basically an exporter of food, but many of our own children are poorly nourished; we have perhaps the largest medical–dental establishment in the world, yet many of our children go without needed professional care. We have a social structure based largely on democratic and Judeo-Christian ideals, yet many of our children are treated unjustly and are denied the affection to which they are inherently entitled.

A certain portion of these unfulfilled needs results from real shortages or major defects in our socioeconomic system that will be with us for many years, but in a great many instances available resources are simply not used. What children need most are concerned adults to help them gain access to the things they require. Someone must see that the environment is free from excessive temperature changes, from fire hazards and dangerous objects, and from those who would do them physical harm or assault their personalities with persecution, sarcasm, or ridicule. Someone must see that medical, dental, or psychiatric attention is available to children when they need it. Someone must help them with their own health behavior and decision making; in some cases they must be told what to do, but more important they need help in learning about their own health needs so they can begin to make their own decisions. In other words, they need (1) school health services, (2) a healthful environment, and (3) the opportunity to become educated in the ways of health.

SCHOOL HEALTH SERVICES

The primary responsibility for the health of American children rests on their parents. Parents are aided in fulfilling this responsibilty by the health professionals and resources available within the community and the school.

4

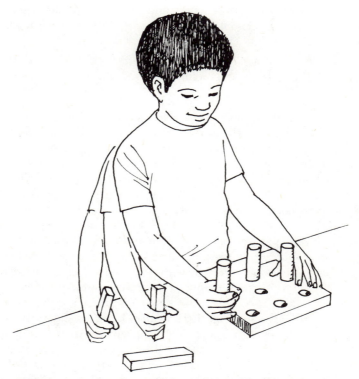

Figure 1.1. A Child Must Learn to Make His Own Decisions.

But other than their parents the most important adults in attending to the health needs of elementary school children are their teachers. Both from a legal standpoint and in accepted teaching practice, teachers function *in loco parentis* to their pupils while they are in school. Teachers share their responsibilty as surrogate parents with the school health service staff (nurses, physicians, dental hygienists) and with administrators, guidance personnel, and others as well. However, because of the relatively large amount of time spent with their pupils, classroom teachers carry the greatest share of the school's responsibility for child health.

Teachers and school health service staff members are better able to discharge their shared responsibility for child health if they are aware of each other's competencies and goals. For example, teachers should know that school nurses and physicians in the United States are legally prohibited from providing definitive treatment of even minor illnesses but are expected to provide emergency first aid care for children who become ill or who are injured at school. Teachers should know that school health professionals

5

seek to prevent disease if possible, to identify departures from health that do occur, to motivate and assist parents of pupils with problems in obtaining needed diagnostic and treatment services through community resources, and to work with teachers and other school professionals in providing appropriate in-school management of children with health problems.

HEALTH SERVICE STAFF

Almost all schools are served by *nurses*. In some schools the nurse is the only school health service professional. Some nurses who work in schools are employed by health departments and do public health nursing in the community as well as school work. Others work exclusively for and in schools. Some of these are permitted and encouraged to visit homes and community agencies in their work with and for children, while others are required by short-sighted administrators or school policies to remain in the school all day. Some nurses are professionally prepared to function as health educators as well as nurses. These nurses, sometimes referred to and certified as *school nurse–teachers*, may assist classroom teachers by giving demonstration lessons or by teaching special units in health education. All well-prepared nurses are able to serve as resource persons to teachers in selecting appropriate content, checking the factual accuracy of instructional materials, and sharing their health knowledge as visitors to the classroom. Other nurses are professionally prepared to perform medical health examinations of children and to assume other functions until recently reserved to school physicians. These nurses are called *school nurse practitioners*. Practitioners often serve several schools, each of which may also be served by a traditional school nurse. In any case the nurse in most schools is the person with the greatest share of the responsibility for building-level planning and conduct of the school health service program, within systemwide guidelines.

Physicians in schools may, like nurses, be employees of either the school system or the public health department. In large school systems the director of the school health service program may be a physician. Like nurses, school physicans are concerned with the development of health-related school policies and practices. Most of their time, however, is spent examining pupils for special purposes, such as assignment to special education classes, or meeting requirements for routine examinations.

Dentists and dental hygienists focus their efforts largely on prevention of dental defects through education and through such services as cleaning and scaling children's teeth and applying fluoride solutions or protective plastic sealants. Dental hygienists, as part of their professional preparation, are educated to serve as classroom dental health educators. In some schools they do so routinely, whereas in others they serve as resource persons at the request of classroom teachers. Dentists and dental hygienists also staff school–community clinics that provide treatment services in some locales.

Screening technicians are employed in some schools to administer and interpret tests designed to detect vision and hearing defects and other problems. In other schools this work may be performed by nurses, teachers, or volunteers. Technicians may be either formally trained or given on-the-job instruction. Those who are well prepared may be helpful as health education resource persons. They are generally less well prepared and paid than teachers or nurses; thus screening is more economically provided through use of these paraprofessionals.

Guidance counselors, crisis room teachers, social workers, psychologists, and *psychiatrists* are mental health service professionals who work in some schools. Of these, guidance counselors and crisis room teachers are most likely to be staff members of elementary buildings, whereas the others are more likely to serve several schools on a part-time basis. A crisis room is a valuable resource to which classroom teachers may send acutely disturbed or disturbing pupils for immediate help and to relieve classroom tensions. The other workers provide counseling or diagnostic and mental health treatment service on more of a continuing or long-range basis.

HEALTH SERVICE GOALS

PREVENTION

The most obvious prevention functions of the school health service staff are to maintain adequate levels of immunization and to identify and exclude from school pupils in the communicable stages of infectious diseases. Regardless of whether immunizations are given in the school or elsewhere, the success of both of these processes depends largely on the education of both pupil and parents as to their importance. The prevention of many chronic diseases depends largely upon alteration of individual life-styles through education and by the development of good exercise and nutrition patterns. Health service workers therefore seek to promote and assist the efforts of teachers and others in health education and to promote desirable school feeding and physical activity programs. In addition they seek to prevent illness and injury through the maintenance of a healthful and safe school environment.

IDENTIFICATION of HEALTH PROBLEMS

Two purposes are served by the identification of children with health problems. First, many health problems can be cured or alleviated by early and adequate medical, surgical, or psychological treatment. Second, children with health defects that cannot be cured or for which prolonged treatment is required may need a modification of school routines or programs. Observation of children, screening tests, and medical examinations are means used to detect health problems.

The value of the elementary school teacher as an identifier, through observation, of children with health problems has been recognized for many years by medical and psychological practitioners and has been demonstrated in research studies. In a classic study eight out of ten children suspected by teachers of having health problems were found to require medical attention.[1] This effectiveness is based in part upon certain built-in advantages that elementary teachers have over others as observers of the health status of children. First among these is their knowledge of normal child growth and development; they know how healthy youngsters of a given age and sex behave, and are thus able to spot possibly pathological deviations from normal. Second, they can be more objective in observing deviations than can the children's own parents, who may view their offspring as perfect in every way. Third, because they interact with smaller numbers of children than do secondary teachers, they get to know how each behaves as an individual when healthy. And finally, as they gain experience and learn more about common health problems, they learn specific signs (things observers see) and symptoms (things children feel and complain about) that are associated with specific disorders.

In short, good health observation by teachers involves continual alertness throughout the school day for

- deviations from behavior normal to a child's sex and stage of development.
- deviations from the way an individual normally behaves when healthy.
- complaints children make about the way they feel.

Because such deviations do not prove that a health problem exists but only that it might, the advice of a medically knowledgeable person, such as the school nurse should be obtained if possible before any drastic action is taken.

One final point merits the highest emphasis. Teachers' knowledge of normality and of the signs of specific conditions and their skills of observation will not be appropriately applied unless they are supported by a genuine concern and sense of caring for children as persons, not merely as pupils who must score higher on the standardized test at the end of the school year. Teachers who care will see things that emotionally detached teachers will miss. This caring attitude, of course, has much to do with the basic warmth and humanness of one's personality; however, this potential is sometimes

[1] Dorothy B. Nyswander, *Solving School Health Problems* (New York: Commonwealth Fund, 1942), p. 34.

8

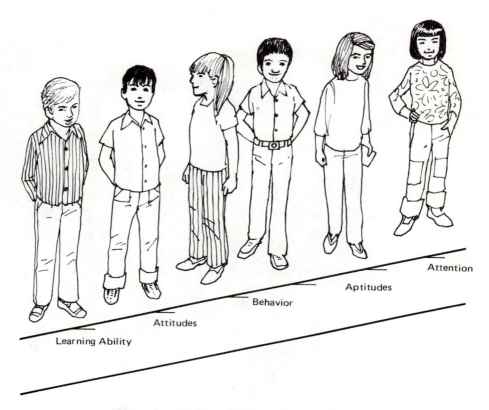

Figure 1.2. "Teachers Have an Objective Yardstick."

not realized until elementary teachers become fully aware of their importance to the children assigned to them. They are not just persons for whom pupils perform academic chores, but important adults who are "fair" and "smart," who can provide hope, encouragement, and reassurance that one is a good, worthwhile child who is becoming a good, worthwhile adult. To a child, a teacher is also someone who keeps others from "picking on me too much" and who can "help me if I get hurt." Although they will try to hide it, school-aged children are painfully aware of their dependent position in life. As teachers become aware of and act to fulfill all aspects of their important roles as adults in the classroom, they not only become more efficient in their official responsibilities but also are more personally rewarded by their work.

Health screening testing is an important means of detecting health problems. A good screening test is a simple, efficient way of separating those who probably have a health problem from those who probably do not. Few screening tests are diagnostic; most of them, like teachers' observations, only indicate which children need a diagnostic examination to determine whether

9

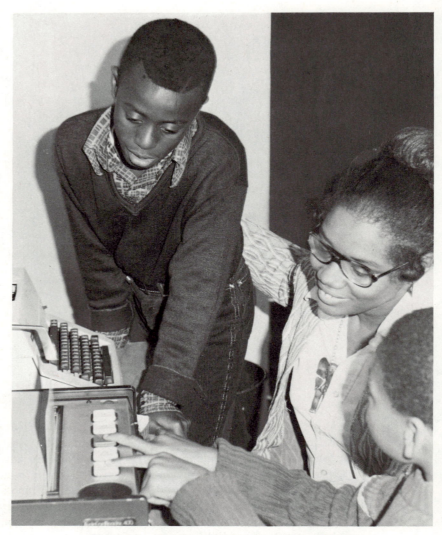

Figure 1.3. "Teachers Need to Care." (Carol Ashton)

a problem actually exists, and, if so, whether some form of treatment is required.

Tests usually administered in schools include those for hearing loss, defects in visual acuity and color deficiency, and periodic checks of height and weight to determine whether growth is occurring on schedule. There are also screening tests to disclose cases of scalp ringworm and tuberculosis where these diseases are prevalent. Many other screening tests are available that are often not used, and new and improved tests are constantly being developed. For example, some schools are now using skinfold thickness measurements to identify fatness—a much more accurate method than height and weight measurements. Testing schedules, the thoroughness with which testing is conducted, and who is assigned responsibility for testing vary from state to state and from school district to school district.

Teachers are called upon to administer screening tests in some schools, but this represents poor use of a teacher's time. Teachers have much more important responsibilities to fulfill. The most important of these is to teach pupils the purpose, nature, and importance of the particular test, and how they can best cooperate as test subjects. This teaching often enhances the accuracy of the test; bright youngsters may cheat on commonly used vision tests, for example. Some tests, like that for tuberculosis, are scary because a skin prick is involved and because bright youngsters with positive tests are quite aware of this before the tests are read. Prior instruction can be reassuring if properly done. Teachers are also often expected to distribute and collect parent permission forms in advance of some tests, to supervise the children during testing, and to keep records of tests given and the results. Much of this essential but mundane work can be done more economically by volunteers or teacher's aides. Another important responsibility that only the teacher can fulfill is to be aware of those screening test results that dictate some immediate modification in classroom management pending medical follow-up. Examples include the provision of preferential seating for those whose tests indicate probable defects in visual acuity or hearing.

Routine health examinations are another way of identifying children with health problems. These are required by laws or regulations in many states and school districts. They may be performed in school by school health service staff members or in outside offices or clinics by the children's own providers of medical and dental care. Studies have shown that, except for the initial examinations required or provided on school entrance, repeat examinations of apparently well youngsters reveal few health problems that were not previously known or that could not be discovered through teacher observation, screening tests, or special medical examinations following serious injury or illness. Therefore, there is a trend away from frequent routine examinations and toward greater reliance on teacher observation, screening tests, and referral examinations.

Teacher responsibilities in connection with routine medical and dental examinations are the same as those they have in connection with screening tests: first, education of pupils as to the purposes and nature of the examinations and how to cooperate in the examination; second, teacher awareness of the implications of examination findings for classroom management of children with defects; third, supervision of children if examinations are done in school; and, finally, responsibility for some of the paperwork involved.

HEALTH REFERRAL, COUNSELING, and FOLLOW-UP

It does no good to discover health problem unless something useful is done about them. The something useful may be medical, surgical, dental, or psychiatric intervention, modification of normal school routine, education of the child as an exceptional person, or some combination of these approaches. In communities where parents are well educated and motivated to care for their children and where they can afford adequate care that is available in the community, simple notification of the parent that a problem is suspected about which a physician or dentist should be consulted is often the only action that is needed. In communities where opposite conditions prevail or in situations where the suspected problem is likely to call for a complex solution, the task of health referral, counseling, and follow-up is likely to be much more complicated.

Joy Cauffman and her associates have shown in referral work that

1. A written note to the parent, followed by a telephone call or some other form of personal communication has optimal impact on referral completion.
2. These contacts are more effective if made by two different school workers, e.g., the nurse *and* the teacher, than by one.
3. Three contacts are not significantly more successful than two.[2]

In a later study, it was found that when poor persons are referred to a specific agency for care, they are more likely to appear there if they are given a specific appointment time to see a specific person in the agency whose name they have been given.[3]

Teachers, in part because they may be able to relate difficulty with school work to a health problem, can often convince parents that children need professional care when the school nurse alone cannot. And a competent school nurse is more likely to know the health care agencies in the community and the persons in them to whom referrals may be made than is a competent teacher. Thus both must often work together to achieve referral success.

In the face of complex problems and difficult family circumstances, mere referral to a source of care is not enough—counseling is called for. Counseling demands a set of skills that are usually attained through education and practice in counseling psychology. Health counseling of parents and pupils is sometimes the primary responsibility of the guidance counselor

[2] Joy G. Cauffman, E. O. Warburton, and Carl S. Schultz, "Health Care of School Children: Effective Referral Patterns," *American Journal of Public Health*, Vol. 60 (Dec. 1970), pp. 1904–1909.

[3] Joy G. Cauffman et al., "A Study of Health Referral Patterns. V. Factors Related to Referral Outcomes," *American Journal of Public Health*, Vol. 64 (April 1974), pp. 351–356.

and sometimes that of the school nurse, depending on whether the problem is basically medical or psychological in nature. The teacher may be consulted independently by the nurse or counselor, or may be invited to participate actively in a three-way counseling session. Counseling may involve any or all of a number of processes. The first of these may be identification or exploration of the problem. Next, a number of possible ways of solving the problem may be proposed, and one chosen. Subsequent sessions may be needed to evaluate progress and modify the plan for solution if necessary. Counseling may be directive, in which the counselor seeks to guide the parent and child to a predetermined course of action, or nondirective, in which the course of action is selected by the counselees. Good counseling is always nonjudgmental; attention is focused on the problem and its solution, not on fault-finding.

Follow-up in the case of a simple remediable health problem focuses on determination of whether or not the agreed-upon solution has been carried out and the problem solved. Has a child with a vision defect been seen by an eye specialist? Do retesting and the child's judgment indicate that corrective lenses have solved the problem? If the problem is complex or irremediable, follow-up efforts may focus on helping the child live with his or her problem by making appropriate adjustments in home and school management. For example, a child with diabetes requires not only continuing medical supervision but also dietary adjustments at home and school, provision for care in emergencies, and informed parents and teachers who neither overprotect the child nor ignore the problems. The whole process may require rather frequent interactions among the parent, teacher, nurse, child, and physician or clinic.

CARE of INJURIES and ILLNESSES

Provision of emergency care for pupils who are injured or who become ill at school is another responsibility shared by health service workers and classroom teachers. The school's basic responsibility is to provide first aid treatment as required, to provide a cot room or other facility in which pupils may rest until taken to their homes or to a source of medical care, and to notify parents of the problem and assist them in assuming responsibility.

The first function of the teacher is to recognize, through observation, the existence of an illness or injury that needs care. Some pupils are stoics who prefer to bear considerable pain and discomfort rather than complain or ask for help. A pupil who comes to school apparently well in the morning may develop a skin rash and fever or diarrhea in the afternoon. Depending upon local school policies and practices, teachers who recognize such problems may be expected simply to refer them to the school nurse or other designated first aid person, or to provide some degree of care themselves. Illnesss and injuries, however, frequently occur when a designated caregiver is absent. Also, the law assumes that in an emergency the teacher will provide the first aid care that is prudent. All prudent teachers therefore prepare themselves to assume this responsibility by taking first aid courses, whether such preparation is legally required or not.

Almost all of the injuries that occur at school, like almost all of those that occur at home, are cuts, scrapes, or bruises of a minor nature. For this reason, practice and policy in many schools dictate that such injuries be cared for in the classroom. If this is the case, first aid kits should be placed in each classroom or in other convenient locations about the school. Ideally, a booklet of approved first aid instructions should accompany each kit. Maintenance of the kits and instructions is usually a responsibility of the health service staff. In some schools this responsibility has been successfully delegated to student monitors. The instructions vary somewhat from district to district depending on local practice and facilities.

Specific parental permission is required before injuries or illnesses of a serious nature are given definitive medical care. A well-meaning school professional who authorized treatment of a child by a physician might be held liable for payment of the bill and might also be sued if the child were harmed by the treatment. The fact that about half of the mothers of United States schoolchildren hold jobs outside the home often makes it difficult to locate a parent who can assume responsibility. Most schools therefore maintain a file of emergency information cards. These cards, which should be filled out annually, contain such information as the names, home and work addresses, and phone numbers of both parents, how to locate the child's physician, and such relevant information as the last tetanus immunization date of the child.

Ill children need a quiet place to rest until their parents can pick them up. They need to be isolated from others because an illness may be communicable. Some have nausea, vomiting, and diarrhea and need equipment and facilities for the care of these signs and symptoms. In addition to notification, parents may need assistance in the transportation of their ill children and advice as to whether watchful waiting or immediate consultation with the child's physician is the preferable course of action.

HEALTHFUL SCHOOL ENVIRONMENT

A major phase of the school's health responsibilities is the provision of a healthful school environment. The laws of all fifty states require that children attend school. During the school year the state, in effect, takes children out of their homes, away from the supervision and care of their parents, and places them in a new environment. From a legal standpoint this mandatory aspect places a heavy responsibility on the schools to provide as safe and healthful a situation as the children's homes. Experience has shown that, although schools usually exceed this standard, continual attention must be given to their environmental conditions if this performance is to be maintained.

DIFFUSE RESPONSIBILITIES

The term *environment* is essentially a complex one whether it is applied to some part of the world of nature or to the more limited realm of the school. A variety of stimuli other than those provided by the task at hand (such as a math problem, for example) affect pupil response and thus academic, social, or emotional development. These include the temperature of the room, the angle and intensity of the light, the noise level, the odors, the feel of the chair and the table or desk, and the general appearance of the classroom. Of perhaps greater importance because of the difficulties involved in its management is the socioemotional environment (sometimes referred to as *school climate*). Do pupils feel generally secure or do they feel threatened? Are school personnel genuinely concerned about the progress and well-being of children or do the children feel ignored? Are children made to feel adequate and successful or overburdened and unworthy? These and other factors sometimes come to the forefront as recognizable problems and on other occasions remain as part of a complex background for other issues; however, in either case they work their persistent effects for better or for worse.

It is somewhat of a misnomer to characterize a healthful school environment as part of a total school health program because the responsibility for the management of as complex an entity as the environment is too widely distributed to fall within the control of any single program. The committee that originally selected the site for the school, the architect who drew up the plans, the city departments that provide the water supply and enforce the air pollution code, the kitchen staff that prepares the school lunch, the superintendent who selects the professional staff and the school custodians, the principals who set policies for school discipline—these are but a few of the many persons who significantly affect the school environment.

THE PERSON in CHARGE

However wide the responsibility for the school environment may be distributed, it is most often the classroom teacher who is in a position to observe or foresee any untoward effects of the school environment on the children. The principal might decide to schedule a class trip for the "graduating" sixth graders, the physical education teacher might decide to wrap up the year with a schoolwide sports day, the parent-teacher club

15

might decide that an award ceremony is in order, and the assistant superintendent might decide to schedule the districtwide administration of standardized achievement tests. Each of these activities could be valuable in itself, but their collective effect might be too much for the average pupil. Although someone is supposed to be coordinating such events, it is easy for the gears to slip a notch at the expense of the children.

Many things in the school environment are supposed to be taken care of. The playground equipment should be in good repair, the fire latches on the doors should work, the heating and ventilation systems should function routinely—but often they do not; the top step of the slide comes loose, the fire latches are chained up by security-conscious custodians, and overpowering paint fumes have been known to come through ventilators. The classroom teacher represents the child's last line of defense against such hazards. And although most of these things call for commonsense action, the development of a professional attitude is required in order to discharge one's responsibility in this area. While on the job, elementary school teachers are not consumers who can assume that the environment is safe and healthy and that people are taking care of things. They are instead part of the management, working professionals with responsibility to see that it is indeed safe and healthy—in other words they are among the persons who take care of things.

Teachers generally have two roles in regard to environmental management. First, they are expected to fix things that they can readily fix. For example, good teachers can often improve interpersonal relations by using conflict resolution techniques rather than blame-setting and punishment to settle pupils' arguments. They can adjust blinds and artificial lighting to improve the visual environment of the room. Second, they can observe environmental problems they cannot fix and report them to those who can do so—the building engineer or principal, for example.

A BROAD SCOPE

Specific aspects of school environment will be discussed throughout the text within the context of particular educational considerations of health topics. The following outline of basic components is intended to serve as an orientation to this broad topic.

1. A safe and healthful physical environment results from attention to
   - *Building construction* appropriate to the school program, the age level of the pupils, and the surrounding community.
   - *Safety*, including provisions for traffic control, fire drills, safe playground equipment, upkeep and supervision, and the like.
   - *Comfort* and *teaching–learning efficiency* through well-designed and

maintained systems to control lighting, acoustics, temperature, humidity, and air movement.
- *Disease control* and *health promotion* by means of adequate and sanitary drinking fountain, toilet, and food service facilities.

2. A healthful socioemotional climate results from attention to
- *Teachers*, professionally prepared, selected, and retained with concern for their ability to develop and maintain good interpersonal relationships with and among children.
- *Administrators* who care more about the growth and achievement of both pupils and teachers than they do about shuffling forms and papers or the fine points of central office policy.
- *Pupil personnel workers* such as nurses, counselors, and attendance officers who view their primary goal as that of finding problems and helping children, parents and teachers solve them.
- *Goals* to which pupils and staff members are committed.
- *Policies* and *practices,* democratically developed and designed, with agreed-upon goals and the welfare of all school members in mind. These include matters of
  — behavior and discipline
  — scheduling
  — homework assignments
  — reporting pupil progress

These two broad aspects of school environment are closely interrelated. Sharing an esthetically pleasing and physically comfortable environment makes it possible for pupils and staff to concentrate on primary goal achievement and personal interactions. A pleasant and stimulating socioemotional environment encourages participation in maintaining and improving features of the physical environment.

SCHOOL HEALTH EDUCATION

In view of the fact that education rather than health care is the main business of the schools, the instructional phase of the school health program assumes obvious importance. Education in a general sense is directed toward the development of long-term living effectiveness. Historically, educational policy makers have repeatedly stated that nothing is more important to this goal than the knowledge (and perhaps the wisdom) needed to preserve and enhance one's health. Without this quality, they say, the other goals of education become meaningless. Thus health was listed as one of the seven Cardinal Principles of Education (1918), was included in the Educational Policies Commission's statement on educational purposes (1938), was cited as important by the White House Conference on Children and Youth (1950), and more recently has been included in the statements of philosophy of countless local school districts.

In all candor it must be recognized that many districts find it easier to make these philosophical commitments than to support them with tangible programs. The general public tends to be heavily concerned with either academic excellence or vocational training, often at the expense of proper attention to the more diffuse goal of healthy living, and within the elementary school both of these competing priorities translate into pressure for proficiency in the "3 R's." Despite these negative aspects, the trend has been toward an increase in the number of strong programs of health science within the elementary school curricula. Particularly helpful has been the growing number of health education supervisors and/or resource teachers hired to assist the regular classroom teachers. Also, attractive textbooks and a wide variety of other effective teaching media designed for health education are becoming increasingly available. Finally, at this writing, there is a growing interest in the prevention of illness, developing particularly within the federal government, that appears to be motivated as much by the threat of rising medical care costs as by humanitarian concerns. Prevention requires education and education is best when it begins at an early age; consequently, the importance of health teaching in the elementary schools is becoming more apparent.

HALLMARKS of HEALTH

Once one accepts the need for a school program of health education, questions arise as to its essential characteristics. There are many different opinions as to the hallmarks of a good program, and any source, including this textbook, is bound to be biased to some degree. However, there are a number of features as discussed in this section that the authors feel have received wide and well-deserved support.

HUMANISTIC EMPHASIS.   The study of health science, perhaps more so than any other subject, requires constant attention to the holistic qualities of human beings. Their important dimensions are all interrelated. Within each person, as in the surrounding environment, "everything is connected to everything else." Not only will poorly nourished children suffer tissue damage, but their ability to give and receive affection will also be altered. Not only will unloved children suffer emotionally, but their physical health and growth will also be adversely affected. The momentous struggles with widespread communicable disease and malnutrition of past decades have left our society with an understandable but excessive emphasis on old-fashioned biomedical concerns. Consequently, modern health education programs tend to stress the emotional and social aspects of health in an effort to bring a proper balance to this situation. The concern for feelings and values thus becomes as important as knowledge and understanding; the concern for personality structure becomes as important as the concern for physical structure. And, most important, the inseparable nature of these human aspects is continually kept in mind.

INTERNALIZED LEARNINGS. Both parents and teachers generally recognize that the knowledge and understanding of health concepts cannot benefit children unless there are corresponding improvements in their everyday health behavior. Often overlooked, however, is the additional need for children not only to act favorably in regard to their health but also to truly believe in what they are doing. Short-term gains in health behavior can be effected through scare tactics, intimidation, or sheer weight of authority, but they are soon lost when the pressure is removed. Children like to make their own decisions; they want to examine some alternatives and discover their own solutions. Well-planned learning activities can accommodate both these natural inclinations and the equally important needs for mature guidance toward favorable behavior patterns. Occasionally, teachers and other school authorities must "lay down the law"; a poorly conceived "discovery approach" could have disastrous consequences when applied to traffic safety, for example. However, enlightened educators accept this practice only as a temporary expedient; they immediately seek to reinforce its shaky motivational structure with the strength that free and open study can provide.

CAREFUL ATTENTION TO SEQUENCE. Once a sound teaching approach has been established, the next priority is the proper organization of subject matter. The task of becoming "health educated" in the best sense of the term involves the development of a workable understanding of the basic factors that affect human well-being such as those related to personality, the human body, and the environment; the formation of favorable attitudes must, of course, take place concurrently with this cognitive understanding. Each maturity level presents new challenges and opportunities to the school program of health education. Preschool children can acquire useful insights related to their own bodies and emotions that can then be used as the formation for more complex learning in the primary grades, which in turn can be augmented at the intermediate level. Children are thus led in stages toward increasingly free and mature decision making. This represents a notable change from the "hygiene" classes of the past that tended to bind children in webs of rules and warnings related to current problems and hazards.

ACCEPTANCE OF CONTROVERSY. Many of the areas of human behavior that tend to produce the most problems and often the greatest opportunities for human fulfillment are also the focus of serious controversy. Examples include many of the issues related to human sexuality, family living, and psychoactive substances (drugs and alcohol). Those involved in modern, comprehensive programs of health education give due attention to these topics, knowing full well that they are often handled poorly by both parents and the mass media. "Due attention" in the elementary school generally implies the building up of good background information and the formation of a constructive approach toward the handling of controversial issues in general. It would seldom be appropriate to push young children toward personal decisions regarding their stand on euthanasia and the lowering of the age for the legal purchase of alcohol. However, much of the ground-work can be laid for the effective coping with such issues in the future. Although individual teachers should not, of course, unilaterally introduce sensitive issues into the curriculum, they have a responsibility to participate in the orderly development of a school program that meets the needs of children in regard to such issues.

EXCITING POSSIBILITIES

The point to all this is that health education does not have to consist of a series of "hygiene lessons." The subject can be approached with an intellectually honest "let's-find-out-about-this" type of attitude in the tone of a good social studies or science unit, and when it is, the possibilities are extremely rich and varied. As evidence of this, one has only to consider the many exciting public issues and controversies that have had health themes. These come to life in the excitement of an "Earth Day" rally, a newspaper story on a new cancer treatment, a TV special on transcendental meditation, or a first-run movie based on the trials and tribulations of a hospital staff.

Of course, many of these intriguing issues are not directly applicable to the elementary school program, but in most cases related topics will be found that will be both interesting and valuable to children at a particular grade level. Third graders are probably not yet ready to discuss the fairness of the fees physicians charge for their services or to examine different approaches to the financing of medical care, but if they are ever to be ready to probe such issues they must first learn about the work done by doctors, nurses, and other health professionals, and this information can be very interesting to them. Children of this age are likewise too immature for any complex study of personality structure; however, they can benefit greatly from a simple unit directed toward discovering "things that make me feel good," and they can do some profitable speculating as to why certain situations make them feel good or bad. A study of the economic and political factors that underlie the food problems of underdeveloped countries would be beyond many elementary children, but they can become very intrigued with the food customs and traditions of the people of other lands and gain valuable insights into their own nutritional needs while gaining a background for a study of the more sophisticated aspects of international food

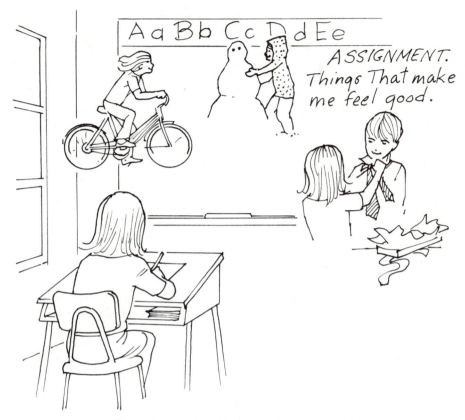

Figure 1.4. "Things That Make Me Feel Good."

problems in later grades. In short, the same qualities that make health issues newsworthy and exciting in the mass media can make health education an exciting subject in the elementary school classroom.

THE SCOPE of HEALTH EDUCATION

At this point one could logically respond to this presentation with the thought "OK, the study of health looks as if it could be very interesting and worthwhile, but where do we start? What is included within the study of health?" The task of defining the scope of health education is complicated by its role as an applied science rather than as a traditional academic discipline. The subject matter of the health curriculum is borrowed freely from the fields of biology, physiology, epidemiology, psychology, anthropology, and in some cases economics and political science. The only criterion for selection is that the content relate to human well-being. This results, of course, in considerable overlap with other subjects, particularly science and social studies, which makes careful planning necessary. This multidisciplinary aspect also creates the opportunity to integrate the study of health either totally or partially with other portions of the curriculum. Whether taught separately or as part of other subjects, certain topical areas are generally considered essential to any health education program. These vary both in substance and mode of organization in accordance with different points of view; however, the following are represented in most health curricula:

1. *Structure and Function of the Human Body*. Because of improper grade placement and uninspired modes of presentation, the study of basic anatomy and physiology has an undeserved reputation as a dull subject. Too often ninth-grade students, for example, with pressing health needs related to adolescent adjustment and sexual behavior have been asked to spend their time learning the Latin names of various bones and muscles. However, the elementary school child typically has a genuine interest in "things" and how they work as well as personal relationships. It is an ideal time to learn some basic concepts about the human body and its functions and thus provide a good foundation for the study of more specific health problems in later grade levels.

2. *The Natural Environment*. This area, like structure and function, may often be taught as part of the science rather than the health curriculum, but regardless of how presented, an understanding and appreciation of man's relationships to other species within the world of nature are essential to a good education in health. Priority topics within this area include food chains, photosynthesis, the nitrogen cycle, and symbiotic relationships.

3. *Nutrition*. Adolescents today often fall prey to various fad diets, spend exorbitant amounts of money on so-called health foods, or simply neglect to make any effort to eat a balanced diet. Often this dubious behavior can be traced to childhood experiences that included far too many imperatives to drink your milk and eat your vegetables. The study of nutrition can be exceedingly interesting and meaningful when the underlying principles are presented in creative ways. Placing the emphasis on the study of food preferences among different persons, subgroups, and cultures is a promising approach. Elementary school children probably hear too much about what they should eat from their parents. What they need most from school is an opportunity to learn why the body needs certain components in preparation for the time when they will be making many of their own choices as adolescents.

4. *Disease*. The study of communicable disease, chronic disease, and allergies has its place when included in proper proportion and with the right emphasis. A study of the basic mechanics of disease and the

body's defenses against disease often leads to improved health behavior on the soundest possible basis. This occurs when individual children make good decisions based on their own knowledge of disease prevention and causation.

5. *Safety.* As almost everyone knows, accidents are the leading cause of death among school-aged children. Learning experiences are needed in this area both to meet obvious immediate needs and to begin the development of perceptual-motor skills, life-long attitudes, and practices related to safety designed to strike a sensible course between carelessness and excessive concern.

6. *Consumer Health.* This area includes the study of health products and services. Young children need to understand the role of physicians, dentists, and their various supportive personnel so that any possible trauma associated with an office visit or hospital stay will be minimized. At the same time they will also be beginning their long-term development of the concepts needed to make their own choices of service as adults and to make political decisions concerning organization and financing of health care.

7. *Psychoactive Substances.* The unconstructive attitudes and misconceptions that often lead to alcohol and drug abuse during adolescence are formed mostly during the elementary school years. This is a prime time to present sound information before children are unduly exposed both to the substances themselves and to undue peer pressure. Beyond this there is the need to build a factual foundation for understanding the broader aspects of drugs in American culture.

8. *Mental Health.* Children need opportunities to develop basic understandings of the factors that affect their behavior and feelings. In particular they need to understand the things that affect their self-concepts or "what I think" and "how I feel about me." Although these topics are related to complex aspects of psychology, they can be put in highly interesting, understandable, and useful forms for the elementary schoolchild.

9. *Human Sexuality.* A number of studies have shown that Freud's latent period is not so latent—that children from 6 to 12 years of age are quite interested in things sexual, but although interested, they are not overwhelmed with sexual problems and concerns. Therefore, in many ways this is a good time to develop basic concepts of sexuality including such topics as reproduction, sex roles, the sex drive, and sex behavior. Although authorities heavily support the presentation of such topics at the elementary school level, what a teacher may actually teach is often severely restricted by the policies of particular school districts.

10. *Family Living.* Although sometimes included as part of sex education, in the opinion of the authors the study of family patterns and interpersonal relationships within the family merits its own identity. When

people marry and begin establishing practices and roles within their newly formed families, their behavior is based largely on their earlier experiences of 20 or so years of family living with their parents. It seems logical to assume that learning experiences in the school program should parallel this "natural" program of education if the most positive results are to be realized. Teachers, school nurses, and administrators often lament "It is the parents who need education—If we could only get *them* back in school!" The logical reply is "You had most of them in school for 10 or 12 years. What did you teach them about family living and parental responsibility when you had the opportunity?"

It is impossible to present a manageable list of health topics without appearing to neglect important areas. The general topic of community health, for example, is important and can be studied as part of each of the ten major headings provided. Thus the government's role in the protection of consumers against impure food can be studied as part of nutrition, the function of the city water department can be included in the environmental or disease areas, and so forth. Dental health can be included under disease or nutrition, and many other common topics can be worked into the curriculum in a similar fashion.

PATTERNS of ORGANIZATION

It would be neither feasible nor desirable to cover all the major topics of a content area as broad as health in every grade level. Just as the "local community" may be emphasized at one grade level in social studies and "faraway lands" at some later year, the health curriculum must be placed in some logical sequence. This task of organizing the content vertically (i.e., from year to year) will be discussed in Part Four along with other curricular aspects. However, a brief overview of the relationship of health to other content areas within the school day, week, or year (i.e., the horizontal organization) is necessary to the understanding of the intervening chapters.

DIRECT INSTRUCTION. The practice of teaching health as a separate and distinct subject with its own daily or weekly time allotment is known as direct instruction. This pattern is both widely endorsed by health educators and often adopted by school districts in which health education enjoys a high priority. The mere fact that health enjoys its own identity and visibility as a curricular area does not, of course, ensure good support or a comprehensive program, but it does tend to facilitate a number of constructive responses. It is not so likely to be ignored by teachers when time becomes tight and "something has to give" as it usually must in today's crowded curricula; the time available can be used for priority health needs because the needs of another subject will not have to be accommodated; financial advantages and consequently more teaching material may be obtained when health appears as "line item" in the budget; occasionally a special health resource teacher, supervisor, or coordinator may become available because of health education's status as a designated content area.

CORRELATED AND INTEGRATED INSTRUCTION. The teaching of identifiable health units or modules as part of other major curricular areas such as science, social studies, mathematics, and so forth is called correlated health instruction. For example, a mental health unit on the self-concept "Getting to Know Me" might appear within the social studies curriculum, or a unit on harmful microorganisms, "Unseen Enemies," might be presented as part of science instruction. The integrated pattern is similar, but here the health content is so finely broken down that identifiable health units do not appear. For example, disease germs might be studied in science as part of a comprehensive unit on one-celled organisms that would include many species of no direct significance to man's health.

With careful planning health can be presented very effectively by use of either of these patterns; however, someone must be designated to review the curriculum to ensure that all needed health topics are included, and the teachers must be made aware of the health education potential of the other subject matter areas as part of their professional preparation if important health concepts are not to be neglected. In most cases a combination of direct, correlated, and integrated instruction works best, with the most clearly identifiable health topics (e.g., "Communicable Diseases," "Psychoactive Substances") taught directly and carefully selected to avoid overlap with related units in science or social studies.

INCIDENTAL INSTRUCTION. Good teachers always remain alert to opportunities to use naturally occurring events to illustrate some aspect of subject matter. Just as the competition among rooms for parental attendance at the PTA meetings might provide impromptu practice in calculating percentages, a breakdown in the school's air-conditioning system might lead to a discussion on one's ability to adapt to temperature change. Such occasions can be used to good advantage and the time spent may often be recovered because a topic covered incidentally may not have to be covered with any intensity when it appears within the planned program. However, incidental instruction obviously cannot be substituted for a planned program in any curricular area. It is by definition unplanned and therefore there is no assurance that essential topics will receive attention in any meaningful sequence. Of course, incidents can be "staged" to create opportunities, but the resulting instruction then ceases to be incidental.

CLASSROOM TEACHER as HEALTH EDUCATOR

The assignment of responsibility for health teaching varies considerably among the nation's elementary schools. In some schools a school nurse–teacher does all the health instruction; in a few districts floating health specialists teach all the health; but by far the most common pattern finds the regular classroom teachers teaching health along with their other responsibilities. This practice is widely endorsed among leaders in heatlh education for a number of reasons. The study of health is focused clearly on human beings and human well-being, perhaps more so than any other subject; within the total realm of education professionals, the elementary teacher is the prime specialist in the teaching of people rather than the teaching of subject matter. Both the subject matter and the methodology of health education cut across traditional currricular areas to draw particularly heavily on science and social studies; once again elementary teachers with their broad training in many content areas and teaching methods are well suited to teach this comprehensive subject.

Occasionally, teachers at the elementary school level shy away from the opportunity to teach health education out of fear that it is something very technical for which they are untrained. The truth of the matter is that it is difficult for anyone to consider himself or herself really well trained in as comprehensive a subject as health. Doctors and nurses, for instance, by the very nature of their training and job responsibilities, are in fact "disease" specialists rather than health specialists; they are very useful members of the health education teams but in most cases their training falls as short of the ideal for health education as does that of the classroom teacher. Health education at its best is the study of the factors that affect human growth and development in the most comprehensive sense. Those who teach health must above all be teachers of people rather than subject matter—thus the most appropriate thing to tell the elementary teacher is "welcome aboard."

REFERENCES

BENDER, STEPHEN. "Health Education in the Elementary School," *School Health Review*, Vol. 3, No. 1 (January-February 1972), pp. 23–26.

BRACY, BONNIE. "Freedom to Think in Elementary School," *School Health Review*, Vol. 5, No. 1 (January-February 1974), pp. 31–33.

FOX, ROBERT S., et al. *School Climate Improvement: A Challenge to the School Administrator.* Bloomington, Ind.: Phi Delta Kappa and CFK Ltd., 1973.

JENNE, FRANK H., and WALTER H. GREENE. *Turner's School Health and Health Education.* St. Louis: C. V. Mosby Company, 1976.

MILLER, C. ARDEN. "Health Care of Children and Youth in America,"

American Journal of Public Health, Vol. 65, No. 4 (April 1975), pp. 353–358.

NATIONAL COMMITTEE ON SCHOOL HEALTH POLICIES. *Suggested School Health Policies.* Chicago: American Medical Association, 1966.

RUSSELL, ROBERT D. *Health Education.* Washington, D.C.: Association of the American Alliance for Health, Physical Education and Recreation, 1975.

SOCIETY OF STATE DIRECTORS OF HEALTH, PHYSICAL EDUCATION AND RECREATION. "A Statement of Basic Belief," *School Health Review,* Vol. 5, No. 2 (March-April 1974), pp. 15–18.

WHEATLEY, GEORGE M., and GRACE T. HALLOCK. *Health Observation of School Children.* New York: McGraw-Hill Book Company, 1965.

WILSON, CHARLES C. *School Health Services.* Chicago: American Medical Association, 1964.

———, and ELIZABETH AVERY WILSON. *Healthful School Environment.* Chicago: American Medical Association, 1969.

part 2

The People

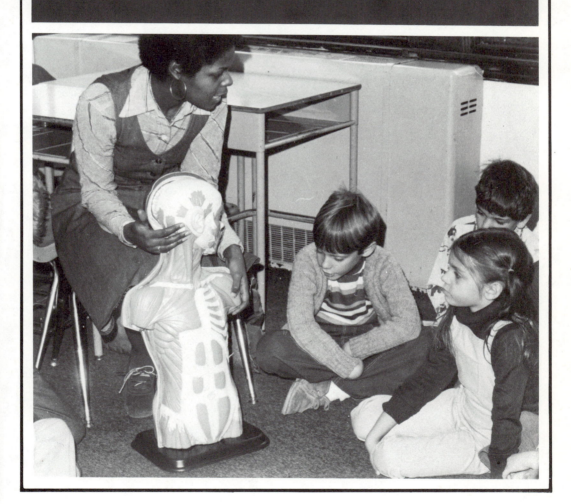

2

Children

A thorough understanding of the characteristics of children is perhaps the single most important requisite of an elementary teacher, and, appropriately enough, considerable attention is given to this basic need within the typical college teacher training program. Because the health status and general school performance of children are so closely interrelated, only a slight change in perspective is needed when one focuses on the task of enhancing the health of children as compared with helping them learn. Although there is no real conflict between these tasks, the rather formidable and persistent pressures for intellectual development that exist in most communities may cause the teachers to lose sight of their roles as guardians of their pupils' health unless a specific effort is made to prevent this lamentable event.

If health is to be promoted, conditions must be created for personal growth. This statement reflects the views of a great many health educators, including the authors, who view growth as the primary characteristic of the healthy person. Physical growth is, of course, a highly visible quality of healthy children, but of equal or greater importance is their growth along other dimensions such as the social, emotional, intellectual, and spiritual. Growth may be defined as a change within an individual that increases his or her ability to function in pursuit of personal or societal goals. According to this view the basic responsibility of teachers is to facilitate growth. This involves arranging a proper environment, providing specific learning experiences, and protecting children from adverse factors that might retard growth or cause regression. If these responsibilities appear to be a simple restatement of the general goals of education, the similarity is intentional. The best way for the elementary teacher to care for the health of his or her pupil is to simply be a good teacher in the fullest sense of the term.

One virtue of a philosophy that equates health with growth and establishes this entity as a primary goal in life is that it provides an integrated concept to guide the efforts of all those who have major responsibilities for the welfare of children. The child's teacher, the family physician, and often a minister, priest, rabbi, or other spiritual leader as well as the parents

31

need to keep the child's overall growth in mind if they are to meet their specific responsibilities. The roles of these "helping persons" obviously differ, but less than one might suspect. Good parish priests, for example, view themselves primarily as spiritual leaders, but if they find that the children of their flock are hungry they often take responsibility for obtaining additional food. Similarly, good teachers may bring great zeal to the task of improving the minds of children but find that their successful advocacy for a school breakfast program was their most important contribution to both the intellectual and physical growth of their pupils. Good parents may assume that their responsibilities are restricted to providing for physical and emotional well-being but find that the intellectual development of their children will be retarded despite the best efforts of the school if the proper stimulation and encouragement are not provided in the home.

TEACHER as FACILITATOR

The most clearly defined responsibilities of teachers within the typical elementary school pertain to intellectual and socioemotional development, and of these the socioemotional is more closely allied with health. Although the physical and spiritual needs of children are certainly no less important, classroom teachers generally have less opportunity to contribute in these areas. However, a basic understanding of all growth dimensions is essential if one is to meet professional responsibilities in any one of them.[1]

INTELLECTUAL GROWTH

Such authorities as Jean Piaget who have spent the major portion of their lives studying intellectual growth have noted, among other things, that the ability to solve increasingly complex problems, the ability to think in the abstract, and the other qualities that compose intellectual ability tend to develop in stages rather than at continuous rates. They have also found that intellectual functioning takes place in response to the need to adapt to specific pressures—in other words, that necessity is truly the "mother of

[1] There have been a number of meritorious attempts to identify the significant dimensions of human existence from the standpoint of health status. The reader is referred to the following:

Steven R. Homel and Thomas Evaul. *The Needs Approach to Health Education.* Bala-Cynwyd, Pa.: The Authors, 1971. (Unpublished materials.)

Howard S. Hoyman. "Rethinking an Ecologic-System Model of Man's Health, Disease, Aging, Death," *The Journal of School Health,* Vol. 45, No. 9 (November 1975), pp. 509–518.

School Health Education Study. *Health Education: A Conceptual Approach to Curriculum Design.* St. Paul, Minn.: 3M Education Press, 1967.

invention." These two observations serve to illustrate the close relationship of intellectual growth with growth along such other dimensions as the physical, social, and emotional where behavior is primarily adaptive in nature and where growth tends to take place in stages. And these observations, of course, should not be surprising if one keeps in mind that these qualities are not merely closely related entities but a single, multidimensional phenomenon.

The interrelatedness of the various human dimensions has been well emphasized in educational literature for many years. Early in this century John Dewey reminded teachers that the "whole child comes to school," not merely his or her brain. The effect of adverse physical, social, and emotional factors on intellectual development is clear and universally accepted. Although they need occasional reminders, virtually all teachers realize that hungry children do not learn well, nor do lonely, anxiety-ridden, or affection-starved children. The converse is equally true and frequently overlooked. Children who do not learn to read when they should often become anxiety ridden, and others who complete school without learning how to count their change and compute percentages often find it difficult to meet their physical needs in our competitive society. Ignorance breeds poverty and poverty breeds illness. Consequently, children need more than food and love if their long-term health needs are to be met. Normal intellectual development is synergistic rather than antagonistic with the general health needs of children.

PHYSICAL DEVELOPMENT

Physical growth and development constitute an exceedingly complex process, with many of its important features still classed as scientific mysteries. The 23 pairs of chromosomes found in the fertilized egg of the newly conceived human being contain literally miles of tightly wound ribbons of DNA (deoxyribonucleic acid) with millions of items of encoded information that provide guidance for every facet of growth and development. Children are in one sense much like fully programmed computers whose internal apparatus handles millions of decisions in a purely automatic fashion. However, despite this complexity, only a few relatively simple external conditions are necessary for the efficient functioning of these "computers." The optimal physical growth and development of children will typically occur if they receive proper nourishment, sufficient rest, and appropriate exercise, and if they are protected from serious disease, injuries, and other adverse environmental factors.

In the average community parents assume the major responsibility for overseeing the conditions needed for the child's physical development. The diet of most elementary school-children is largely controlled by their parents, as are their rest, sleeping habits, and medical care. The teachers are involved with all these factors to a much lesser degree. But however limited the role of teachers may be, their responsibilities are important, and in school districts that serve poor rural areas, the urban ghetto, and other economically depressed areas they may assume major proportions. Regardless of whether these responsibilities are small or large, the elementary teacher needs a general understanding of the basic features of this important process.

BASIC CONCEPTS.[2] Anyone who spends much time with children soon realizes that they are different—although thoroughly human they are not miniature adults. Clothing manufacturers, for example, have long since found that children have shorter legs and a larger head in proportion to the trunk than do fully grown persons. They also require more food in proportion to their size, especially more protein, in order to provide for both growth and energy. Throughout the day they function much like human dynamos, yet they tire more rapidly than adults and require more rest and sleep.

These differences reflect the basic truism that physical growth, like growth along other dimensions, takes place in stages, with each stage characterized by certain reasonably well-defined features. To a certain degree children become different persons as they enter each new stage, yet these differences follow a reasonably predictable pattern. In other words, growth is an orderly process. In terms of its most visible aspects, for example, the male infant adds an average of 10 pounds to its weight and 16 inches to its length during its first year. These are tremendous annual gains that normally exceed those of any other year of the child's life, and the figures for the female are only slightly smaller. Both sexes settle into a more moderate but still rapid rate of growth during their preschool years. This rate decelerates further to a period of slow growth by the age of six and continues at a stable pace during most of the elementary school years until the preadolescent spurt begins at approximately age 10½ for girls and 12 for boys. Growth then continues at a much faster rate for perhaps 2½ years before slowing once more to a moderate pace for the balance of adolescence.

These external gains in height and weight are paralleled by internal changes leading to increased strength, endurance, and coordination that interact with intellectual and socioemotional factors to provide the children of each maturity level with their own distinct qualities. But regardless of how orderly the growth occurs in terms of averages or "typical" children, individual children may vary greatly within the normal range in terms of both the time they enter a new growth stage and the eventual level they attain with respect to height, weight, motor coordination, or other qualities

[2] The material in this section is taken largely from Frank H. Jenne and Walter H. Greene, *Turner's School Health and Health Education* (St. Louis: The C. V. Mosby Company, 1976). For a more thorough treatment the reader is referred to Chapter 13 of this source.

within a specific stage. Groups, classes, or grade levels, for example, tend to display predictable qualities, yet each individual is different, and therein lies much of the fascination of any people-oriented occupation.

FACILITATING PHYSICAL GROWTH.   The elementary teacher's specific responsibilities in regard to the physical growth and development of his or her pupils may be organized in the traditional health program categories of education, services, and environment. And although services and environment are generally of more importance, the process of helping children learn about their bodies and how they grow may well have the heaviest impact on their well-being over the long term. As will be shown in Chapter 4, children display high interest in their own physical growth throughout all their elementary school years. This natural interest pattern may be used to involve children in a study of the basic features of growth leading to the development of positive attitudes and favorable health habits.

The teacher's responsibilities within the realms of health services and environment are somewhat more of a preventive nature than are those pertaining to health education. Injury and disease are two potent enemies of normal growth and development that the classroom teacher can do much to prevent. When these misfortunes do occur the teacher can help the child receive proper care, usually by referral to the school nurse or occasionally by the prompt administration of some simple first aid procedure. Poor nutrition, which sometimes is so severe as to result in clinically defined malnutrition, is another condition that may appear in the children of any classroom and necessitate referral action by the teacher. There is even preliminary evidence that severe emotional stress can retard a child's physical growth—a very plausible hypothesis considering the close functional relationship of the neural and endocrine systems. These and other aspects of the classroom teacher's role regarding physical growth and development will be discussed in further detail in successive chapters dealing with the body, nutrition, disease, and mental health.

SPIRITUAL GROWTH

Most Americans hold some type of belief in God, a creator, or some powerful force that does not readily lend itself to scientific analysis. As Howard Hoyman maintains,

> . . . a truly healthy person continues to ask the big questions about life; and . . . he sees his life in part as a spiritual odyssey, in which he seeks and strives to relate himself and his life meaningfully to his neighbor, his society, the world, the universe and *his* God.[3]

[3] Howard S. Hoyman, "The Spiritual Dimension of Man's Health in Today's World," *The Journal of School Health,* Vol. 36, No. 2 (February 1966) p. 54.

The various believers generally maintain that their version of metaphysical force plays a strong and direct part in the affairs of mankind, and although the skeptics may deny the existence of the outside power, they cannot discount the real effects these beliefs have on human behavior. But however strongly teachers may view the importance of spiritual matters, they generally find that they can do little for the spiritual well-being of their children, at least in any direct way. Such efforts soon run afoul of parents of atheistic or agnostic persuasions who deny or question the very existence of a spiritual dimension, or incur the wrath of spiritually inclined parents who may feel that the basic tenets of their children's faith are somehow being undermined by the teacher's views. Even were it not for the rather complete ban imposed by the legal doctrine of the separation of church and state, public school teachers would find it difficult to act very directly on spiritual matters.

Despite these obstacles, the child or teacher with strong religious or philosophical beliefs cannot leave them at the schoolhouse door. These beliefs exist within the classroom regardless of how scrupulous an effort one might make to ignore them. The teacher thus incurs responsibilities in this area even though they must be passive ones. The right to freedom from persecution for one's personal beliefs is a near-universal American value; elementary teachers thus have a mandate to make their pupils aware of this fact and to create an environment within the classroom in which this point of view will prevail. In terms of service, teachers have a particular responsibility toward those children whose beliefs may be in conflict with the majority views of the community and who may need adult intervention to protect them from untoward peer pressure or ridicule.

Those teachers who have managed to come to terms with the spiritual side of their lives either through church participation or through other forms of spiritual endeavor sometimes wish that they could do more in a direct way for this dimension in the lives of their pupils. One possible outlet is provided by the fact that most well-organized philosophies, religious or otherwise, provide guidance for ethical behavior and effective interpersonal relationships. Preaching, prayer, and rituals are generally inappropriate in the public school classroom. However, teachers with strong beliefs will never find themselves in a spiritually sterile environment. Although they may not be able to tell people what they believe, they can do something better—they can show them.

SOCIOEMOTIONAL GROWTH

Because of their close relationships, social and emotional growth will be discussed as a single entity. Emotional growth is basically concerned with intrapsychic matters, particularly with how children think and feel about themselves as persons and how they respond internally to stress, whereas

36

social growth deals with interpersonal matters, mainly with how children act toward other people in various situations. However, emotional growth as well as social growth takes place almost entirely in a social context. For better or worse, children tend to use their parents, teachers, peers, and other significant persons in their lives as "mirrors" in their efforts to see into their own personalities. Children who are continually at odds with those around them are almost invariably at odds with themselves; conversely, children who suffer from inner conflicts with their emotions will almost surely be impaired in their social relationships. Moreover, such emotionally disturbed children often need a specific type of social interaction, as in the client–therapist relationship, in order to correct their condition.

GROWING PERSONS. Carl R. Rogers, one of the leaders of humanistic psychology, poses the rhetorical question "Can Schools Grow Persons?" and proceeds to answer in the negative, explaining that "only persons can grow persons." He suggests that the schools must ". . . ensure that the employed personnel in our schools—those known as administrators, teachers, supervisors, professors, counselors, research workers, budget directors, etc., etc.— are first and foremost persons in their own right." [4]

Here Rogers both highlights the importance of school personnel in fostering the personality growth of children and suggests a basic approach to the accomplishment of this task. The most essential ingredient is an environment of other healthy personalities, and the personality of teachers is particularly important because children tend to depend rather heavily on them for emotional support during their elementary school years. Furthermore, the health of teachers' personalities cannot become manifest if they are continually threatened or otherwise undermined by hostile administrators or jealous colleagues; thus the health of the entire school system as a social organization becomes important.

Many severe critics of the schools, such as John Holt in his book *How Children Fail* [5] and Charles E. Silberman in his *Crisis in the Classroom,* [6] have made it clear that schools do not always provide desirable conditions for personality growth. Somewhat in response to this criticism—and perhaps because of a gradual improvement in the training level of teachers and in their working conditions in regard to reduced class size and relief from many nonprofessional tasks, together with a general shift toward a more humanistic philosophy—the performance of public schools in this area appears to be generally improving in what is clearly a very welcome trend. The school's role as the child's first real challenge outside the family and the neighborhood play group has always made it a major factor in person-

[4] Carl R. Rogers, "Can Schools Grow Persons?" *Educational Leadership,* Vol. 29, No. 3 (December 1971), pp. 215–217.
[5] John Holt, *How Children Fail* (New York: Dell, 1970).
[6] Charles E. Silberman, *Crisis in the Classroom* (New York: Random House, Inc., 1970).

ality formation. More recently, the continuing trends toward single-parent families and families with both parents working outside the home have caused an even greater proportion of the child-rearing burden to be shifted to the elementary school.

A GUIDING THEORY. The personality of the teacher as a factor in the emotional environment of the school will be discussed in some detail in the following chapter. Here, the emphasis will be placed on personality development process as it takes place within children. The depth and complexity of the human personality make it both a fascinating and a frustrating subject to study. The relatively young discipline of psychology has made a noble effort to provide a scientific explanation of personality structure and functions, but thus far the best it can offer is a few reasonably well-supported theories. Theories are by nature tentative and to some degree unreliable, yet they can still be quite helpful in their provision of a logical framework on which teachers can organize and give some meaning to the behavior they observe in their pupils. Teachers who make the effort to organize what they know and believe about children into a coherent point of view will generally find that they will act with more confidence and consistency in the classroom. These qualities have value in themselves over and above any improvement in the accuracy of the insights that support them.

One of the difficulties involved in deriving any useful guidance from psychological theories is that initially they seem to present a bewildering variety of conflicting views. A closer examination will usually reveal, however, that the great variety actually represents many variations of a limited number of themes and the conflicts represent differences in emphasis or focus rather than substantial contradictions. For example, if a curriculum consultant is concerned with the planning of a new math sequence for the elementary grades, then Piaget's theory, which focuses on the intellect, might be very helpful. School psychiatrists concerned with helping emotionally disturbed children are often trained in Freudian theory, which arose out of the therapeutic process. To make or break specific habits such as overeating or cigarette smoking, a behavior modification approach based on Skinner's behaviorism would be a logical choice. Finally, when one is seeking guidance for the nurturing of normal personality growth, there is considerable merit in reviewing general theories espoused by Carl Rogers, the late Abraham Maslow, and others of the humanistic school of psychology. Maslow in particular offers a comprehensive theory of personality focused on the concept of mental health as opposed to illness.[7]

MASLOW'S THEORY. Of all the personality theorists, Maslow provided perhaps the most optimistic view of children. Conventional Freudian theory

[7] See Abraham H. Maslow, *Motivation and Personality* (New York: Harper & Row, 1970), for a thorough treatment of his views on personality.

tends to describe children as erotic little hedonists whose main task, in terms of personality, is to learn to subjugate and redirect their instincts into socially acceptable directions. Skinner, on the other hand, conveys the impression that children enter the world as blank tablets, or perhaps blank computers, who may be programmed by the experiences fed into them to produce any pattern of characteristics that the "controllers" deem most desirable. Like the Freudians, Maslow attaches considerable importance to the innate tendencies of children or "instinctoid" needs as he terms these factors; however, he views these tendencies as basically good things to be nourished and encouraged rather than bad things to be suppressed or redirected. And, like Skinner, he is also greatly concerned with environmental influences, particularly how children are treated by other persons, but he sees this treatment not so much a molding influence as it is a culturing medium that facilitates wholesome personality growth provided that it contains the proper elements in the proper proportions. Parents, teachers, and other helping persons thus become analogous to gardeners who can either stunt growth by poor management or help children develop their unique potential by meeting their needs.

Within this general scheme the needs of children can be identified by the type of behavior they display, such as affection seeking, attention seeking, and so forth. The particular needs that a child manifests represent not only an imperative to the adult, that is, something to fulfill, but also a useful clue to the child's current maturity level—an indicator of personality growth. Maslow organizes human needs into categories that are in turn organized into a hierarchy. From lowest to highest these are as follows:

- *Physical Needs.* The newborn child is essentially a little bundle of physical needs. Later, he or she will seek love and recognition, but for now the child's behavior is motivated by the need for food, warmth, and a certain degree of physical activity. As these obviously essential needs are met, the child begins to mature physically and emotionally, and a new category, the security needs, emerges.
- *Security.* Within the first few months of life children begin to show a preference for certain stable features in their environment. They want people to be around—the same people, or at least people who handle them in similar ways; they want to be fed with some degree of regularity; they want a solid, dependable surface on which to sleep or play. Should they be injured, frightened by loud noises, scalded by hot bath water, or otherwise mishandled too frequently, they will become fearful, insecure, and retarded in personality growth, but if properly cared for they will begin to demonstrate an increasing need for affection.
- *Affection.* The fearful, threatened, neglected child will tend to view people as merely a class of mechanical objects to avoid or perhaps to use or manipulate if they show some promise of relieving his or her desperate plight. The secure child, however, will come to view people as something

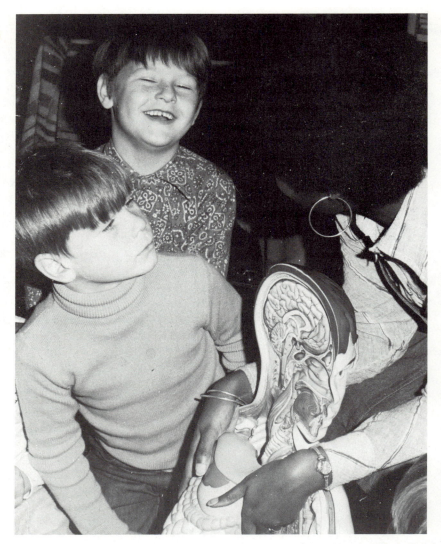

Figure 2.1. Helping Children Develop Their Unique Potential by Meeting Their Needs. (Carol Ashton)

special—objects of value who can make them feel good just with a word or touch. Much of their behavior will now be directed toward seeking such expressions of affection from the significant people in their environment.

- *Esteem.* One might think that secure, loved, and well-cared-for children would be content to merely bask in their fortunate situations, but Maslow maintains that a new set of needs will emerge within such children that will cause them to seek social recognition and self-esteem. Affection is not

40

enough; they now want to be regarded as worthy, competent persons both by themselves and by others. Most healthy, emotionally stable elementary school pupils display these tendencies as they work hard at various tasks to gain recognition from parents, teachers, and peers.

Self-actualization. In a favorable environment in which the developing person is able to gain satisfaction and recognition from the accomplishment of meaningful tasks, he or she develops a feeling of general competence and acceptance—a feeling of "I'm OK—I'm going to make it." With the basic personal needs now well fulfilled they tend to fade in urgency; with no personal "hang-ups" to impede them, such persons now tend to invest their full talents and energy in tasks and causes out of a sense of genuine concern and caring—not merely for personal profit and prestige.

As with all personality theories, one should not try to read too much precision into Maslow's scheme, particularly with regard to identifying specific maturity stages. In general, it is possible to see behavior patterns related to these need categories emerge in the general sequence Maslow describes. However, complete gratification rarely occurs; thus the emergence of the next categories commonly takes place after only partial satisfaction of the lower categories. According to Maslow,

> . . . most members of our society who are normal are partially satisfied in all their basic needs and partially unsatisfied in all their needs at the same time. A more realistic description of the hierarchy would be in terms of decreasing percentages of satisfaction as we go up the hierarchy of prepotency. For instance, if I may assign arbitrary figures for the sake of illustration, it is as if the average citizen is satisfied perhaps 85 percent in his physiological needs, 70 percent in his safety needs, 50 percent in his love needs, 40 percent in his self-esteem needs, and 10 percent in his self-actualization needs.[8]

As also implied in this description, Maslow believes that anything close to complete self-actualization is a rare phenomenon. In a conclusion that many of his readers find irritating, he views the average person as falling short of the ideal in terms of mental health. He, in effect, provides us with useful guidance and direction, but not with a realistic goal for any but the most fortunate persons.

APPLICATIONS. It is one thing to accept a particular theoretical approach as logical and true but it is quite another to draw useful implications from it for the solving of real-life problems. Perhaps one reason theory seems to fail so often and to serve new teachers less well than commonsense solutions or folklore is that the teachers expect too much of it. Theory is no substitute for experience; the crucial part of a teacher's training occurs in those

[8] Ibid., pp. 53–54.

situations that involve face-to-face contact with children. However, theory can provide a logical framework for the development of one's own unique approach to teaching; it can be particularly helpful for the development of ideas to try, hypotheses to consider, when unusual problems are encountered. Maslow's views tend to support a number of useful ways of interpreting the nature of children and the teaching process. A few of the major implications are as follows:

1. When children encounter difficulties at school it is very logical to look for factors within the immediate situation as one seeks to analyze the problem. Perhaps the learning materials are inappropriate, perhaps the room is too noisy, or perhaps the child has some specific weakness in learning ability. These are logical starting points, but one should also consider what may or may not be happening outside of school. The physical, security, and affection needs are more basic and tend to take priority over the needs for esteem and self-actualization that are prime motivators of formal learning. Consequently, Maslow reminds us to also ask, "Did the child have breakfast?" "Is some gang or bully threatening physical violence?" and "Does anyone really care about this child?" These questions are rather obvious, but they are too often forgotten in many school situations.

2. Each child is unique. Long ago, Henry Thoreau reminded us that a child who does not seem to keep pace with the group may be listening to the "beat of a different drummer." Skinner would contend that schools can educate for diversity if they deem it to be wise—or for conformity if this trait offers more advantages. But Maslow would say that the diversity, the uniqueness, is ingrained in each child and that the teacher's only choice is to help it mature and develop or inhibit it at the risk of damaging or at least stunting the child's personality. Children are not clay to be molded, but living organisms that must follow their own unique pattern of growth.

3. Maslow sees no conflict between personal and societal needs. The best way to help children develop into socially responsible adults is to help them meet their own personal needs. The individual who succeeds in this endeavor will soon become more concerned with the needs of others. Conversely, the individual who develops into a person who feels chronically threatened, affection-starved, or incompetent will tend to be nonproductive or even dangerous to society.

4. Like other humanistic psychologists, Maslow views humans as qualitatively different from the balance of the animal kingdom—we are not merely smarter or blessed with more dextrous hands for the use of tools, we have very different needs. Human beings in general have great intellectual ability, artistic sensitivity, and a capacity for affection that can embrace the whole human race. As a central task, each person is motivated by innate factors within the personality to fully develop

his or her combination of talents. Therefore, the traditional academic and artistic skills also represent pathways to the ideal of self-actualization. Although interpersonal skills are important and too often neglected in the typical school, each child also needs effective guidance in the traditional subjects. It is difficult for a sixth grade pupil to feel "lovable and capable" if he or she has not yet learned to read.

The humanistic approach does indeed place definite emphasis on personality development. And this development is not viewed as the mere prevention of emotional problems but rather as the active encouragement of each child's unique personality as an important educational goal. It also typically requires the development of the more common academic skills that are included as parts of one's personality. There is no call for a radical change in educational goals but simply for a small but vital change from the traditional educational approach. Teachers are asked to view each child as an individual with unique potential—with integrity that must be respected and that often takes the form of wanting to do things "my way" when "I am ready." The task of helping children develop the complex skills needed for effective living in modern society without doing violence to this integrity represents the fundamental challenge of the teaching process.

REFERENCES

ERIKSON, ERIK H. *Childhood and Society*. New York: W. W. Norton & Co., Inc., 1963.

HOLT, JOHN. *How Children Fail*. New York: Dell, 1970.

HOMEL, STEVEN R., and THOMAS EVAUL. *The Needs Approach to Health Education*. Bala-Cynwyd, Pa.: The Authors, 1971. (Unpublished materials.)

HOYMAN, HOWARD S. "The Spiritual Dimension of Man's Health in Today's World," *The Journal of School Health,* Vol. 36, No. 2 (February 1966).

JENNE, FRANK H., and WALTER H. GREENE. *Turner's School Health and Health Education*. St. Louis: C. V. Mosby Company, 1976.

LUGO, JAMES O., and GERALD L. HERSHEY. *Human Development*. New York: Macmillan Publishing Co., Inc., 1974.

MASLOW, ABRAHAM H. *Motivation and Personality*. New York: Harper & Row, 1970.

MUSSEN, PAUL, JOHN CONGER, and JEROME KAGAN. *Child Development and Personality*. New York: Harper & Row, 1974.

ROGERS, CARL R. "Can Schools Grow Persons?" *Educational Leadership,* Vol. 29, No. 3 (December 1971).

SILBERMAN, CHARLES E. *Crisis in the Classroom.* New York: Random House, 1970.

SMART, RUSSELL, and MOLLIE SMART. *Children,* 3/e. New York: Macmillan Publishing Co., Inc., 1977.

_____. *Readings in Child Development and Relationships,* 2/e, New York: Macmillan Publishing Co., Inc., 1977.

STARR, BERNARD D., and HARRIS S. GOLDSTEIN. *Human Development and Behavior.* New York: Springer Publishing Co., Inc., 1975.

STONE, L. JOSEPH, and JOSEPH CHURCH. *Childhood and Adolescence.* New York: Random House, 1972.

3

Teachers

Thus far, this book has focused on the professional decisions teachers make during the course of their work, that is, on the more formalized policies and procedures they establish with respect to the management of the classroom and their conventional teaching responsibilities. The important effects that these and other actions taken by the teacher have on the health of children quite properly receive considerable attention by parents, administrators, and other persons involved with schools; however, the equally potent effects that the behavior of children have on the health of teachers tends to receive far less attention. Virtually all teachers find their jobs to be both physically and emotionally stressful. Many of them leave the profession after a few months or a single "hellish" year, and many of those who remain suffer from a variety of stress-related health problems. In an effort to characterize the burdens that produce these untoward effects, two prominent authorities in school health offer this somewhat whimsical description:

> By the end of your day you've made as many decisions as a Fortune 500 executive. You've directed as many comings and goings as an air traffic controller at O'Hare. You've walked X miles around the school, treating your feet like those of an umpire who calls a 27-inning game. Your vocal cords have been worked out not unlike those of Beverly Sills in a rehearsal. Your eyes have performed like those of a Tiffany gem cutter. The physical energy you have expended would wear out a construction worker, and the mental stress and strain matches that of a family doctor except that he sees one person at a time, and by appointment only.[1]

Although the analogies are perhaps overdrawn, the general tone is accurate in terms of the activities of typically busy, overburdened teachers

[1] Vivian K. Harlin and Stephen J. Jerrick, "Is Teaching Hazardous to Your Health?" *Instructor,* Vol. 86, No. 1 (August/September 1976), p. 55.

who are surviving and even thriving in their work. The situation is much more grim, however, for many of the less fortunate types who, because of inexperience or chronic adjustment problems, find themselves in constant emotional strife with 25 or 30 immature personalities in the tight little world of the self-contained classroom.

ILLNESS in the CLASSROOM

When these very real pressures produce or contribute to illness within the teacher, whether it is some exotic emotional syndrome, the latest version of influenza, or something as mundane as low back pain, many serious possibilities arise. Most obvious, of course, is the reciprocal effects on the health of the children. Ill teachers can spread disease germs and personality defects with equal ease, although the "incubation period" for emotional pathology may be a bit longer. A less noticeable but equally important hazard is the long-term erosion of academic progress among the children that illness-related teaching inefficiency can produce. Should these problems cause the teacher to resign in favor of other employment, the community becomes the loser, for there is little evidence to suggest that it is only the poor teachers who are "weeded out" by this process. On the contrary, it appears that in the classroom, as on the battlefield, the good people are the first to fall, as the more sensitive and idealistic young teachers wilt under the pressures of classroom reality. Herbert M. Greenberg in his book *Teaching with Feeling* describes a somewhat extreme but nonetheless valid example of a new teacher with a middle-class background who finds herself unable to adjust to an inner city school:

> . . . she had failed. And failed quite miserably, with humiliation. She could not handle the children. They drove her to tears. She couldn't stand the constant fighting and the destructiveness. Second graders, pushing over desks in anger—cursing each other at the drop of a hat, spontaneously screaming out four letter words—Miss Barnes' whole being rejected having to face this kind of experience as a daily occurrence. Other behavior of the children was just as upsetting. Miss Barnes had had it. She quit. She felt a complete sense of relief. It was over. Thank God. Never again.[2]

Since the time this example was recorded both the training of teachers and the situation within the inner city have improved to some extent. But teachers still drop out, and it is not only inner city children who push them to this extreme act. Many such teachers survive or even benefit from their classroom traumas and successfully adjust to other less stressful work,

[2] Herbert M. Greenberg, *Teaching with Feeling* (New York: Macmillan Publishing Company, Inc., 1969) , pp. 70–71.

but others never really find their occupational niche. They thus forsake their chance for a meaningful career, and a serious personal as well as a societal loss is the ultimate result.

Stress, of course, does not invariably lead to illness. Both the human body and the human personality possess remarkable capacities for adaptation. In terms of physical threats, for example, first-year teachers typically miss more days work because of colds and flu than do their more experienced colleagues whose years of exposure to children have apparently stimulated their immunity mechanisms to provide added resistance to upper respiratory infections. In a similar fashion postural muscles firm up and vocal chords strengthen in response to the hours of desk work and class discussion that teaching entails. These internal adjustments to physical stress are typically matched by appropriate changes in the young teacher's health behavior. It soon becomes apparent that comfortable shoes are essential and that an adequate breakfast reduces the prospects of midmorning fatigue and/or headaches. In their college days prospective teachers may have found it convenient to skimp on sleep and doze through a few classes in the often passive role of a student. Once on the job, however, they generally find it very painful to provide a full day's leadership to active children without a full night's sleep. The physical demands are thus accommodated in fairly routine fashion. When breakdowns occur, they more commonly result from the unique emotional burdens of the teaching task.

SOURCES of STRESS

As the examples cited have shown, teaching can be a hazardous profession. Many new candidates drop out; many others barely manage to survive only to condemn themselves to years of dissatisfaction. However, there is a much brighter side to this situation; the very factors that produce these unwholesome effects in some young candidates also provide the challenges that stimulate personal growth in others. A closer look at the particular type of stress involved in teaching can better prepare one for coping with these worthy adversaries.

SOCIAL INTERACTION

The layman generally thinks of teachers as persons who first and foremost must know their subject matter and whose main problems occur when they fail to have the answer to some child's question. In actual fact, of course, the challenge of teaching lies in the ability to live in contact with children 5 or 6 hours a day, 5 days a week. Most mothers are at their wits' end by the end of the summer with only two or three young children in their households; however, teachers must spend the major portion of the year with 20 or 30 children. And schools for the most part accept all who wish to enter; they have few of the built-in selection factors that produce a high degree of homogeneity in the groups commonly found in summer camps, youth organizations, and Sunday school classes. Consequently, the average elementary teacher typically faces a wide variety of personality types, each with a unique combination of assets and liabilities.

The task of helping each pupil accomplish the various formal learning tasks would be a significant challenge even if it were all that was required, but young children demand much more from their teachers. They want help for personal problems ranging from unfair bullies to hopelessly knotted shoelaces; they want considerable sympathy for the problems that cannot be readily solved; they want encouragement for each little task and praise for each little achievement; and they want the affection that their own home provides, or perhaps fails to provide. In other words they want their teachers to be parents. This desire is in many ways unrealistic but this does not stop the pupils from trying to place teachers in this role, and these efforts take their toll.

This contact with children is the most sustained and intense social interaction associated with teaching; however, there are other persons who have important effects. Perhaps the most important of these persons is the teacher's immediate superior, the building principal. Lillian Bernhagen, past president of the American School Health Association, describes this importance as follows:

> If the teachers work in a school with a principal who cares, who works with the kids, cooperates with the faculty, and creates a supportive environment, then those teachers will most likely be positively reinforced, and emotionally will feel rewarded . . . . But if teachers have a principal who criticizes and never compliments, and who creeps around corners rather than being open, then morale will drop and teachers become emotionally exhausted and starved for positive reinforcement. Not long after comes the physical manifestation of frustration and stress.[3]

This point of view is supported by objective research such as that by Leonard D. Ponder and Cyrus Mayshark, who investigated the relationship between the organizational climate and the health status of teachers and found that teachers working in schools with open organizational climates took fewer days of sick leave than those working in closed climates. An organization with an open climate in this case was defined as "an energetic, lively organization which is moving toward its goal and which provides social needs satisfaction for its group members."[4] Although this study was

[3] Harlin and Jerrick, op. cit., p. 57.
[4] Leonard D. Ponder and Cyrus Mayshark, "The Relationship Between School Organizational Climate and Selected Teacher Health Status Indicators," *Journal of School Health*, Vol. 44, No. 3 (March 1974), pp. 122–125.

relatively modest in scope, encompassing only 20 schools, its results are in agreement with the mainstream of authoritative opinion. In speaking of the threats to the emotional well-being of teachers posed by their evaluation by the principal and other school authorities, Greenberg states:

> Our feelings about ourselves are very sensitive to negative evaluation from persons in authority. Our self-feeling may be shattered—our self-confidence shaken, our liking for our ourselves dissolved and replaced with self-hate, self-dislike and self-dissatisfaction.[5]

Although principals and supervisors with direct authority over teachers have perhaps the greatest effect on the teachers' emotional adjustment of any of the adults associated with the school, others such as parents, colleagues, school nurses, and custodians all represent potential sources of support or additional burdens to endure, depending upon the personalities of the individuals involved and the way they interact with any particular teacher.

VALUE CONFLICTS

In addition to the need to adjust to an environment of diverse personalities, teachers must also adjust to the philosophical environment of a particular school. Although principals, teachers, and community members all may be pleasant and reasonable human beings, they may have strong and conflicting views about the nature of teaching and the general management of school affairs. New teachers, for example, may be accepted at the personal level, but if they are not understood and accepted for what they are trying to do professionally all manner of difficulties may arise. A school district has a right to exert a certain degree of control over the type of subject matter taught, the methods of presentation, and the criteria used to determine if a particular teacher is performing satisfactorily. Teachers have a parallel right to expect both a certain degree of freedom to work out their own individual teaching approaches and a measure of respect for their judgment as to how specific topics or situations should be handled. They also need appropriate support and encouragement for the work they are doing in the classroom.

A number of factors exist that make significant discrepancies between these two sets of expectations almost inevitable. The most important of these factors pertain to the different personal concepts and value systems that produce differences in interpretations and perceptions of the various situations involved. Such philosophical issues seem harmless enough when discussed in the college classroom or when faced by a curriculum committee struggling to draft a statement of philosophy, which is too often

[5] Greenberg, op. cit., p. 122.

filed away and forgotten soon after the ink dries; however, the "crunch" comes when supervisors and principals must make their evaluation of the work of individual teachers and their subsequent recommendations as to retention, tenure, and promotion. Perhaps even more crucial are the judgments that must be rendered when parents or colleagues complain about a particular teacher's work or behavior. Such pressures cause this abstract issue to crystallize into concrete actions with important effects on real people.

One might expect that there would be a sufficient consensus on the important elements of the educational process to support a universally accepted definition of a good teaching job, particularly in view of the effort that has been directed toward this task. Yet the differences are perhaps greater than ever. Larry Cuban, who is, among other things, a veteran inner city teacher, points to an extreme but nonetheless common interpretation:

> The good teacher is the authoritarian veteran whose very glance throws a blanket of silence over a class; the "poor" teacher is the one whose class can be heard down the hall . . . . Many principals, supervisors, and colleagues rate teacher competency by the answer to the single question: Can he keep them quiet? It is stupid but it is true.[6]

Cuban also reports the words of an older principal in the process of comparing the teachers of her generation with recent candidates. She appears to move one step up the scale from the concept of teacher as policeman to teacher as active lecturer as she states:

> "Give me a teacher . . . who can really teach . . . . I want a gal who is on her feet in front of the class talking to the children. Someone who has her class in the palm of her hand. The children will be so interested that they wouldn't want her to stop talking. That's teaching." [7]

Neither of these views is in accord with the concept of the teacher as a guider of activity that prospective teachers generally acquire on the campus during their training. Most teacher training programs advocate an approach focused on the activities of the learners, not the teacher. This approach also generally includes an emphasis on relating to each child as an individual in terms of his or her total personality as opposed to lock-step instruction directed solely toward academic goals. And of course it must be recognized that the approach one acquires in training may not be all that workable in any given teaching situation, nor will it always be compatible with the personal characteristics of any given candidate. The ultimate result of this situation is that new teachers are exposed to a number of

[6] Larry Cuban, *To Make a Difference: Teaching in the Inner City* (New York: The Free Press, 1970), pp. 41–42.
[7] Ibid., p. 43.

diverse models of teaching effectiveness, none of which is likely to be wholly satisfactory. The confusion is often compounded by the fact that any or all of these models may contain internal inconsistencies. People who advise teachers do not always mean what they say. Consider, for example, the ambivalence of the type of communication that teachers sometime receive from their principals:

1. Be more creative in your teaching. Find new ways of involving your students in the learning process. [But] Be sure to follow the teacher guidebooks so all classes will be approximately at the same place at all times during the year. And as you know, the standardized test scores will be used in measuring your teaching effectiveness.
2. Learning should be fun and exciting not routine and boring. [But] A good teacher always keeps his students highly motivated and his classroom quiet and under control.[8]

Few principals would incorporate such inconsistencies into a single statement; however, it is not at all unusual for the components of such "double-binding" imperatives to be issued on separate occasions during the course of a single school year. And principals are not the only persons guilty of making contradictory demands on teachers. Parents often call for tight discipline—so long as their children are not chastised or punished. School boards call for more individualized instruction but fail to raise the tax money necessary for smaller-sized classes. School nurses warn teachers that only physicians can diagnose illnesses but then ask that children not be sent to the nursing suite unless they are really sick.

Most new teachers begin their work with considerable enthusiasm. They feel that it is important—that it greatly affects the lives of their pupils—and almost everyone connected with the schools tends to agree on this point. However, they are often not provided with any clear indication of what they are expected to accomplish and how they are to accomplish it. Fortunately, most teachers resolve this difficult situation and complete satisfying careers, but this task is not easy.

LIMITATIONS of ADJUSTMENT

The problems described in the preceding section are very real and very common; however, one compensating factor is that few teachers encounter all of them in the same teaching situation. For example, few teachers must endure the combined effects of an inadequate training program, a classroom full of problem children, and an inept school administration. Strength in anyone of these external factors can spell the difference between an

---

[8] Howard G. Garner, "How to Prevent a School from Becoming Schizophrenic," *Journal of School Health*. Vol. 42, No. 9 (November 1972), pp. 556–557.

impossible first year and a tolerable one. Good professional training can enable a teacher to at least survive any poor teaching situation; helpful, supporting principals and supervisors can compensate for many inadequacies in one's background; and, although the bad groups of children receive more notice, there are also many other good groups where the emotional dynamics seem to fall into place to make the teaching job relatively easy. But in most situations, of course, these factors are neither very good nor very bad but fall at some point between the extremes to pose a challenging but manageable adjustment problem for the teacher. However, as will be described in the following section, *adjustment* is perhaps not the proper term, for it is sometimes accomplished by means of costly compromises.

PROFESSIONAL DETACHMENT

Some teachers learn to detach themselves emotionally from their work to an excessive degree. They lower their expectations; they too readily accept the fact that it is impossible to do all they would like to do for each child; they learn to restrict their workload by getting papers corrected and scores recorded in class; they never question the curriculum as established by committees and handed down by supervisors; they resist most efforts directed at constructive changes and spend little if any energy working on their own innovations; they learn not to worry so much about the personal problems of individual children, maintaining that little can be done for them; when they leave the school they are usually through with school concerns until the next morning; in fact, they are often able to sell life insurance or pursue some other part-time business enterprise in their spare time.

In its worst form this pattern of adjustment tends to produce reasonably content, satisfied, but generally uncaring teachers—and children with a host of unmet needs. Such situations have led to the scathing indictments of American schools by John Holt, Charles Silberman, and other critics of American education as mentioned in Chapter 2. But before one condemns this behavior too vehemently it is well to consider the more positive side of detachment. A certain degree of this quality is probably essential to the emotional health of most teachers if they are to function at the best possible level. Although such extreme examples as these are useful in illustrating a point, they are not commonly found in real life. Many teachers are able to withdraw to a point that enables them to function effectively yet still retain a significant degree of involvement. However, like any defense mechanism, this serves best when not overused.

SUITS of ARMOR

The late Sidney M. Jourard's general views on defense versus growth seem to apply quite clearly to the new teacher's task of dealing with his or her emotions. Anything as challenging as teaching must also be to some extent threatening. In speaking of such situations, he states:

> . . . threat opens options. It can spur defensive maneuvers that are themselves barriers to life, and it can promote enlarged awareness and greater competence. If every time a person was threatened, he put on a heavier suit of armor, then in time he would be immobile—safe but out of touch. If he could postpone defensive maneuvers long enough, he could act in ways that further his growth.[9]

Jourard's phrase "safe but out of touch" appears to quite accurately describe the teachers who make excessive use of defense mechanisms. There are many "suits of armor" available to those who wish to insulate themselves from the lives of children. Among the more common are the following:

1. *Social Distance.* This is achieved by remaining aloof and staying with the planned schedule at all times; above all, not engaging in any frivolous activities—don't smile until Christmas.
2. *Harsh Discipline.* This is used to solve problems by force, either force of personality such as browbeating or intimidation or physical force where permitted.
3. *Game Playing.* This takes various forms but in each case the children become actively involved in irrelevant activity such as long rows of easy arithmetic problems or the copying of each spelling word 20 times. Movies unrelated to the course objectives are another possibility.

MOVING TOWARD the IDEAL

Most teachers are forced to resort to compromising adjustment tactics on occasion to preserve their emotional well-being and get themselves through difficult situations. The general style, the routine mode of operating, of even the best of teachers is no doubt contaminated to some degree by these mechanisms that serve the teacher but do little for the children. There is, of course, a better way, a sounder basis, but it would be irresponsible to give the impression that any simple formula exists for the development of an ideal teaching style leading to an optimal rate of academic progress for the children, and, more to the point, maximum emotional growth for both children and teacher. No clear agreement exists as to even the basic characteristics of such a happy state, much less as to how to achieve them. And if such a formula should ever be devised, it almost surely would apply differently to each and every teacher. But although the goal remains elu-

[9] Sidney M. Jourard, *Healthy Personality* (New York: Macmillan Publishing Co., Inc., 1974), p. 174.

sive, there are some promising leads that can give direction to one's career-long task of professional growth.

INVOLVEMENT

Perhaps the best general advice for the achievement of a meaningful teaching career is to *be* a teacher, rather than to merely *act like* a teacher. This does not happen overnight; the process begins when the new teacher starts to attack problems, opportunities, and situations rather than to withdraw from them. If the class is not behaving well, if many children are "goofing off" (which in more genteel terms becomes "off-task behavior"), then one must do something about it rather than merely hope the situation will correct itself. This may involve changing the assignment, changing the working arrangements, conducting a general discussion with the class to seek a solution, or, on occasion, an emotional outburst together with some disciplinary measures. If one type of action does not succeed, then try another. If a child seems unhappy and upset, ask him or her about the source of the problem. Perhaps you can help; if not, the child will benefit from the knowledge that you care.

EMOTIONAL EXPRESSION

Closely related to the concept of involvement is the humanistic concept of self-disclosure. Although professional restraint is necessary in many situations, teachers tend to overuse this isolating device. Greenberg cites a number of myths that cause teachers to carry burdensome façades rather than to act as real persons in the classroom. Among these are the "myth of calmness" and the "myth of moderation." [10] The first of these myths insists that the teacher not display any of his or her real feelings or moods. No matter how joyous or angry, these feelings, too, must be hidden, disguised, "controlled." The "myth of moderation" insists "that the mentally 'healthy' person has no problems that can't be dealt with mildly, has few conflicts, and rarely experiences extreme or strong feelings." In summing up his case for freer expression of teacher emotions, Greenberg states:

> It is difficult, if not impossible to deny pressing needs of one's own, while attempting to meet the needs of others. A teacher who expresses his own feelings, moreover, sets a climate in which children's feelings are also acceptable and understood. [11]

Probably the most important benefit arising from this type of behavior is the avoidance of the practice of pushing negative emotions below the

[10] Greenberg, op. cit., pp. 25–27.
[11] Ibid.

surface where they typically function as "hidden agendas" and cause problems that defy solution simply because the root causes remain inaccessible to examination and correction. When emotions are revealed, the way is cleared for constructive solutions. As one dedicated teacher reveals,

> If I see it's going to be a lousy day because everybody's in a lousy mood [I don't want to] pretend it's going to be an okay day. I don't tell them, "Let's be happy today, have fun." Sometimes I say the opposite. (Laughs) I say, "I'm very unhappy today and we're not gonna have fun, we're gonna work." They pull me out of it. And when they're in a lousy mood, they don't hide it. They certainly let me know it.[12]

INTEGRITY

We often hear that each child is unique—that each child has something special to offer—but tend to overlook the fact that each teacher is also a unique personality. Each teacher brings a particular pattern of strengths and liabilities to the job and responds to the experience of teaching in a way different from that of any other teacher. One teacher, for example, might have a "knack" for teaching language arts but have to struggle to do a merely adequate job in mathematics. Another might relate better to the children who are bright and perhaps bored, as compared to a colleague with a special ability to motivate those who have problems keeping up with their classmates. This does not mean that teachers should ignore their weaknesses, but that they need to develop a classroom teaching style that is valid in terms of their particular pattern of qualities.

Actually, the development and refinement of this unique style is a never-ending process. As teachers allow their real selves to function in the classroom and as they find out who they are in that situation, there "is a merging of the professional activities of the teacher with his total life situation. The teacher is alive in the fullest sense, a being with self-consistency and structure, but also fully growing and becoming."[13]

LEARNING

Perhaps the most commonly overlooked benefit of teaching as a career is the opportunity it provides for one's maturation and growth as a person. Human learning for the most part takes place in a social context, and teaching perhaps more than any other occupation immerses one in an environment of people. New teachers generally enter this challenging arena for some combination of the desire for personal gain and the need to per-

[12] Studs Terkel, *Working* (New York: Pantheon Books, 1972), p. 492.
[13] Clark Moustakas, *Teaching as Learning* (New York: Ballantine Books, 1972), p. 33.

form a useful service. However, the better teachers soon find that teaching is not a one-way street; they find that they can learn much from their children, pertaining both to school matters, and more importantly, to life itself. Children are obviously very naive about many things, but they are also amazingly insightful about many other matters, and their emotional reactions to many of life's problems and opportunities are often more constructive than those of adults. Also, in contrast to many adults, most elementary children have not yet "learned" to hide their true feelings and thus to present false impressions.

If the teacher can establish the proper classroom climate, many good things become possible. As Clark Moustakas states:

> In an atmosphere of freedom and trust where individuals are involved, fully accepted and respected the group becomes its own best resource and serves as the primary basis for emerging insights and for the resolution of problems. . . . Once the leader fulfills his initial responsibility, the group functions on its own and he becomes a learner too.[14]

Those who accept Alexander Pope's observation that "The proper study of mankind is man" [15] should never find their classroom lacking for learning resources.

Children not only provide cognitive stimulation to adults but also, when things go well, serve to meet some of the deepest emotional needs of adults. In discussing his concept of "generativity" Erik Erikson observes:

> The fashionable insistence on dramatizing the dependence of children on adults often blinds us to the dependence of the older generation on the younger one. Mature man needs to be needed, and maturity needs guidance as well as encouragement from what has been produced and must be taken care of.[16]

When viewed in these terms, teaching becomes something more than another stressful occupation; it offers an opportunity to achieve a state in which the borders between one's personal and professional life blur and self-actualization begins to take place.

COMMITMENT

A final word of caution is in order. Like other types of behavior that gratify deep personal needs, teaching can be habit forming. Some new teaching

---

[14] Ibid., p. 207.
[15] Alexander Pope, *An Essay on Man* (Epistle I, 1. 290).
[16] Erik H. Erikson, *Childhood and Society* (New York: W. W. Norton & Co., Inc., 1963), pp. 266, 267.

candidates react adversely and are forced to leave. Others teach for years without any sense of commitment; they can take it or leave it. But still others, after a few good years, find that they are not common ordinary persons anymore; somewhere along the line they have become teachers. As one such person describes his feeling about his work,

> I run into people who say how much they admire what I do. It's embarrassing. I don't make any judgments about my work, whether it's great or worthless. It's just what I do best. It's the only job I want to do. . . . This is my life. I just am.[17]

REFERENCES

CUBAN, LARRY. *To Make a Difference: Teaching in the Inner City.* New York: The Free Press, 1970.

ERIKSON, ERIK H. *Childhood and Society.* New York: W. W. Norton & Co., Inc., 1963.

GARNER, HOWARD G. "How to Prevent a School from Becoming Schizophrenic," *Journal of School Health* (November 1972).

GREENBERG, HERBERT M. *Teaching with Feeling.* New York: Macmillan Publishing Co., Inc., 1969.

HARLIN, VIVIAN K., and STEPHEN J. JERRICK. "Is Teaching Hazardous to Your Health?" *Instructor,* Vol. 86, No. 1 (August/September 1976).

JOURARD, SIDNEY M. *Healthy Personality.* New York: Macmillan Publishing Co., Inc., 1974.

MOUSTAKAS, CLARK. *Teaching As Learning.* New York: Ballantine Books, 1972.

PONDER, LEONARD D., and CYRUS MAYSHARK. "The Relationship Between School Organizational Climate and Selected Teacher Health Status Indicators," *Journal of School Health,* Vol. 44, No. 3 (March 1974).

SCHLOSSER, COURTNEY D. *The Person in Education: A Humanistic Approach.* New York: Macmillan Publishing Co., Inc., 1976.

TERKEL, STUDS. *Working.* New York: Pantheon Books, 1972.

TRAVERS, ROBERT M. W. The Making of a Teacher: *A Research-Based Plan and Manual for Students.* New York: Macmillan Publishing Co., Inc., 1975.

[17] Terkel, op. cit., p. 493.

part 3

The Subject

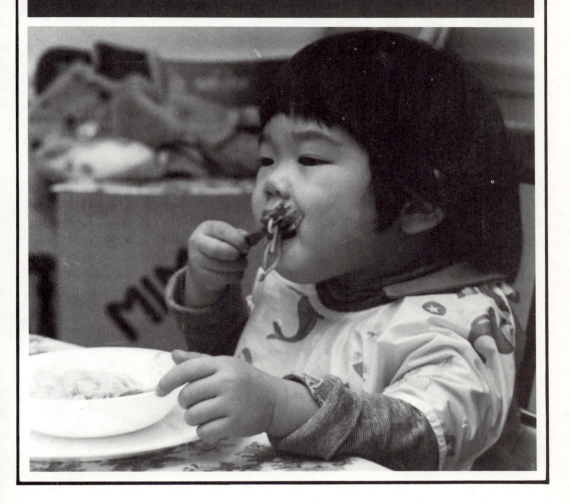

Bones, Flesh, and Sinew— The Human Body

In the eyes of the anatomist a human being is a body that somehow possesses a mind that helps it function and go about its business. The psychologist, of course, would see it differently—a human being is essentially a mind, a personality, that happens to reside within a body that helps it carry out its decisions. At this point a philosopher is likely to come along and scoff at this debate as a meaningless exercise, for on the basis of his logical analysis he might very well conclude that mind and body are one and the same. This somewhat esoteric issue manages to cause some practical problems for health educators who advocate the study of the human body as part of the health curriculum. They often run afoul of educational theorists who protest that "it is the whole child who comes to school—mind, body, spirit, personality and whatever—you should not be breaking him into isolated segments for study." This may be true in one sense, but even though we must always remember the human being's interrelatedness we must at times concentrate on single aspects or dimensions if our study is to remain manageable.

MODERN-DAY ATTITUDES

Once this hurdle is passed, we soon encounter another potent obstacle that threatens to distract and stifle even the most elementary study of human anatomy and physiology, namely, the irrational squeamishness and distaste that most persons, within our culture at least, exhibit toward many of the basic bodily functions. One of the authors can remember his fifth grade teacher with pointer in hand tracing the path of food on a large chart of the digestive system. She started out well enough with the mouth, esoph-agus, and stomach, but became increasingly ill at ease as our imaginary meal made its way through the small intestine, the ascending colon, the transverse colon, and the descending colon—at this point with a quick flour-ish of the pointer she explained that the food was then "passed off." Although there was probably no great need for a unit on defecation, we fifth graders could have used a few more details.

Excretory functions are not the only aspects that Americans seem unduly sensitive about. Our concern over how to discuss sexual functions with other adults, much less children, is tantamount to a national neurosis; nudity often evokes unwarranted prudishness; we are taught that body odors are something that should never exist, and many girls come to believe that it is very unladylike to do anything that might produce perspiration. These points are not presented as a rejection of our modern standards of privacy and personal hygiene but only to bring some balance to the situa-tion. Every teacher knows that most parents prefer that their children learn to keep themselves clean and odor free. But what is sometimes over-looked is that this emphasis on cleanliness can be carried to a point where it represents an attempt to deny that we have a body rather than an effort to give it proper care.

Depending upon one's choice in philosophy, our body either defines our total being—after, all, what are brain cells other than physical entities—or at the very least represents a very prominent part of our existence as a person. Therefore, acceptance of our body is an important part of acceptance of ourselves. Abraham Maslow, in describing this quality as observed in per-sons of outstanding mental health, states:

> The first and most obvious level of acceptance is at the so-called animal level. Those self-actualizing [mentally healthy] people tend to be good animals, hearty in their appetites and enjoying themselves with-out regret or shame or apology. They seem to have a uniformly good appetite for food; they seem to sleep well; they seem to enjoy their sexual lives without unnecessary inhibition and so on for all physiological impulses . . . . [They have] a relative lack of the disgusts and aversions seen in average people and especially in neurotics, e.g. food annoyances, disgusts with body products, body odors, and body functions.[1]

These "disgusts and aversions" held by average people are obviously going to be part of our culture for a long time, but Maslow certainly implies that the time has come to ease off a bit in this apparent aesthetic overkill.

This national tendency for bodily denial seems related to a more tangible obvious problem in national attitude and behavior toward the human body. The average person's preoccupation with "covering up" many bodily

---

[1] Abraham H. Maslow, *Motivation and Personality* (New York: Harper & Row, 1970), p. 156.

attitudes and imperfections often contributes to a neglect of fundamentally important bodily needs. Somehow we are raising and educating children in such a manner that as adults they place more value in underarm deodorants, mouthwashes, and cosmetics than they do in nutritious food, exercise, sufficient rest, or regular medical and dental care. Each person owns what is, in one sense at least, the world's most miraculous machine, yet people are more interested in giving it a "Sunday shine," a cheap wax job, rather than the important maintenance and sustenance it requires for top efficiency.

EDUCATIONAL NEEDS

The reasons for these dubious attitudes and unconstructive behavior patterns are difficult to determine; it seems clear, however, that many of them are carryovers from earlier generations who were forced to rely on superstitions and folklore rather than scientific knowledge as they tried to understand and care for their bodies. The effective education of elementary schoolchildren in this important topic requires some direct training and supervision in related health behaviors such as those in posture, rest, and exercise; a direct attack on feelings and values by means of appropriate affective techniques; and the development of a sound knowledge and understanding of the basic structure and functions of the body. This last task, the development of knowledge and understanding, is not likely to produce any immediate impact on health behavior but will ordinarily exert a long-range influence in years to come.

ILLUSTRATIVE CONTENT

The traditional way to organize the study of the human body is to consider each of the organ systems in turn. Although this approach tends to produce a fragmented view, it does feature logic and simplicity. More generalized topics, however, such as the body's general efficiency and adaptability or lack of adaptability to modern life, its evolutionary history, and a comparison with other organisms represent more promising topics for either introducing the topic or culminating the study, that is, putting the pieces together after studying the separate systems. In this section some of the more interesting subtopics will be highlighted in order to acquaint the reader with some of the possibilities of this curriculum area.

GENERAL CHARACTERISTICS

The human body, in comparison either with other members of the animal world or with machines, possesses many unique and remarkable qualities.

The relatively large brain sets humans apart in terms of intelligence and learning ability. The upright posture frees the hands to develop into highly dexterous instruments that in terms of overall performance remain much more versatile than the most sophisticated machines. Much of this dexterity is attributed, oddly enough, to the human thumb with its unique arrangement that permits it to work in opposition to the fingers. The capacity for skilled movement, that is, for voluntary action, is wondrous and too often taken for granted, as are the intrinsic functions of the internal adjustment mechanisms that monitor such tasks as digestion, energy metabolism, posture maintenance, and so forth.

ORIGIN of the BODY

According to the widely endorsed theory of evolution, the human animal evolved into its present form from simple beginnings in approximately 500 million years. This theory is based on the concepts of genetic variation, mutation and natural selection. Unique combinations of genes during reproduction and modification of genes by such factors as cosmic rays and various chemicals produce variations among the offspring of any species that give some individuals more survival value than others. These better-endowed individuals then survive to maturity and pass their traits on to their progeny in a constant process of refinement. One interesting sidelight to this scheme is that mankind's cultural and technological progress has brought natural selection on the basis of physical fitness or intelligence to a standstill; one doesn't have to run fast, fight hard, or even be very intelligent to survive long enough to produce children these days. Consequently, the basic characteristics of the human body have remained largely unchanged since the emergence of Cro-Magnon man about 40,000 years ago. Geneticists worry about the perpetuation of defective genes among humans, but thus far any problems seem to be offset by good medical care and other compensating factors.

The alternate version of the origin of man is of course the story of the Creation as described in the book of Genesis. Some school districts have prescribed that this religious version must also be discussed out of consideration for those who subscribe to a literal translation of the Bible. However, an Indiana court recently ruled that the teaching of the Genesis interpretation violated the constitutional separation of church and state and therefore should not be presented in public school textbooks. This is perhaps unfortunate; although unscientific in any conventional sense, the biblical version opens up some interesting possibilities for discussion, as shown in this excerpt:

> So God created man in His own image; in the image of God He created him; male and female He created them. God blessed them and said to

64

them, "Be fruitful and increase, fill the earth and subdue it, rule over the fish of the sea, the birds of heaven, and every living thing that moves upon the earth." [2]

The concept of man in the image of God is a fascinating one, as is his apparent mandate to take dominion over the earth. Regardless of one's belief concerning his origin, human beings and their bodies appear as marvelous entities worthy of careful study.

ORGANIZATION OF THE BODY

The human body is an intricate organization of cells, tissues, organs, and organ systems. A basic understanding of cell physiology makes many of the grosser functions and malfunctions of the body more understandable. Cells generally can live only in a fluid environment where certain conditions such as oxygen, pressure, temperature, and acid–base balance (pH level) must not vary beyond close limits. The circulation of the blood and the elimination of wastes are essential to this task. Either heart failure or kidney failure will produce cell death that, if extensive enough, will kill the whole organism.

A few cells such as blood cells float freely; however, most body cells are connected to other similar cells to form tissues; both the shape of the individual cells and the nature of their arrangement within tissue are related to the functions they perform. Thus skin cells are flat and thin and are arranged much like shingles on a roof, whereas muscles are long and thin and arranged in parallel bunches or shelves. Organs are composed of tissues arranged to facilitate a particular function; thus the heart is seen basically as a muscular sack that relaxes to fill with blood and constricts to pump it on its way; it is lined inside and out with skinlike tissue and nerve components that enable it to both respond to outside stimuli and provide its own innervation (stimulus). The heart itself forms part of a larger organization, the circulatory system, with its vast network of arteries, veins, and capillaries.

THE SKELETAL and MUSCLE SYSTEMS

The bones of the skeleton provide support for the body and, in the case of the skull and spinal column, protection for more delicate organs. Much of the skeleton consists of softer cartilage at birth, for only these soft portions can grow. As the bone matures, the spaces between individual bone cells become filled with deposits consisting mainly of calcium phosphate,

[2] *The New English Bible* (Cambridge: Cambridge University Press, 1970), Genesis 27–28, p. 2.

which become hard. Bone growth then ceases, but the bone cells continue to live and among other functions stand ready to repair the bone in case of a fracture. Some of the cartilage remains in its original form and serves as pads between the joints. The joints are generally surrounded by ligaments that form joint capsules lined with membranes that secrete a lubricating fluid. Other ligaments form bonds that help hold the joint together.

The muscles are attached to the bones with another type of connective tissue—the tendons. The long, parallel muscle cells, are arranged in groups called motor units that contract or relax in unison as directed by nerve impulses. The strength and speed of a particular muscle contraction are controlled by the number of its units that are brought into action and may range from the powerful lifting action of the quadriceps (on front of the thighs) to the delicate movements of the eye when reading. During vigorous exercise the muscle cells involved contract frequently, requiring considerable internal chemical activities; oxygen and nutrients are consumed and carbon dioxide and acid wastes are produced, thus making heavy demands on the circulatory system to deliver the needed materials and remove the waste products.

THE NERVOUS SYSTEM

The form and motion of the body as largely determined by the skeleto-muscular system provide a natural starting point for its study, but the question arises as to "Who gives the orders and how do the muscles know when to contract?" The answer begins with a consideration of our 12-billion-element (cell) computer, the human brain, and although the computer analogy is inevitable the computer still has a long way to go in the thinking and perception realms if it is to approach human standards.[3] The brain is still so complex as to be virtually unfathomable, but although there is still much for scientists to discover, a wealth of information is available. The upper portion of the cerebrum is highly developed in humans, and perhaps more than any other single feature, gives us a chance to fulfilll the Book of Genesis's mandate to dominate the earth. Here, reasoning, memory, and the interpretation of sensory stimuli (perception) take place; also, both sensory and motor maps of the entire body can be found.

Although the initial decision for movement (e.g., whether to wait, walk, or run) comes from the cerebrum, the infinitely complex instructions to the muscles are stored at the next lower level, in the cerebellum. Once the recording process is completed, as when one learns to walk or swim, the skill is "learned" and remains available in the cerebellum, awaiting the signal from the cerebrum. This decision-making ability is facilitated by

[3] See, for example, Fred Hapgood, "Computers Aren't So Smart," *The Atlantic,* Vol. 234, No. 2 (August 1974), pp. 37—49.

the body information network, which features a highly unique category of cells called sensory receptors. These microscopic structures are designed to fire off a signal (nerve impulse) when their particular stimulus happens along in the environment; prominent examples include those in the retina of the eye, the cochlea of the inner ear, the taste buds of the tongue, the proprioceptors within the muscles, and the wide variety of receptors in the skin. Interestingly enough, all this variety of stimuli reaches the brain in nerve impulses of the same form; the cerebrum must sort out all this incoming material and give meaning to it. This it does with high efficiency except in occasional mixups as when a blow to the head is interpreted as stars and bells as well as physical force.

At the lowest portion of the brain, the brain stem, one encounters a miraculous set of feedback devices that monitor several critical factors that affect the safety and functional efficiency of the body and trigger needed adjustment without the owner of this complex system ever knowing about it. When the glucose level of the blood dips too low, impulses are sent to the adrenal glands for the release of epinephrine, which subsequently causes stored glucose to be released; when carbon dioxide levels get too high, the respiratory rate is caused to increase; when the body temperature rises unduly, sphincters (valves) are activated, allowing more blood to go to the skin where water is released as perspiration that evaporates to produce a cooling effect. The sensory receptors that trigger these changes, together with their network of nerve fibers, compose the autonomic nervous system. Human efforts to make similar electronic devices, servomechanisms, to monitor his industrial processes have been highly successful even though they are still primitive in comparison to the corresponding system each human being possesses.

THE VISCERA

The internal organs of the body as found in the abdominal and thoracic cavities are somewhat analogous to the engine room of a ship: air, fuel, and water are fed in, and heat, energy, and waste products are taken out. The digestive system begins the processing of food, with the mechanical action of the teeth and the stomach together reducing the incoming meal to a homogeneous liquid in the manner of an electric blender. The chemical action of the enzymes of the small intestine works on this uniform solution and breaks the food molecules down into simple components that are able to pass through the intestinal wall and into the bloodstream. This newly absorbed material is first routed through the liver, where certain impurities are filtered out and some further processing takes place; then these simple sugar and fat molecules, vitamins, minerals, and amino acids (protein components) are distributed throughout the body to nourish cells. The unused portion of the food is, as the author's fifth grade teacher explained, "passed off." The number of bowel movements a person has per day or week is an individual matter. True constipation rarely occurs. It is better prevented by adequate intake of fluids and fibrous foods than treated by use of laxatives.

As the muscular diaphragm under the rib cage pulls down and the muscles between the ribs pull up, the chest expands and air is sucked into the lungs and down into the innermost chambers, the alveoli, where only a thin membrane separates it from the circulating blood. Here, because of the law of partial pressure, oxygen passes into the bloodstream and carbon dioxide passes out. This fresh, red, newly oxygenated blood is collected in the vast pulmonary vessels that merge into a single vein leading to the heart, and is further distributed to the body by the heart. On each swing around the body, one-sixth of the blood is shunted through the kidneys, where the waste products of cellular activity are filtered out and piped to the bladder for periodic evacuation as urine.

THE SKIN

The many complex functions that the skin performs commonly go unappreciated by the average person, who simply assumes that it is a relatively inert covering material. Actually, this thin layer of tissue is teaming with activity, the most basic of which is the continual production of new cells in the lower layers to compensate for the constant shedding of cells from the surface. The cells at the surface of the skin are already dead or dying, as cells require a fluid environment for their survival. This process of cell death is retarded to a degree by a waxlike film that develops over the entire skin surface as a result of secretions from the sweat glands and sebaceous glands; bacteria reside in this film and cause few problems unless they are allowed to accumulate in creases and crevasses to multiply and produce unpleasant odors. This can be prevented with appropriate bathing; however, the scrubbing of the skin can be overdone to the point that the constant disruption of the film will cause excessive drying and cracking.

Few bacteria or even few chemicals can penetrate the dense cellular structure of the skin, thus making it an ideal protector against infection. The many sweat glands that are often functioning even when the skin appears dry, together with the rich capillary beds that may be filled with blood or drained according to the demands of the situation, serve as highly efficient regulators of body temperature. Specialized sensory receptors, including those sensitive to heat, cold, pressure, and pain, are distributed throughout the skin, thus making it a highly effective sensory organ. Relatively more receptors are found in critical areas like the fingertips, thus facilitating finely coordinated movements. Skin color results from a wide variety of chemical and physical factors, most important of which is the pigment, melanin, which is largely responsible for the tanning capability of light skin, for the basic color of dark-skinned persons such as Negroes, and for the freckles that many persons have. Dark skin serves as protection against the ultraviolet rays of the sun and thus helps to prevent cancer and premature aging of the skin.

THE ENDOCRINE SYSTEM and GROWTH

One of the most consistent results in studies of children's interests has been their preoccupation with their own physical growth.[4] Although many factors are involved in growth; the most dramatic role appears to be played by the ductless (endocrine) glands. The thyroid gland located near the "Adam's apple" releases hormones that regulate the body's general rate of activity or metabolism. The pituitary gland located just under the cerebrum releases, among many other secretions, human growth hormone (HGH), which determines the rate of linear growth and thus largely controls height. If children deficient in HGH are identified early in life, treatment is now possible to stimulate growth and thus prevent some cases of dwarfism. Excessive growth is not now treatable, however.

At approximately 9 years of age in girls and 11 years of age in boys, the pituitary gland releases hormones (gonadotropins) that stimulate the gonads to begin secreting their own endocrine products: these are testosterone, produced by the testes in boys, and estrogens, produced by the ovaries in girls. These hormones first produce a rapid preadolescent growth spurt, then stimulate the development of the typical male and female physical sex characteristics, and finally serve to terminate growth 5 to 7 years later as the bones become completely ossified. Girls are typically taller than boys between the ages of 9 and 10; however, the boys pass the girls in height between the ages of 13 and 14.

The great range of differences in the timing of the growth process is something that upper elementary children should come to understand in order to prevent undue concern among early or late maturers. The general rate of growth throughout childhood seems largely determined by genetic factors that affect the flow of HGH. The factor or factors that affect the timing of the release of the gonadotropin and thus the preadolescent growth spurt are still unknown. Interestingly enough, the late-maturing children often exceed in adult height those that mature early. This is because the HGH has a longer period of time to exert its influence on the temporary cartilage of the long bones before the gonadal secretions stimulate full ossification.

[4] Ruth Byler, et al., *Teach Us What We Want to Know* (New York: Mental Health Materials Center, Inc., 1969) .

CHILDREN'S INTERESTS as RELATED to the HUMAN BODY

The extensive study of the health interests of children conducted by Ruth Byler and her associates provided additional support to the widely accepted observation that children are intensely interested in the structure and inner workings of their bodies. This investigation, which involved over 5,000 children in the schools of Connecticut, yielded results that closely paralleled those of similar efforts using subjects from other sections of the country. Representative findings and in some cases verbatim quotes of children are presented in this section in an effort to provide the reader with some concept of the general range of children's interests in regard to the human body.[5]

KINDERGARTEN THROUGH GRADE TWO

• Kindergarten children ask: How does my body get made? How does God get your heart in there? How do you get bones in your body?
• Second grade children ask: What does my brain look like? How many atoms are in our bodies?. . . How do my legs bend? . . . What is your heart made of? How does it beat blood?

GRADES THREE AND FOUR

• Interest in the details of the entire body, conspicuous in grade two, rises steadily in the third and fourth grades. Children want to know all about the body, how each separate part got there, how it looks, what it does it . . . .
• Third graders ask: How do I grow? What is important in my body? . . . Does my heart look like a valentine? What shape are bones?
• Fourth graders ask: I am nine years old and small. Do you think I will be six feet tall? . . . Why are people so different? Why don't we have two of everything?

GRADES FIVE AND SIX

• Children in grades five and six express high interest in the body. They want to know all about it, the wonders of how it is made and its functions. In both grades questions are numerous about the organs, especially the heart and brain. Questions about puberty began in the fifth grade and increased in the sixth.
• Fifth graders ask: How does a body grow? . . . What is [are] skin, body tissue, dimples, freckles, beauty marks, fingernails, a hernia, hiccups? Why do we have hair? . . . .

[5] Ibid.

• Sixth graders say: Why does everyone like me take on the human form and not some other form? What makes the body go? You have everything you need, but what pushes it so it will operate and you start living?

TEACHING APPROACH

The overall goal that guides both the general planning and the specific teaching decisions in this content area is the development of an awareness and an appreciation of the beauty and the marvelous complexity of the human body. Involvement in the subject matter is sought in this particular health area more so than are specific behavioral outcomes.

BEHAVIORAL CHANGE

The fact that the implications for health behavior related to the study of the human body per se are not so obvious as they might be in the study of tobacco and alcohol, for instance, does not mean that they are of no importance. Actually, it is possible that good teaching in this area might have more long-range effects on good health practices than will the applied health areas. The child who through effective visual aids or microscopic study comes to appreciate the delicate and complex structure of the lungs, with the blood-and-air communication through gossamer membranes and the tireless cilia that undulate like tiny fields of grain in their efforts to sweep out impurities, is likely to think twice before applying noxious tars and gases to these structures through the use of cigarettes. The same thing applies to a study of the nervous system with its billions of cells and its unfathomable intricacies; many who fully understand this are reluctant to "gum up" such efficient machinery by abuse of drugs.

Of course, it is much easier to talk of "marvelous efficiency" or wondrous complexity" than it is to create learning situations where such conceptualization will take place. But it helps to realize that involvement, awareness, and appreciation are needed rather than thoroughness and deadly accuracy. Many a child has been "turned off" with a "pre--med" type of approach, with too many charts to fill in with too many Latin terms. The study may be started on topics where good teaching materials are available, whether it is the nervous system, the digestive system, or evolutionary development. If the children become genuinely intrigued with the heart and blood vessels, don't terminate their study merely to stay on schedule; let them go as far as their interest carries them. They can catch up on the other topics next time the human body comes around in the curriculum.

71

TECHNIQUES and APPROACHES

As implied in the teaching suggestions provided earlier in the chapter, the general techniques for science teaching are most applicable. Preference should be given to real materials in the form of tissues and organs from the butcher shop, pond water for study, frogs for dissection, and so forth; good audiovisual material, particularly films of living material and processes, is an acceptable second choice.

The opportunities for correlation and integration with other subjects are many and varied. The human body has been the prime subject of much artistic endeavor throughout history. One interesting topic within this area is the efforts of such masters as Leonardo DaVinci and Michelangelo to learn anatomy as an aid to their work. Also, a review of art through the ages shows how popular notions of the ideal feminine figure or male physique tend to change. Within the social studies curriculum, the sometimes weird ideas of Galen, the ancient Roman physician, and their even more surprising acceptance as the final authority through the dark ages make a fascinating study, as does the later work of Vesalius, who risked the flaming wrath of the medieval church to make human dissections and write the first modern medical text.

Thus to the artist the human body is often a thing of beauty and always a subject of interest; to the scientist it is the end product of 500 million years of evolutionary refinement, the highest form of life known; to the theologian it is the image of God and the temple of the spirit; to the average child it is simply me, my person. In any case it is something very worthy of study and appreciation.

SUGGESTED LEARNING ACTIVITIES

The following suggestions are presented in an effort to demonstrate how the content described in the preceding section might be translated into effective classroom learning activities. They were designed to accommodate a wide variety of classroom groups provided that proper selection and adaptations are made according to the needs, interests, abilities, and maturity level of the particular children involved.

- Ask your students to dip one of their fingers or thumb into poster paint, then ask them to complete some tasks, such as picking up an object, writing on the chalkboard, etc., without using the freshly painted finger. Have the students select different fingers to determine which is the worst to lose. Following the activity, have the children complete the following statement: "I learned that_____."
- While studying the various cultures around the world, have the stu-

dents make comparisons of human characteristics of today with those of the past (e.g., height, weight, life span). Using the time period you are studying (e.g., 1492–1978), make a mural depicting the characteristics as they differ over the years.

- Have the students draw pictures of how they think people on Mars look. Do they have physical characteristics similar to ours?

- Divide the class into small groups and hand out tinkertoys. Have them build a house and a human being with the toys. Have them explain how these two structures are similar.

- *The Bionic Arm.* Cut two pieces of wood and join them together with a hinge joint. Cover the top side with a piece of black elastic tape and the bottom side with white elastic tape, using one to indicate the biceps muscle and the other to indicate the triceps muscle. As the two pieces of wood are brought together, you can see the alternate shortening and lengthening of the two muscles. With the use of a metric tape measure, have the children measure how much the muscles shorten and/or lengthen. (If you have a skeleton, this can be shown with the particular bones and muscles you wish to indicate.)

- Using a model skeleton, have the students name the various bones by placing name tags on them. If you do not have a skeleton, use a Halloween skeleton.

- To find out how students feel about a beautiful and efficient body, have them complete the following continuum by putting their initials at a point on the line that best indicates how they feel:

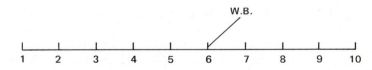

Danny Doubtful   Ginney the Greek

Danny Doubtful

(The body doesn't matter at all)

Ginney the Greek

(A healthy happy body is the pathway to happiness.)

- Take a piece of yarn and extend it across one side of the room. Have the children cut out pictures and/or draw those foods and exercises that will make for a healthy heart and hang these on the line with clothespins.

- To show the children how the blood flows through the heart, take a calf heart and pour red-colored water through the right chambers and then through the left ones to show how the blood flows through the heart.
- The above activity can also be done by cutting out a heart from large pieces of construction paper and coloring and labeling it. Fasten it to the floor and then make a tape recording of the various functions of the chambers, muscles, valves, etc. Have the children walk through the heart while listening to the tape recording.
- To show the children how fat deposits build up on the arterial walls, take the cardboard cylinder from toilet tissue rolls and progressively build them up on the inside with different-colored clay. The stages should indicate the beginning of hardening of the arteries. As you squeeze the tubes together, they will show the failure of blood to get through and supply the necessary nutrients to the various organs.
- Make a big paper cutout of a skeleton or use a Halloween skeleton. Next to it, make a big cutout of the side view of the brain. For the three sections of the brain—cerebrum, cerebellum, and medulla—prepare different-colored pieces of yarn with name tags of the body functions that each section controls (e.g., breathing—medulla). Have the students tack the yarn to the part of the body that is regulated from this part of the brain.
- Have a child lie down on a large piece of paper while another child traces his or her body. Then have them fill in the torsos with various bones, organs, etc., that you specify. This can be progressive as the various lessons in the unit develop.
- Have the children do a sensory walk. Make dyads (one student is blindfolded and the other acts as the guide); have the children walk around outside in the school area that you have indicated and use their senses of touch and smell to learn about things that they may not have been familiar with before or may have taken for granted.
- *Movement.* Help the students become aware of their bodies by acting out the different ways that they can react to the following directions:
  — show me all the different ways your body can stretch.
  — show me all the ways you can relax your body.
  — show me all the ways you can make your body small.
  — show me all the ways you can make your body tall.
  — show me all the ways that you can make your body
     turn around.
- On the window sill or bookshelf, place a brightly decorated container (e.g., a coffee can) with a sock placed on its open side. Place items in the container that the children can identify through touch and smell (e.g., lemon, onion). Change the items frequently.
- To make the children aware of how their pupils will dilate and con-

strict, use a pocket flashlight and carefully flash it on the students' pupils. The children will notice how the variation of light makes the pupil size change.

- With an opaque projector, make silhouettes of each student's head (side view). Have the students make a collage on the silhouette of cut-out pictures, drawings or printed words to describe what makes up good skin care.

- Have the students make a scrapbook based on their physical growth and development during the school year. Using the metric system where appropriate, record such items as height, weight, waist size, number of teeth, and a particular muscle size; also include drawings of their hands and feet. At the end of the scrapbook conclude with the statement: "I discovered that_____."

SUGGESTED RESOURCES

The learning resources listed in this section are a selected sample of materials with which the authors are personally familiar. Appropriate grade levels have been included when these were indicated by the source.

BOOKS

Health: Decisions for Growth
Harcourt Brace Jovanovich, Inc.
757 Third Ave.
N.Y., NY 10017
(Grades 1–6)

Health for All
Scott, Foresman and Co.
Glenview, Illinois 60025

How We Are Born
How We Grow
How Our Bodies Work
And How We Learn
Joe Kaufman
Golden Press, New York

Moving, Moving, Moving About
(6–8 year olds)
Scott, Foresman and Co.
Glenview, Illinois 60025

FILM

Take Joy
(Teacher's guide and dittos included)
American Cancer Society
Contact your local chapter

FILMSTRIPS

Body Basics
(Grades 5–8)
Guidance Associates
757 Third Ave.
New York, New York 10017

Health Decision for Growth
(Grades 1–6)
Harcourt Brace Jovanovich, Inc.
757 Third Ave.
New York, New York 10017

KITS

An Early Start to Good Health
(4 Units—Grades K–3)
American Cancer Society
Contact your local chapter

Epilepsy School Alert Kits
Local Epilepsy Foundation

PUZZLE

Heart Puzzle
American Heart Association
Contact your local chapter

HEALTH SERVICE ASPECTS

Most school health service professionals recognize the potential benefits health education offers for the prevention of health problems through study of the structure and function of the human body. They are therefore ready and willing to help teachers plan instructional units and find useful materials, and even to assist in classroom activities. In turn, they need the assistance of teachers in identifying problems through health observation and other appraisal activities, and in the referral and follow-up of problems thus discovered.

GROWTH PROBLEMS

Growth screening is part of the health appraisal program in many schools. Children are weighed and measured periodically. Present weights and heights may simply be compared with children's own past records, or they may be plotted on complex growth charts to determine whether growth is occurring as it should. Any case of growth failure is then investigated medically to determine the basic cause and, if indicated, appropriate management. Possible causes of growth failure include not only HGH and thyroxin deficiencies but also diabetes, malnutrition, and a variety of acute illnesses. Early and adequate treatment of a few basic causes of growth failure sometimes results in catch-up growth. Instances of treatable growth failure are rare, however, and most are detectable as easily through observation as through screening. It is therefore questionable whether growth screening is worth its cost in professional time in terms of its medical value. On the other hand, the interest created when children weigh and measure themselves as part of a teaching unit on growth can be of considerable value.

The fact that extremely tall or short stature rarely indicates a medical problem needs to be emphasized when teaching about growth. Doing so and providing sympathetic understanding and protection against peer ridicule of short and tall youngsters may help them preserve healthy self-images. Extremes in weight also often arouse more concern than is warranted. One child may be chunky and another thin not because of over- or undernutrition, but because that is the nature of their genetically predetermined body builds. Both overly fat and undernourished children are characteristically less physically active than their peers, and undernourished pupils are also likely to show signs of fatigue and to perform poorly in academic subjects. As Erik Erikson points out, the most striking characteristic of healthy elementary school age children is their extreme industriousness. In the early elementary years pupils tend to tire rather quickly but they also recover quickly with a brief rest or change in activity.

POSTURAL and ORTHOPEDIC PROBLEMS

Healthy musculature and skeletal alignment is indicated by good posture and balance in the way children stand, sit, run, and walk. What constitutes

77

good posture varies with a child's stage of development and with the strength and tone of the abdominal muscles. Children normally enter elementary school with heads tilted slightly forward, because their heads are larger and heavier than those of adolescents in relation to the size and strength of the rest of their bodies. Their tummies normally protrude, as do their rear ends, and the inward sway of their lower backs is normally exaggerated. Their upper backs are quite straight, however. Knock-knees are common in preadolescence. In standing, running, and walking, the feet usually toe-out slightly. In sitting, children often contort themselves into all sorts of weird positions, but for the brief periods of time that their short attention spans permit they can sit and work comfortably at a desk with their backs straight, shoulders parallel to the floor, and feet flat on the floor, provided that the furniture fits.

Teachers can do three things to promote good posture. First, they can show children how to sit, stand, and walk correctly. Second, to the extent that their classrooms are equipped with a range of furniture sizes, they can provide seating to fit each individual. Third, they can provide exercises to strengthen and tone abdominal and back muscles and otherwise promote good posture. These include sit-ups, climbing exercises, and walking across the room with a book balanced on the head.

Elementary children with awkward running or walking gaits, or with standing or sitting postures abnormal for their age group, should be referred to the school health services for investigation. Causes include body structural defects that require orthopedic attention, such as having one leg shorter than the other or scoliosis (a spinal curvature that causes one shoulder to be lower than the other). Other causes include poorly fitted shoes and imitation of the poor posture of an admired peer or adult. In some schools, the health service or the physical education teacher conducts a formal posture screening program. In other schools, detection of postural defects depends on teacher observation and/or periodic health examinations.

SENSORY DEFECTS

Some children of normal or better intelligence have difficulty in learning because of defective visual or auditory acuity. Others of normal or better intelligence and with adequate vision and hearing have difficulty in interpreting what they see and hear. Still others are unable to communicate and live in private worlds of their own.

VISION PROBLEMS. Most defects of visual acuity are not preventable, a notable exception being defective night vision, which is prevented by adequate vitamin A intake. Most are medically correctable, usually with the use of lenses. An exception is color vision deficiency, which is vocationally but not educationally handicapping.[6] Special education programs for blind and partially sighted students, or the use of special equipment and techniques with them by regular teachers in regular classrooms, often result in striking educational achievement when medical intervention fails. Effective mainstreaming requires that special equipment and consultant help be made readily available to the classroom teacher, however.

There is available only one highly valid and reliable screening technique for the detection of defects in visual acuity in school children. This method is called the Modified Clinical Technique.[7] Unfortunately, this test battery must be administered by ophthalmologists or optometrists. The other tests available, such as the Snellen test chart and various testing machines, can be administered by nurses, screening technicians, teachers, or adult volunteers with relatively little training. Although useful, these simpler tests, like teacher observation, refer many children for professional eye care who do not need it, and fail to refer many who do. Most school systems rely on the less complicated screening test and on teacher observation.

Teacher observation for signs of visions defects is complicated by the fact that many early elementary children are normally farsighted; they see things well at a distance but poorly close up. This condition is often outgrown during the elementary school years. Its prevalence is one reason for printing early-grade materials in large type. Observable signs and symptoms of possible vision problems include

- holding books too close or too far from the eyes.
- shutting or covering one eye.
- rubbing the eyes excessively.
- squinting or frowning when reading.
- difficulty in reading.
- squinting to read.
- crossed eyes (this is a serious sign).
- red eyes.
- complaints of eye discomfort, inability to see well, or headaches, dizziness, or nausea after prolonged reading or other eye work.[8]

Many overreferrals that might otherwise result from teacher observation can be prevented by sending children to the nurse for appraisal before a referral is made.

[6] J. M. Lampe, M. E. Doster, and B. B. Beal, "Summary of a Three Year Study of Academic and School Achievement Between Color Deficient and Normal Primary Age Pupils: Phase Two," *The Journal of School Health*, Vol. 43 (May 1973), pp. 309–310.
[7] Henrik Blum, Henry B. Peters, and Jerome W. Bettman, *Vision Screening for Elementary Schools: The Orinda Study* (Berkeley, Calif.: University of California Press, 1959).
[8] Adapted from Joint Study Committee, *Teaching About Vision* (New York: National Society for the Prevention of Blindness, Inc., 1972).

HEARING PROBLEMS. Many cases of hearing loss are preventable. Children need to be taught that hearing is endangered by sticking anything in the ear canal, even a cotton-tipped stick. Blows to the ear or exposure to loud noise can also endanger hearing. Infections can result in either temporary or permanent hearing defects. The viral common cold, which is not preventable and is curable only by time, often results in a temporary hearing loss. Some permanent losses due to viral infections such as rubella are preventable by immunizations. Permanent loss sometimes results from bacterial infections of the middle ear (the usual cause of earache). These losses are often preventable through the early detection and medical treatment of earache. Elementary-age children are much more subject to ear infection than they will be later.

School health service professionals rely primarily on pure-tone audiometer screening coupled with teacher observation to detect hearing loss. Audiometer tests are usually administered by the nurse or a trained screening technician. Those whose first test indicates a hearing loss are usually retested a week or so later to minimize overreferrals due to colds or other temporary losses. For the same reason it is good practice to test those observed by teachers to have signs or symptoms of hearing loss before they are referred for medical care. Pupils who complain of earaches should be referred at once without testing, however.

Some otherwise permanent hearing losses can be partially or wholly corrected by medical or surgical intervention and/or by use of a professionally fitted hearing aid in selected cases. These more or less treatable losses are typically the result of problems in the outer and middle ear structures. Other losses, those resulting from damage to the inner ear structures or the auditory nerve or brain, are typically not amenable to medical intervention or use of a hearing aid. Although these losses are not correctable through medical intervention, special education programs provide training that equips these youngsters both for further education and with job skills.

Observable indications of possible hearing loss in elementary age children include

- failure to respond to sounds from behind the pupil.
- speaking too softly or too loudly.
- mistakes in pronunciation.
- giving inappropriate responses to questions.
- asking to have questions repeated.
- inattentiveness.
- mistakes in copying dictation.
- scholastic achievement below the pupil's ability level.

LEARNING DISABILITIES. Some children whose academic achievement is lower than their potential and who do not necessarily have impaired vision or hearing or come from socially disadvantaged homes, have specific learning disabilities to which descriptive labels are assigned. The label *dyslexia* is

80

assigned to those who have difficulty in reading, while *dyscalculia* is used to describe difficulty in arithmetic, for example. These children often perceive letters, words or numbers in reverse order, and find it difficult or impossible to copy geometric figures correctly. They are also often described as *hyperactive* or *hyperkinetic;* that is, they are more than normally overactive for their age, are unable to concentrate on a given task, and are therefore annoying to their peers, their parents, their teachers and themselves.

Causation of these and other specific learning disabilities has not been definitely established. Some workers who believe that these problems are caused by organic brain damage or by psychological insults diagnose such children as minimally brain damaged or as having minimal brain dysfunction. Others blame these problems on developmental disorders which may be overcome with time or by application of special education techniques. Still others deny that the affected children have problems; instead, they assert them to be individualists who are victims of unrealistic expectations held by parents, teachers and society as a whole. Whatever the explanation is, most children identified as learning disabled are boys, and such children also tend to come from middle and upper class homes where expectations tend to be high.

Children with learning problems are usually first identified by teachers or parents who observe their struggles and frustrations as they try to learn or sit still long enough to complete a task. In far too many cases a diagnosis is made by the child's physician acting alone. Ideally, diagnosis is based on both medical and psychological tests and examinations, because root causes may be physical or psychological in nature. Thus, treatment may involve either medical or psychological therapy. Much controversy surrounds the use of either drugs or dietary controls in case management, however.

There is no substantial disagreement that proper home and school management of learning disabled children is crucial. Most authorities agree that firm, predictable and consistent treatment is required. These children need to know, even more than other youngsters, exactly what behaviors and achievements are expected of them. They need consistent rewards for achievement and consistent penalties for failure. An open environment in which choices abound is to be avoided. Most classroom teachers would probably prefer that all learning disabled children be placed in special education classes. Estimates of their numbers range from one in every twenty children upward, however, and to do so would place a large fiscal burden on the schools. The best that can be hoped for in most schools is that the most disturbed cases will be placed in special classes and that resource help will be made available to regular teachers in dealing with the rest. Many of them do overcome their problems and achieve success both academically and in the world of work.

AUTISM. Children who have extreme difficulty in communicating with others may be labeled *autistic.* Autism is considered a psychosis because these children seem to live in an imaginary world of their own. All autistic children can also be classified as learning disabled, but unlike other learning disabled children many of them are mentally retarded. Authorities now tend to believe that the basic cause is organic brain damage rather than psychological trauma.

Autistic children are usually identified as such during infancy and before they enter school. Some are very passive, others are loud, and some play incessantly with favorite objects such as blocks which they arrange in meticulous rows or piles. They pay no attention to others. If they talk, they talk to themselves, not others.

In the school years, autistic children may learn to like and respond to other people. With the help of skilled and dedicated teachers those who are not too severely retarded may grow well enough to hold down jobs and maintain some sort of social relationships. The outlook is poor for those who have failed to talk by the time they enter school, and many of these are institutionalized. Guidance at home and school of the more hopeful cases requires the continued interdisciplinary teamwork of special educators, neurologists, pediatricians and various rehabilitation therapists. Treatments may include medication and behavior modification techniques.

ENVIRONMENTAL ASPECTS

PHYSICAL ACTIVITY RESOURCES

It is apparent that healthy physical growth and development and good posture depend on good nutrition and on vigorous and appropriate physical exercise. School food service programs will be discussed in the next chapter. The nature and value of elementary school physical education and activities vary widely.

Some elementary schools are served by physical educators; others are not. The more desirable situation prevails in schools with well-planned physical education curricula taught directly by well-prepared specialists. Next best is a school in which a physical educator serves as a consultant to classroom teachers who are then responsible for teaching and supervising physical activities. Least fortunate are schools in which no professional physical education assistance is available. Teachers in such schools may prepare themselves to some extent for activity leadership by taking the courses offered for elementary teachers by most college physical education departments. In general, children in grades K–3 need large-scale activities—running, climbing, and throwing big balls and the like. Activities designed to improve posture are also helpful. They are not ready for competitive games. Boys and girls play well together. In the upper elementary grades, boys and girls prefer to separate for play. Motor coordination and eye–hand coordination improve. They are ready to learn and refine physical skills. They are ready to form teams and play complex competitive games.

School grounds should be designed to provide separate activity areas for younger and older pupils and suitable equipment for both groups. Younger children need a variety of play equipment—swings, climbing apparatus, and large pipes to crawl through, for example. Older children need large spaces and equipment for such games as softball and basketball.

PERSONAL HYGIENE FACILITIES

Toilet, handwashing, and drinking fountain facilities are often provided for and connected directly with each kindergarten and first grade room in modern elementary schools. These self-contained facilities make it easier for teachers to supervise and instruct children in their proper use. In schools where fountains are placed in the halls and large central toilet rooms are provided, younger pupils may go thirsty and soil themselves rather than leave their own room and risk harassment by older children. Regardless of the location of these facilities, fixtures of appropriate size should be provided. Facilities should be attractive and clean to invite use, and should meet sanitary plumbing standards. For example, a sanitary drinking fountain emits water from a jet located at an angle above and to one side of the bowl. This arrangement prevents contamination of the drinking water outlet if the drain is clogged by chewing gum or paper.

LIGHTING

Lighting that is too dim has not been proven to harm the eyes, but glaring sunlight that is much too bright is believed to be potentially harmful. Lighting should be of an intensity and quality that make the performance of visual tasks as comfortable to the eyes as possible. In some modern classrooms, the intensity of artificial light is controlled by automatic dimmer switches; in most rooms the teacher controls it by switching lights on and off as needed. Sunlight intensity is usually controlled by teacher and pupils who close or open window shades as conditions warrant.

The quality of classroom lighting is improved when a mixture of light sources is used. Fluorescent lighting alone is somewhat boring. Shiny surfaces, such as high-gloss varnished desk tops, reflect light as discomfort-causing glare, whereas rough and flat finished surfaces, such as a rough masonry wall decorated with flat paint, diffuse light to promote eye comfort. In general, all room surfaces should be pastel or off-white to reflect equal amounts of light and thus help prevent distracting shadows on books or other work surfaces.

In addition to controlling natural and artificial light within the room, teachers and pupils can cover glare-producing wall surfaces with artwork. If an area in the room is badly lighted, work surfaces can be moved from that area. Dirty light fixtures or those with burned-out bulbs should be called to the attention of the principal or custodian. Artificial lights should be turned off to conserve energy when they are not needed.

NOISE

Noise is unwanted sound. The intensity of noise within an elementary school is unlikely to damage hearing unless the school is located near an airport. Classroom noise is often annoying and distracting, however. Noise from a nearby highway, railroad, or factory can be partially blocked by erecting an earthen mound or by planting trees and shrubs between the noise source and the school building. Noise originating from the gym, band room, kitchen, or other source within the school can be blocked by isolating such rooms in a separate wing of the building and by providing separate air ducts for them.

Noise originating in a classroom can be reduced or made less annoying in several ways. One way is to carpet the floors and hang fabric drapes that absorb noise within the room. Other approaches are aimed at reducing the amount of noise generated within the room. For example, when teachers speak softly, pupils tend to speak softly also. Audio equipment should be operated at the minimum loudness level that enables those within the room to hear. Considerable noise not so subject to control is generated in open classrooms, but work group noise can be partially blocked by isolating each work area with tall storage furniture or movable screens.

AIR CONTROL

School rooms must be adequately ventilated to remove annoying odors. Temperatures must be adjusted to enable occupants to teach and learn in comfort. As is true of light and noise control, air control affects comfort and efficiency more than it affects physical health. Teachers and pupils in most schools are able to control temperature and ventilation only by opening and closing windows or by complaining to the custodian or engineer. The thermostats in some schools can be adjusted by the teacher.

Metabolic rates are more rapid among elementary pupils than adults; thus pupils are more comfortable at lower room temperatures than are teachers. In addition, women prefer warmer temperatures than do men. Thus conflicts over temperature adjustment are most likely to arise between elementary pupils and their female teachers. Teachers can accommodate their pupils to some extent by wearing sweaters and by physically moving about the classroom more than their pupils do.

Classroom temperatures of 68°F to 72°F are generally recommended.

Adequate ventilation and comfort at these temperatures require air movement that is barely perceptible. Air control equipment in some schools includes mechanisms for air cleaning, so that in the presence of unhealthful outside air pollution it may be better to leave windows closed. Some city schools ban outdoor physical activity when pollution levels are high.

REFERENCES

BANTA, JOHN V. "Early Recognition of Orthopedic Problems in Childhood," *Journal of School Health,* Vol. 44, No. 1 (January 1974), pp. 38–40.

BEALS, RALPH L., HARRY HOIJER, and ALAN R. BEALS. *Introduction to Anthropology.* New York: Macmillan Publishing Co., Inc., 1977.

EISNER, VICTOR, and LAURENCE B. CALLAN. *Dimensions of School Health.* Springfield, Ill.: Charles C Thomas, Publisher, 1974.

GROLLMAN, SIGMUND. *The Human Body.* New York: Macmillan Publishing Co., Inc., 1978.

GRUNBERG, ELEANOR. "Color Deficient Versus Color Blind," *Journal of School Health,* Vol. 43, No. 2 (February 1973), pp. 135–139.

HAMMOND, PETER B. *An Introduction to Cultural and Social Anthropology.* New York: Macmillan Publishing Co., Inc., 1978.

HENDERSON, P. *Disability in Childhood and Youth.* London: Oxford University Press, 1974.

HOEBEL, E. ADAMSON. *Anthropology: The Study of Man.* New York: McGraw-Hill Book Company, 1972.

JENNE, FRANK H., and WALTER H. GREENE. *Turner's School Health and Health Education.* St. Louis: C. V. Mosby Company, 1976.

MASLOW, ABRAHAM H. *Motivation and Personality.* New York: Harper & Row, 1970.

MOREHOUSE, LAURENCE E., and AUGUSTUS T. MILLER. *Physiology of Exercise.* St. Louis: C. V. Mosby Company, 1971.

MORHOLT, EVELYN, PAUL F. BRANDWEIN, and ALEXANDER JOSEPH. *A Sourcebook for the Biological Sciences.* New York: Harcourt Brace Jovanovich, Inc., 1966.

NOURSE, ALAN. *The Body.* New York: Time Incorporated, 1964.

PARK, CLARA C. and LEON N. SHAPIRO. *You Are Not Alone.* Boston: Atlantic Monthly Press, 1976.

TANNER, JAMES M., and GORDON RATTRAY TAYLOR. *Growth.* New York: Time Incorporated, 1968.

WILSON, CHARLES C. *School Health Services.* Chicago: American Medical Association, 1964.

WOODFORD, CHARLES. "A Perspective on Hearing Loss and Hearing Assessment in School Children," *Journal of School Health,* Vol. 43, No. 8 (October 1973), pp. 572–577.

5

Food and Drink—
Sustenance

Eating should be a simple activity. Many factors in our modern society tend to make the task easier than ever before—and to this optimistic situation we as human beings bring durable, adaptable digestive and assimilative organs that were designed to see us through far harsher times than any of us are likely to experience. Those who feel times are difficult should consider how it probably was when humans, as a distinct species, were just getting started. Reay Tannahill, in her fascinating book *Food in History*, speculates on this point:

> It was roughly four million years ago—some authorities say thirty million—when the ape-into-man transmutation began, and it is generally accepted that the change was set in motion by a shortage of eggs, nestlings and fruit which drove the ape down from his familiar habitat in the trees to forage in the grasslands. He found lizards and porcupines, tortoises and ground squirrels, moles, plump insects, and grubs, and took to them with such enthusiasm that, in time, he almost wiped out a number of the smaller species.[1]

When the eggs and the fruit become so scarce that you must leave your tree and forage in the grasslands—that is a real food crisis! Although the accuracy of these events and their specific sequence must remain largely conjecture, this episode does serve to illustrate some fundamental truths concerning human eating habits. The first of these pertains to man's omnivorous diet. Carnivorous species are in dire straits when game is scarce and grazing species are in trouble when the annual grass crop fails, but humans, with their complex enzyme system, high intelligence, and versatile arms and hands for climbing, digging, and tool making, have a variety of eggs, fruits,

[1] Reay Tannahill, *Food in History* (New York: Stein and Day, 1973), pp. 12–13.

animals, insects, and grubs available as food. This adaptability has led to the domestication of animals, the development of agriculture, the discovery of modern methods of processing, preserving, and transporting foods, and the study of nutrition itself so as to leave less to chance in the task of obtaining nourishment.

These cultural achievements are better known than are the many built-in physiological advantages. One of these, which many persons might gladly surrender, is the capacity to store food as fat as a hedge against possible shortages in the future. In the old days it was feast or famine, and a layer of body fat added greatly to one's survival capability. And it is not only fat that can be stored; the body has a remarkable system of reserves for many essential nutrients and a mechanism for breaking down less essential tissue for its components when real starvation is threatened. Persons who fail to take in enough of a given nutrient on a particular day first draw upon their tissue reserves. If the deficiency continues long enough, tissue depletion occurs and less essential tissue is broken down in a process that can often be recognized by laboratory tests; at this stage biochemical lesions being to appear. The person may still feel as good as ever; even more nutritional abuse is necessary before the onset of the chronic fatigue, sleeplessness, and digestive disturbances that signal functional changes.[2]

One final mechanism that should be mentioned because of the present concern about nutritional education is the human organism's apparent innate tendency to select the foods needed for good nutrition. Experiments have shown that children, when given a choice of a wide variety of foods, will generally select a well-balanced diet. And today a government-instigated policy of food enrichment and supplementation now serves as further insurance against poor nutrition. Iodine is added to salt, vitamins A and D are added to milk, B complex and iron are added to bread and flour.

Despite the complaints of the average food shopper, economic factors present no serious threat to the average American's ability to obtain the proper foods. The situation for those genuinely poor is another matter; however, the majority of Americans enjoy a rich diet. Per capita consumption of beef and chicken, for example, is approximately twice what it was in the "good old days" of 20 years ago. People tend to complain loudly about the prices but they keep buying the food. When they must cut expenditures, the cuts come in other areas that are normally less well publicized.

With all of these advantages it is difficult to be poorly nourished in the United States today, but millions manager to place themselves in this category. The recent Ten State National Nutrition Survey of 24,000 families throughout the United States revealed that "Americans easily obtain their caloric needs but frequently fail to meet all their nutrient needs."[3] Al-

[2] A. M. Thomson, "The Diagnosis of Malnutrition in Well-Nourished Communities," *American Journal of Clinical Nutrition,* Vol. 4 (1956), p. 647.

[3] Phillip L. White, "New Thoughts on Dietary Practices," *School Foodservice Journal,* Vol. 27, No. 9 (October 1973), p. 50.

though this study was focused primarily on low-income groups, a number of middle- and upper-income families were also included for comparison purposes, and, interestingly enough, many persons in these groups were also shown to be malnourished or at risk of becoming malnourished. This phenomenon of poor nutrition among the higher-income brackets has been shown in older students. One study of 114 college women, for example, revealed almost one-third of this group to have essentially no tissue reserves of iron.[4] Another interesting finding is that adolescents are often shown to have poorer diets than younger children.[5]

The general conclusion to which most of this evidence leads is that in a nation of plenty there are a surprising number of malnourished people. Despite all of the advantages of the human species and the specific cultural and technological advantages of the present-day United States, there are still serious nutritional problems. There are reasons for this apparent contradiction that provide direct implications for school health programs.

Most disturbing is the fact that much of this poor nutritional status is caused by genuine poverty. The findings of the major study of 1968, *Hunger, U.S.A.*,[6] provided firm evidence of this that was confirmed by the more recent Ten State National Nutrition Survey.[7] The percentage is not great, but there are some Americans who simply cannot afford to eat properly. Consider the first-hand report on such a case:

> Near the Canadian border my husband and I sat in a log cabin home of a Sioux Indian and watched one cold boiled potato being divided among seven family members. It was all the food available for an aged man, a three-year-old child, two young adults and three school-age children. This single potato provided only a morsel for each, and they ate slowly.[8]

This is surely an extreme case, but there are many extreme cases and one is too many. Many average American wage earners will maintain that they cannot afford to feed their families properly in these days of rising prices. What they mean is that they are eating less roast beef and more hamburger casseroles. They probably have little understanding of or feeling for what real hunger is.

However, malnourishment also exists among those who can afford good food. Simple ignorance is part of the story, but if that were the only prob-

[4] D. E. Scott and J. A. Pritchard, "Iron Deficiency in Healthy Young College Women," *Journal of the American Medical Association,* Vol. 199 (March 1967), pp. 897–900.

[5] Henrietta Fleck, *Introduction to Nutrition* (New York: Macmillan Publishing Co., Inc., 1971), p. 261.

[6] *Hunger, U.S.A.: A Report by the Citizens' Board of Inquiry in Hunger and Malnutrition in the United States* (Washington, D.C.: New Community Press, 1968).

[7] White, op. cit. p. 50.

[8] Myrtle R. Real, "What It Is Like to Be Hungry," *School Foodservice Journal,* Vol. 27, No. 5 (May 1973), p. 31.

lem the solution would be relatively easy. The really difficult obstacles are provided by a fascinating complex of emotional, cultural, and, to some extent, political problems. The study of these factors constitutes a fascinating part of a thorough program of nutrition education.

CHILDREN'S HEALTH INTERESTS as RELATED to NUTRITION

Ruth Byler and her associates, in their extensive study of children's health interests, reported expressions of concern for nutrition from all grade levels; however, the frequency and intensity was somewhat lower than for other health topics. The fourth grade represented, perhaps, an exception. There, the children tended to ask many relatively complicated questions concerning this topic. A few representative findings and questions are included in this section.[9]

KINDERGARTEN THROUGH GRADE TWO

• In response to the question "What is good health?" kindergarten children respond in part: You eat lots of vegetables and fruits and no coffee. . . . You take vitamin pills. They also ask: Why do some things taste bitter and some sweet and some things smell awful?

GRADES THREE AND FOUR

• Both groups show interest in foods, but the fourth graders much more so than thirds, and they ask more complicated questions than do thirds.
• Third graders ask: How do food and other things make you healthy? What kinds of liquids should you drink to keep healthy? How much milk? Water? . . . How do people get fat? . . . Where does food go from your mouth?
• Fourth graders ask: How do you make different kinds of food? How can you be sure to eat the right things to make you grow? . . . Do carrots help you see better? Is fish good for the mind?

GRADES FIVE AND SIX

• Nutrition does not seem an area of great concern. A few questions deal with proper diets and what causes a person to become fat.
• Fifth graders ask: What foods are the best foods for a person to eat? What foods are bad for you? Are sweets bad for you because they cause tooth decay?

[9] Ruth Byler, Gertrude Lewis, and Ruth Totman, *Teach Us What We Want to Know* (New York Mental Health Materials Center, Inc. 1969).

ILLUSTRATIVE CONTENT

The study of nutrition within the modern health curriculum is more than a consideration of vitamins, minerals, proteins, and the basic four. This restricted approach has been used for years with little demonstrable impact on eating behavior. Immediate improvements in eating habits can probably be achieved only through a "training" type approach where the food habits of children are directly monitored, as in the cafeteria, with food diaries, award systems, and so forth. However, the long-term educational objectives seem best served if children are helped to understand the emotional and cultural significance, and hence the underlying dynamics, of food behavior. This can be achieved if such content is presented in appropriate terms according to the maturity level of the pupils involved.

THE CULTURAL SIGNIFICANCE of FOOD

The relative abundance of food and the freedom from fears of famine and starvation among the majority of present-day Americans and members of other modern nations tend to be taken for granted; however, this comfortable situation is the exception, not the rule, for the majority of the world's population. Whereas malnutrition in rural poverty pockets and inner-city ghettos within our own country may receive considerable publicity, thousands of children starve in remote villages in Asia and Africa, oftentimes with little world-wide attention. During the recent African drought, for instance, an estimated 100,000 perished in Ethiopia alone.[10] Currently, there is serious doubt that famine can be averted in India despite vigorous relief efforts.

Historically, freedom from famine is a comparatively recent phenomenon even among the more highly developed countries. In terms of bountiful harvests, America has been perhaps the most blessed of all nations, yet many of the older generations can remember the depression days of the 1930s when they learned first hand what it was like not to have enough to eat. In other countries the historical experience has been more severe. In Russia, for example, 3 million persons starved during a famine in 1932–1933, and many of the American-Irish are descendants of immigrants who fled the potato famine that took a million lives between 1846–1849.[11] Thus from both a geographic and a historical standpoint the current American complacency about food is unique and unusual.

Although obtaining food is not a conscious problem for modern Amer-

[10] Claire Sterling, "The Making of the Sub-Saharan Wasteland," *The Atlantic Monthly*, Vol. 233, No. 5 (May 1974), p. 100.
[11] William H. Sebrell, Jr., and James J. Haggerty, *Food and Nutrition* (New York: Time Incorporated, 1967), p. 178.

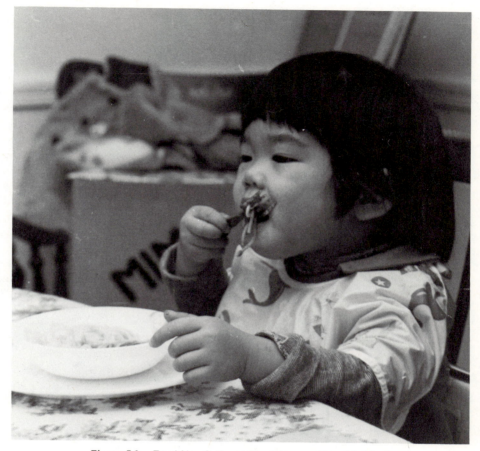

Figure 5.1. Food Has Cultural Significance. (Carol Ashton)

icans, it has been one of the dominant tasks in the cultural history of the human race; a generation of relief does not wipe out the customs, traditions, and fears of this struggle. The anxiety of hunger, the delights of the feast, the thankfulness of the harvest remain a vital part of our lives. The elemental nature of food as a need and the normal hunger pangs every child suffers in infancy and childhood have served to add emotional impact to these cultural traditions. Feeding time to the infant means a pleasurable relief from tension and its first meaningful interaction with another person. To the child the availability of food means that someone cares; to the mother it becomes the hallmark of responsible parenthood so much so that public health authorities have had to conduct campaigns to discourage the harmful overfeeding of children. The net result is that food acquires emotional and symbolic values that affect people's behavior in ways out of proportion to its basic importance.

91

FACTORS AFFECTING FOOD PREFERENCES

Most children, when given suitable opportunity, will select a good diet without any instructions. Although this ability has some significance, it seldom operates under real-life conditions. In the original experiment the various foods were presented in a way to make them look as similar as possible; the same type of dish was used for all items and garnishes or decorative elements were omitted. Thus mashed potatoes competed with plain ice cream, not with a chocolate sundae. Modern advertising and packaging techniques tend to distort this natural choice mechanism and often the less nutritious foods such as soft drinks and party snacks are given the heaviest sales promotion.

Food preferences are conditioned also by a wide variety of other positive and negative stimuli. The classical example is the lifelong aversion to a food that may have been contaminated or may have been eaten prior to the onset of an unrelated digestive disorder. A similar situation occurs when an upset child is forced by a well-meaning parent to eat a particular food; the child may come to dislike this item for the rest of his or her life.

Conditioning does of course work both ways. Parents often provide

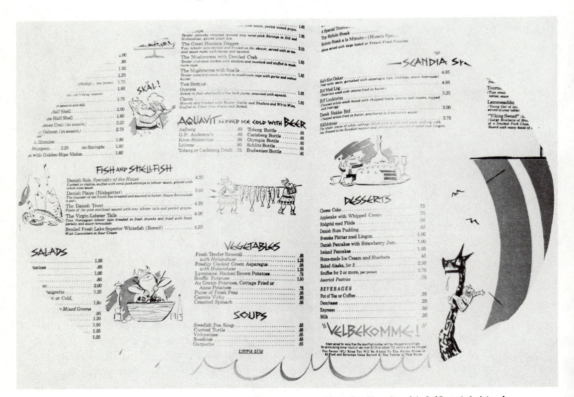

Figure 5.2. Food Preferences—How Do You Decide? (Carol Ashton)

cookies, candy, or other sweet items as reward for good behavior, in which case the natural appeal of the treat is greatly enhanced by the warmth and praise of the parent. The foods that are traditionally offered during festive occasions such as Thanksgiving and Christmas often pick up special allure by virtue of the pleasant holiday mood, the good fellowship, and perhaps the anticipation of presents.

Ethnic food patterns are another potent factor in food choices and tend to be internalized along with habits of speech, dress, family roles, and other aspects of one's total cultural heritage. These patterns have their historical roots in the natural flora and fauna of the original homeland but are often carried by families to other parts of the world. Although most persons enjoy having an exotic meal occasionally, they prefer the meals of their childhood.

Cultural tradition is strong, but so too is the impact of modern technology and changing conditions. In recent years the old ethnic patterns appear to be giving way to a new, distinctly American way of eating that some nutritionists term the "all-day snack." With working mothers becoming more common and more and more activities for children and youth taking place outside the home, fewer families are able to assemble for meals on any regular basis. Phillip White, in reviewing the findings of the Ten State National Nutrition Survey, describes this changing pattern:

> Food habits have indeed changed drastically during the past 25 years. Traditional meal patterns still linger among older people and those who are able to hold on to culturally or ethnically defined patterns. But the general shift is to highly individualized, unstructured modes of eating.
>
> Three square meals are a thing of the past. We are now a mini-meal, snacking society.[12]

This new trend carries at least two important implications for modern families. First, the family that fails to have any meals together as a total group has lost an important opportunity to develop unity and cohesiveness; this loss is difficult to compensate for in other ways. Consequently, some parents make a special effort to get everyone together for the evening meal regardless of outside activities. Where this has proved impossible, a few of the more Spartan types have even tried to get everybody up early enough for a big family breakfast. When these efforts are made, children can help greatly to make the idea work when they understand its value.

The idea of a snack-type meal pattern is disturbing to many traditional nutritionists, but the key to accommodating this trend is expressed by the food editor of *Family Health* magazine. "If snacks form 30 per cent of the day's food intake, they should supply 30 per cent of the day's nutrient needs." [13] From a purely nutritional standpoint there is nothing wrong

[12] White, op. cit., p. 50.
[13] Elizabeth Alston, "Snacks: The American Way of Eating," *Family Health,* Vol. 5, No. 1 (January 1973), p. 27.

with eating several small portions throughout the day; it certainly represents an improvement over the too-common pattern of eating little throughout the day, then having an excessively large evening meal. However, the snacks need to be just as carefully selected for their nutritional value as is the mealtime menu. Intelligent snacking calls for a more thorough knowledge of nutrition on the part of each family member than the old pattern where one good meal planner could presumably keep the whole family eating well. Beyond this, of course, is the importance of each member placing some value on a balanced diet. In theory, a snacking pattern means each person, including children, must take more responsibility for his or her own nutrition; this is not without its advantages.

NUTRITIONAL NEEDS

According to one source there are at least 45 and possibly as many as 50 known essential nutrients.[14] Despite years of research, nutritionists still cannot agree on an exact number. It is surprising how often another essential element is discovered. One might ask how the human species survived all these centuries ignorant of many essential food elements. Most of the 45 known elements are abundant in common foods, so that only a relatively few such as iron, calcium, and vitamin C require special attention. Nutrients may be categorized into three groups that provide food energy or calories, i.e., carbohydrates, fats, and proteins, and three nonenergy groups, i.e., vitamins, minerals, and water. Water is somewhat unique in that it provides mainly for such supportive activities as transporting materials, facilitating chemical reactions, and providing for temperature control; it sometimes is not classed as a food. A true nutrient can function in the body in three ways:

1. It may provide the body with fuel, which, when oxidized, releases energy for its activities.
2. It may provide materials for the building and upkeep of body tissues, both the skeletal structure and the soft tissues of the body.
3. It may provide the materials that are necessary to regulate body processes or that the body can use to synthesize its own regulatory substances.[15]

Although any of the three food categories that have caloric value can satisfy the body's energy requirements, the carbohydrates, i.e., the sugars and starches, are best suited to serve this need. Excessive reliance on fats or proteins with their more complex residue of waste products tends to place a strain on the excretory system: carbohydrates oxidize much more cleanly. Within this group the starches offer advantages over sugar foods as they are

14 Nevin S. Scrimshaw and Vernon R. Young, "The Requirements of Human Nutrition," *Scientific American*, Vol. 235 (September 1976), pp. 51–64.
15 Fleck, op. cit., p. 35.

more likely to include vitamins and minerals; examples that incorporate both these features are whole wheat or enriched bread, many of the breakfast cereals, and, surprisingly enough, the potatoes, which are quite a good food when not buried in butter, gravy, or grease, as in potato chips. Some sweet and sugary foods are probably essential if one is not to feel unduly deprived, but it is generally good to minimize these items. Soft drinks and candy, for example, usually represent "empty calories," i.e., calories with no other nutrient value. Unless one is very active these items contribute either to poor nutrition or to excess weight, and constitute a dental hazard as well. A small amount of fat in the diet is essential to good health, but most persons eat far too much of this "caloric dynamite." Lumberjacks working in a cold climate need lots of butter and bacon; most other persons would do well to cut their fat intake.

During digestion, proteins are broken down into amino acids, of which 23 are known to exist, including eight essential ones that the human body cannot synthesize. Human body cells use these amino acids to produce "tailor-made" proteins for the body tissue and for enzymes to regulate body processes. These proteins are important to two of the three main functions of foods. No single vegetable source can provide all eight essential amino

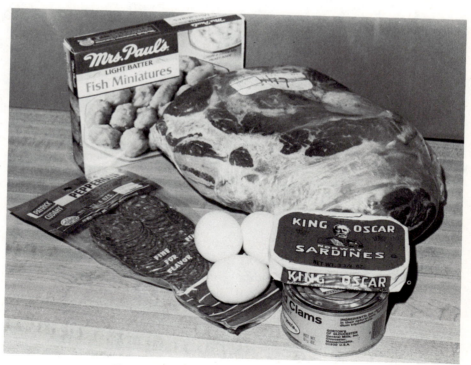

Figure 5.3A. The Meat Group. (Carol Ashton)

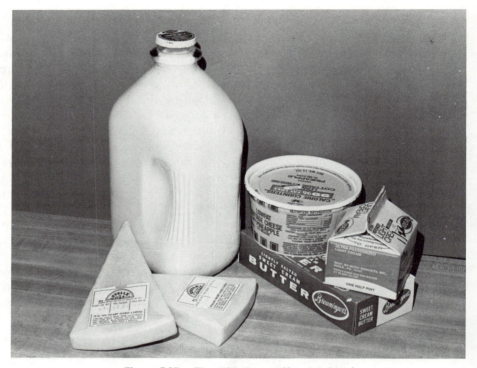

Figure 5.3B. The Milk Group. (Carol Ashton)

acids, but most animal sources, including meat, milk, and eggs, do contain all eight. Thus the safest policy is to include one animal source each day.

Of the minerals, calcium and phosphorus are needed in large amounts. Dairy products meet these needs quite readily for most persons, but milk avoiders should be encouraged to substitute other dairy products. This normally is not too difficult, as one enterprising teacher taught her class to sing to the tune of "Row, Row, Your Boat":

> Drink, drink, drink your milk
> Or eat a piece of cheese.
> Ice cream, too, is good for you,
> Eat any kind you please.[16]

Primary grade children will enjoy this song, although it may be a "bit much" for sophisticated fifth and sixth graders.

Sodium and chlorine are also needed in large amounts; the normal use

[16] Patricia Steiner, "Menu Pocket Packs Nutrition Education Wallop," *School Foodservice Journal*, Vol. 27, No. 10 (November-December 1973) , p. 44.

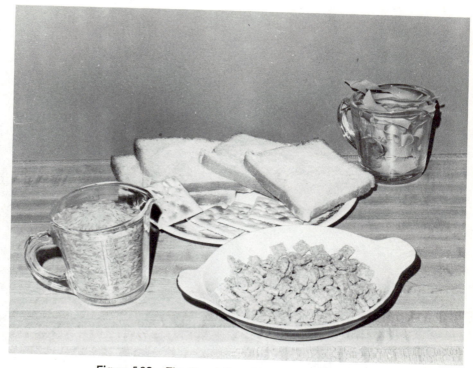

Figure 5.3C. The Bread–Cereal Group. (Carol Ashton)

of salt for seasoning supplies these amounts except under unusual conditions as when excercising in severe heat. Iron is needed in relatively smaller amounts to facilitate oxygen transport in the blood. Leafy green vegetables are the classical source of iron, but because of higher prices and changing habits these are fading somewhat in popularity; therefore, much of the average person's iron comes in the form of enriched bread and cereals. Menstruating females, however, need more iron; thus menstrual education should include suggestions for girls to include six to seven eggs per week in their diet or get additional iron from some other source.

People who eat too few fruits and vegetables may become deficient in vitamin C. It is well to use one good source of this nutrient each day. Most persons get an adequate supply of vitamins A and D as a supplement added to milk; the B complex vitamins are added as a supplement to enriched breads and cereals. Large amounts of the fat-soluble A and D vitamins are highly toxic, because they accumulate in body fat. Excessive amounts of the water-soluable vitamins such as B and C are not considered dangerous, although some painful urination and an added risk of kidney stones were reported in persons taking astronomical amounts. Persons deficient in vitamin C, as many persons are, will naturally benefit from taking 50 times the recommended allowances; however, there is little evidence to show that they would not have done just as well with one times the recommended amount.

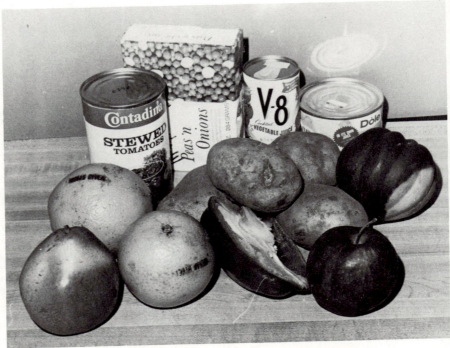

Figure 5.3D.   The Vegetable–Fruit Group. (Carol Ashton)

CONTROL of OBESITY

Obesity, or excess body fat, is a public health problem of major proportions. Excess body fat in adults is associated not only with a number of chronic diseases such as atherosclerosis but also with a weakened self-concept as well. Related research data also show that fat children generally become fat adults, particularly if they remain overweight throughout adolescence. Fatness that begins just prior to the adolescent growth spurt and ends during this time is of little or no importance. Also, overweight adults who were not fat as children are much more successful in their efforts to reduce and maintain their weight loss than are those who were overweight during childhood.

The factors that contribute to the problem of obesity are many and complex: modern improvements in transportation and other labor-saving devices have reduced caloric expenditures while parents still force food on their children; food acquires symbolic value and becomes a means of compensation for various types of need frustration; advertising pressure encourages indulgence in snack foods; and, finally, advocates of fad diets belie the seriousness of the problem by promises of a quick and easy solution. The root causes of obesity extend deep into American life-styles and

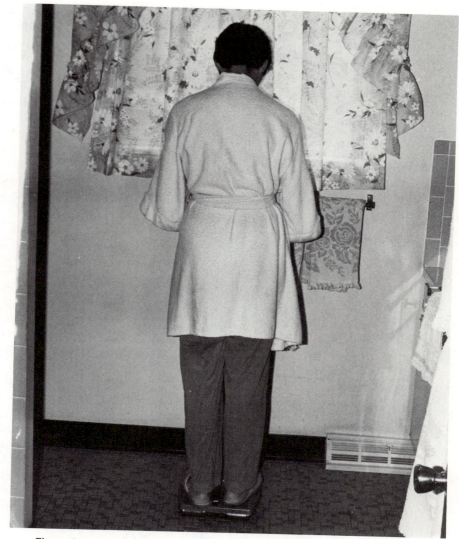

Figure 5.4. Weight Control Requires Regular Attention. (Frances Greene)

education alone will not provide a solution; however, it can help by making individuals more responsive to those persons and influences that encourage obesity control.

The most important concept to the understanding of obesity control is that of energy balance. Everything the body does requires energy whether it be internal functions such as the pumping of blood or the digestion of food, or external work such as washing the dishes or mowing the lawn; this energy cost is measured in calories. On the other side of the ledger every morsel of food has a specific energy value whether it be a leaf of lettuce, a

99

spoonful of sugar, or a piece of roast beef; these energy values are also measured in calories. Whenever a person takes in 3,500 more calories than the body expends in activity, a pound of fat appears, whether this average is accumulated over a period of 24 hours or 24 months. Likewise, whenever a 3,500-calorie deficit is accumulated, a pound of fat is lost. The basic accuracy or validity of this concept is so overwhelming as to make the exceptions and qualifying factors of no practical consequence. However, adult dieters accept this principle about as readily as a religious fundamentalist accepts Darwinian evolution; they seize upon any shred of evidence that will discredit it, and they receive support and encouragement from all manner of health hucksters who cash in on this national problem.

Although the concept of energy balance requires some elaboration and interpretation for its full understanding, its basic principle should be continually stressed: when intake exceeds energy expenditures a weight gain results. Of course, some foods are more calorically dense than others; thus an ounce of margarine has approximately twice the calories of an ounce of bread, sugar, or lean meat. Likewise, some activities are more calorically costly than others; thus five minutes of running will expend more calories than 5 minutes of walking or cycling. Also, different activities with the same energy cost can vary widely in their appeal or tolerability; most persons find 30 minutes of cycling much more pleasant than 30 minutes of calisthenics, for example. Similarly, different foods with the same energy cost can vary considerably in the satisfaction they provide; many dieters have learned to include high-bulk food in the form of salads and melons, for instance, to give a feeling of fullness without providing excessive amounts of calories. Thus the applications and strategies vary, but the principle remains the same.

The specific role of exercise as a factor in obesity control is another important concept that is poorly understood by the general public. This confusion is based upon two facts that appear to contradict one another. Exercise is a poor way to reduce; one must exercise all day to lose a pound of fat; this is generally true. However, exercise is a good way to *control* obesity; active people are less fat than sedentary people; this is also generally true both in childhood and in adult life. Most persons who decide to reduce want to take off in a few weeks excess fat that they may have taken months or years to accumulate. The only way this can be done is by a drastic reduction of intake; the effects of exercise are too slow. However, exercise is very important to the lifelong task of weight maintenance at the desired level. Persons, for example, who add 30 minutes a day to their daily routine add at least 70 calories per day to their expenditures. A year later, they will weigh 7 pounds less than they otherwise would have, provided that their eating habits remain unchanged. And, contrary to popular folklore, added exercise generally does not increase the appetite of the overweight person.

Most children of the elementary school grades are not so concerned about their weight as are typical adolescents with their exposure to the pressure of dating, competitive athletics, and similar factors. This provides an opportunity to teach the simple concept of weight control before many natural emotional barriers to the truth develop. It is difficult, for example, to teach 16-year-old girls anything about weight control for they "know it all already." They read about the "egg diet" in the Sunday supplement of the newspaper, or spend $2.00 for a paperback edition of *Dr. Quick's Inches-Off-Now Plan,* or have found a supply of amphetamines or diuretic pills. If they had been given the opportunity to develop clear concepts and sound values related to this topic during their pre-adolescent years, they might be far less susceptible to such nonsense.

SUGGESTED LEARNING ACTIVITIES

The following suggestions are presented in an effort to demonstrate how the content described in the preceding section might be translated into effective classroom learning activities. They were designed to accommodate a wide variety of classroom groups provided that proper selection and adaptations are made according to the needs, interests, abilities, and maturity level of the particular children involved.

- Have the children make collages of themselves using pictures of foods that they have selected from various magazines. Have them discuss their collages with the rest of the class and then display them throughout the room.

- Have the children join two coat hangers together and from each of the four corners display pictures representing the four food groups. They may take their hanger of food ideas home to show members of their families the necessary foods needed in our daily diet.

- Have the children design their own placemat, using their name and illustrations indicating nutritional foods, good eating habits, etc. They may use these placemats in school or at home. Cover them with laminating material or cellophane if available, so that they can be wiped off when soiled.

- When studying foreign lands, have the children taste and prepare the foods of these countries' cultures (e.g., China: rice, bean sprouts, etc.). If the various foods cannot be prepared in the classroom, bring the foods in already prepared. This activity can also be used for foods that are eaten during the various holidays throughout the year.

- Have the students write a TV commercial regarding the proper utilization of the new labels appearing on food containers. If possible, present it on one of the local channels.

- Have the students design puppets representing various foods (e.g., Carol Carrot, Lucy Lettuce, Tommy Tomato) and write a play regarding the four food groups and their value. If practical, have the children put on the play during the school lunch periods.

- *Junk Sack.* "I'm a junk collector and in my sack I have many of the junk foods that many of us use everyday." Have a cloth sack with various empty containers and packages of foods that do not have any nutritional value. Students will select an item and tell the other students why this item is poor in nutritional value.

- Many of our snack foods are nutritionally healthy but orally hazardous to our teeth. On the following continuum, have the students write their favorite snack food at a point indicative of its status. After all of the children have entered their favorite snack food on the continuum, have them discuss whether their snacks are orally healthy or orally hazardous to their teeth, and why.

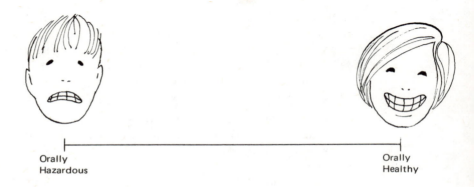

Orally
Hazardous

Orally
Healthy

- For one week, have the students go through the cafeteria lunch line and see if they can select a balanced lunch with items from the four food groups (for those students who bring their lunch, try to encourage them to participate for the week or evaluate their own lunches). If they reach the cashier with a balanced lunch, they are allowed to select a reward coin from an egg carton. The various colored reward coins represent privileges the children have earned for their proper food selection. Select your rewards to best fit interests of your students.

- When having parties, (e.g., birthday, Halloween) or snack breaks in school, encourage the children to have nutritional foods (e.g., raisins, apples, apple juice, bran muffins).

- Have the students eliminate junk foods from their diet for one week. For every junk food that they avoid, have them donate a nickel for the food avoided. The money that is collected will be donated to an appropriate organization (e.g., UNICEF).

- Have the children work with the school's dietitian in designing and planning the school's lunch menu for the month.

- Have the students bring in short advertisements and articles related to weight and figure control. Divide the class into small groups and assign each group the task of evaluating a number of the weight loss schemes in light of what they know to be true. Assemble the class and ask a representative of each group to report on both the soundness and the weakness of the proposals they considered.

- Have the students make a list of the ten foods that they enjoy eating the most. Next to each food place a code letter to identify on what basis they made their selection: parents eat it (P), eat it because my friends do (F), eat it because I saw it advertised on TV (A). Conclude the activity with the following statement: "I discovered that the foods I eat_____."

- Ask each child to place the following items (name them one at a time or have them on the chalk board or paper) in the boxes according to their feeling as to its importance, 1 being the most important and 15 the least important. Only one item may be placed in each box, and all boxes must be filled. Answers may be changed at any time that the activity is going on.

peanut butter   soda   cupcakes
apples   candy bar   chicken
hamburgers   fruit drink   cereal
lettuce   eggs   cheese
green peas   hot chocolate   raisins
                         (with water)

1.	2.	3.
4.	5.	6.
7.	8.	9.
10.	11.	12.
13.	14.	15.

SUGGESTED RESOURCES

The learning resources listed in this section are a selected sample of materials with which the authors are personally familiar. Appropriate grade levels have been included when these were indicated by the source.

BOOKS

A Guide to Good Eating
National Dairy Council
6300 North River Road
Rosemont, Illinois 60018

Buy and Buy
Food and Consumerism
9–13 years old
Building #7
Mailing Room
Research Room
Cornell University
Ithaca, New York 14853

Choose Your Calories by the Company They Keep
Ruth Leverton
National Dairy Council
6300 North River Road
Rosemont, Illinois 60018

Food Is More Than Just Something to Eat
U.S. Department of Health, Education, and Welfare
Public Health Service
Food and Drug Administration
5600 Fishers Lane
Rockville, Maryland 20052

McDonald's Nutrition Pack
McDonald's Action Packs
Box 2594
Chicago, Illinois 60690

The Thing the Professor Forgot
U.S. Department of Agriculture
Consumer Information
Pueblo, Colorado 81109

CURRICULA

General Mills, Inc.
General Offices
Teacher's Guide to Nutrition
9200 Wayzata Blvd.
Minneapolis, Minnesota 55440

Little Ideas
3–5 years old
National Dairy Council
6300 North River Road
Rosemont, Illinois 60018
(or your local council)

Big Ideas
6–12 years old
National Dairy Council
6300 North River Road
Rosemont, Illinois 60018

FILMS

Read the Label—Set a Better Table
Modern Talking Picture Service
2323 New Hyde Park
New Hyde, New York 11040
(also available from many of your FDA offices)

The Big Dinner Table
Grades K–3
National Dairy Council
6300 North River Road
Rosemont, Illinois 60018

FILMSTRIPS

Nutrition for Young People
Grades 5–8
Guidance Associates
757 Third Ave.
New York, New York 10017

Too Much of a Good Thing
Marsh Films
Shawnee Mission, Kansas 66208

GAMES/ACTIVITIES

Four Food Groups for Better Meals (Bingo)
Superintendent of Documents
U.S. Government Printing Office
Washington, D.C.

Nutrition with Games
Grades K–9
Nutrition Education Service Center
Montclair State College
Upper Mt. Claire, New Jersey 07043

Yardstick for Nutrition
(Packet of vitamins, iron, and calcium)
Cornell University
Ithaca, New York 14850

KITS

Breakfast USA
Age 7–9
Kellogg Company
Home Economics Services
Battle Creek, Michigan 49016

POSTERS

Flannelboard Stories
Set of four stories (e.g., "Ollie and the Orange")
Sunkist Growers, Inc.
Box 7888
Valley Annex
Van Nuys, California 91409

Food Mobile—Foodway to Follow
American Institute of Baking
Nutrition Education Department
400 E. Ontario Street
Chicago, Illinois 60611

National Apple Institute
(free posters and teaching aids)
2000 P Street N.W.
Washington, D.C. 20036

Versatile Vegetables
Green Giant Company
Home Services
5601 Green Valley Drive
Minneapolis, Minnesota 55437

RECORDS

Alexander's Secret
Grades K–2
Cereal Institute, Inc.
135 South La Salle Street
Chicago, Illinois 60603

CONSIDERATIONS for the SCHOOL ENVIRONMENT

Most schools participate in the federal–state school feeding program. Through this program schools receive subsidies that enable them to offer breakfast, midmorning milk snacks that may include crackers or fruit, and/or the traditional noon lunch. The present goals of the program are
  • to improve the nutrition of children.
  • to provide nutrition education.
  • to provide social education.

Whether or not these goals are achieved in a given school depends on how well planned and run the program is and on the extent to which teachers and food-service staff members cooperate in working toward the educational goals. Given favorable conditions, school kitchens can and do turn out nutritious, attractive, and palatable food, and some programs can and do serve as effective learning laboratories.

NUTRITIONAL CONSIDERATIONS

School breakfasts and lunches are required to meet certain nutritional requirements if they are to be eligible for the subsidies paid by the U.S. Department of Agriculture through the designated state agency. *Breakfasts* must include milk, bread or cereal, and either a fruit or full-strength fruit or vegetable juice. Schools are encouraged to serve a meat or meat substitute as often as possible. *Lunches* must meet Type A standards: milk, meat or a meat substitute, vegetable and/or fruit, bread and butter or margarine. On average, lunches are expected to provide a third of the daily dietary allowance established by the National Research Council. *Milk,* in addition to its use with meals or as a snack, may also be sold to children who choose to bring their own lunches. One intent of the program is to make possible a good deal of flexibility in menu planning without sacrificing nutritional quality.

There have been numerous studies of the values of school feeding programs. One study of the effect of school lunches failed to show improvement in growth or hematocrit (iron levels) among school lunch patrons.[17] The classic Iowa Breakfast Studies [18] showed that an adequate breakfast results in improved attitudes and performance of tasks. These favorable results have been confirmed in several other studies that also showed improved nutritional intake status, fewer complaints of late morning hunger pains and headaches, and improved classroom behavior. Decreased tardiness and absenteeism result, where school breakfast and milk snack programs exist.

David Paige and his associates [19] have identified a genetically caused deficiency of the enzyme lactase in a small proportion of black children. These youngsters suffer from gas and diarrhea when they drink milk, and thus dislike this wholesome food. They can enjoy and obtain equivalent nutrition from cheese or yogurt—products in which lactose has been fermented.

The nutritional quality of the lunches that children bring from home varies considerably. Although milk may be brought from home, it is usually less costly and more convenient for children to buy it at school. Some children bring nutritionally worthless artificially flavored fruit drinks instead. Milk, fruit or raw vegetables, and meat or cheese or peanut butter sandwiches provide the nutritional equivalent of a Type A lunch. The nutritional quality of lunches brought from home can be judged either by unobtrusive adult observers or by the children themselves after instruction. Lunch quality can then be improved by direct instruction of both pupils and parents, if indicated. In poor neighborhoods, the use of economical meat substitutes such as peanut butter can be stressed.

Nutritious food served in school will be eaten if it is acceptable to the children. One way of judging acceptability is to observe which foods go into the garbage container as the children return their trays. Rejected foods can be either eliminated from future menus or offered again in a better-prepared or more attractive form. Another way of improving acceptance is to provide pupils with copies of menus for the week or month.

[17] David M. Paige, "The School Feeding Program: An Underachiever?" *The Journal of School Health,* Vol. 42 (September 1972), pp. 392–395.
[18] Cereal Institute, *A Complete Summary of the Iowa Breakfast Studies* (Chicago: The Institute, 1962), pp. 57–59.
[19] David M. Paige, T. M. Bayless and C. C. Graham, "Milk Programs: Helpful or Harmful to Negro Children?" *American Journal of Public Health* Vol. 44 (January 1974), pp. 8–10.

They can then decide when to patronize the school food service and when to bring food from home, depending on their likes and dislikes. An even better method is to involve committees of pupils to assist the food service manager in menu planning. The committee can survey all the pupils to determine food likes and dislikes. They can identify dishes preferred by ethnic groups. What they plan, with the help of the food service manager, is limited only by federal guidelines and the ingredients supplied to the school.

Meaningful pupil involvement in school menu planning can occur only in school buildings that have their own cafeterias and kitchens. In some systems, food is prepared in a large central kitchen and brought to many satellite schools prepackaged for individual service, as are airline meals. This system offers no freedom of choice, but it is economical and it does make food service possible in schools without kitchens. In most schools where there is no cafeteria, pupils eat at their desks.

SOCIAL CONSIDERATIONS

Federal guidelines require that if food service is offered in a school it must be offered to all pupils. Service must be provided free or at a reduced price to those pupils judged by the school district to be unable to pay. Practices and policies vary, but teachers may be asked to help identify the poor pupils and to collect breakfast, milk, or lunch money from those judged able to pay. Care must be taken to hide the identity of poor pupils from the others to avoid embarassment.

Maintenance of a relaxed yet well-disciplined and relatively quiet atmosphere while eating is always a problem. Teachers need to get away from their pupils at times, and some collective bargaining contracts recognize breakfast or lunch as one of those times. Thus mealtime supervision is sometimes turned over to nonprofessional aides who are rarely as competent as teachers in maintaining relaxed discipline.

Whichever system of supervision prevails, pupil instruction in acceptable mealtime behavior is essential. This can be discussed and demonstrated in the classroom. Pupils can be involved in developing and enforcing appropriate rules through peer pressure. They can and should be involved in cleaning up after themselves. They can help decorate the cafeteria. Discipline can be improved by eating at small tables, at each of which an older pupil serves as host and helps maintain order.

In addition, the lunchtime routine should provide for visits to the toilet and for handwashing prior to eating. Neither the lunch hour nor preparation for it should be hurried. If play follows lunch, the time at which play starts should be specified so that pupils have adequate time for a relaxed, unhurried meal first. Children also should be taught to either rinse their mouths (swish and swallow) or eat some detergent food such as an apple or raw carrot after eating.

HEALTH SERVICE CONSIDERATIONS

American elementary school pupils are generally better nourished than are high school students, particularly girls. The probable reason is that adolescents are less responsive to adult controls and that adolescent girls are more susceptible to fad diets. The prevalence of overeating, undereating, and diets deficient in food quality will vary from place to place, but at least one or two children in each classroom are likely to show some evidence of poor nutrition.

THE FAT CHILD

Many children become fat for a year or two at the beginning of adolescence and then outgrow their fatness as their height increases. Such transient fatness is regarded as normal. Children who were fat as babies and remain fat throughout childhood and adolescence are likely to remain fat throughout their adult lives in the absence of successful intervention. Mayer's research leads to the conclusion that abnormal fatness during the elementary school years results more from lack of exercise than from overeating. Fat children typically eat the same amount of food or even less than their non-fat peers.[20]

It is not easy to distinguish those who are so fat as to warrant treatment. Some children appear chunky because of their genetically predetermined body builds but are not really too fat. A child may be "overweight" according to a height–weight sex table and yet not be fat, because the excess poundage is made up of muscle, not fat. A screening test now recommended for the detection of fatness among school children is the measurement, by use of a special caliper, of the thickness of a double fold of the skin and its underlying fat taken over the triceps muscle—the muscle at the rear of the upper arms, above the elbow.

Minimum normal triceps skinfold measurements, as provided by Mayer for boys and girls, are shown in Table 5.1.

Fatness is a matter of degree, and whether or not one is too fat is a matter of medical judgment. Also, a reducing diet and exercise regimen should be individually prescribed by a physician. Therefore, children suspected of being obese by school screening programs should be referred to their usual sources of medical care for diagnosis and treatment. Once this is done, the school can cooperate in the treatment plan by supervising

[20] Jean Mayer, *A Diet for Living* (New York: David McKay Co., Inc., 1976), pp. 110–118.

110

TABLE 5.1

MINIMUM NORMAL TRICEPS SKINFOLD
THICKNESS IN MILLIMETERS BY
AGE AND SEX*

Age in Years	Boys	Girls
5	12	14
6	12	15
7	13	16
8	14	17
9	15	18
10	16	20
11	17	21
12	18	22

1 Adapted from: Jean Mayer, **Overweight—Causes, Cost and Control,** Englewood Cliffs, N.J.: Prentice-Hall, Inc., 1968, p. 34

dietary practices at school and by providing opportunity and motivation for prescribed exercise.

In some schools, nurses and physical educators cooperatively sponsor reduction clubs for obese students who have the permission of their physicians to join. These clubs feature motivational nutritional education and activity sessions. Every week or two, members may be weighed. This should be done on the same scales at the same time of day, with the bladder empty, and in the same state of undress, to assure reliability. Rewards may be given for failure to gain, and for the achievement of weight loss.

Beyond medical referral and the establishment, if possible, of a reduction club, one authority states:

> Perhaps teachers can help most by taking a personal interest in the child, not his (her) obesity, listening to his (her) feelings and problems; sharing his (her) confidences; accepting him (her) as he (she) is. . . .[21]

THE BREAKFAST SKIPPER

The socio-emotional climate in elementary classrooms during the morning hours would be more pleasant and educationally productive if all parents provided a good breakfast and encouraged children to eat it, or if breakfasts and midmorning snacks were served in the school. Unfortunately, many children do not have these opportunities. And, like some adults, some

[21] Charlotte M. Young, "The Fat Child," *Today's Education,* Vol. 60, No. 3 (March 1971), p. 50.

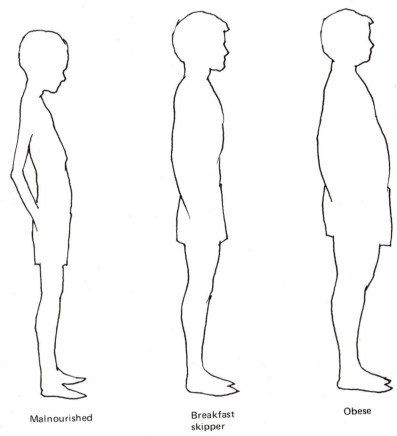

Malnourished   Breakfast   Obese
                      skipper

children lack the appetite to eat before they have engaged in some form of activity.

Questioning of children who show signs of late morning lethargy or misbehavior or who complain of nausea, headaches, or stomach pains may reveal lack of breakfast as a probable cause. The solution may be simply a parent–child conference aimed at promoting better home breakfast patterns. A good breakfast need not follow the traditional American pattern. A tuna fish, cheese, or peanut butter sandwich may be more acceptable to some children than cereal, toast, or eggs.

THE MALNOURISHED CHILD

Except in areas where grinding poverty prevails, cases of severe deficiency of one or more vital food elements are rare. Such cases are difficult to diagnose. A simple screening test for iron deficiency (the hematocrit test) exists, but is rarely administered in schools because it requires withdrawal of a blood sample. Malnourished children may be of normal weight, or even fat, as well as thin, and many children are thin because that is their geneticly dictated body build. Observable signs of malnutrition may be absent, but such signs often include

- poor skin color or tone.
- wrinkled or cracked skin.
- dryness or yellow spots on the skin.
- extreme lethargy or irritability.
- red or dull and vacant eyes.
- dull or excessively dry hair.

These clues are quite general and could easily be symptomatic of other illnesses, but medical attention is called for in any event.

REFERENCES

ALSTON, ELIZABETH. "Snacks: The American Way of Eating," *Family Health,* Vol. 5, No. 1 (January 1973), pp. 27–30.

CAREY, JOYCE. "Dietary Factors and Atherosclerosis," *Journal of School Health,* Vol. 44, No. 9 (November 1974), pp. 511–513.

DUNNING, H. NEAL. "Nutrition Labeling—A New Educational Tool," *School Health Review,* Vol. 5, No. 3 (May-June 1974), pp. 12–15.

FLECK HENRIETTA. *Introduction to Nutrition.* New York: *Macmillan Publishing Co., Inc.,* 1976.

HAYDEN, EUGENE B. "Breakfast and Today's Lifestyles," *Journal of School Health,* Vol. 45, No. 2 (February 1975), pp. 83–87.

MAYER, JEAN. *A Diet for Living.* New York: David McKay Co., Inc., 1976.

PAIGE, DAVID M., and GEORGE G. GRAHAM. "School Milk Programs and Negro Children: A Nutritional Dilemma," *Journal of School Health,* Vol. 44, No. 1 (January 1974), pp. 8–10.

PUNKE, HAROLD R. "Caffeine in America's Food and Drug Habits," *Journal of School Health,* Vol. 44, No. 10 (December 1974), pp. 551–562.

REAL, MYRTLE R. "What It Is Like to Be Hungry," *School Foodservice Journal,* Vol. 27, No. 5 (May 1973), pp. 22–32.

ROBINSON, CORINNE H. *Fundamentals of Normal Nutrition.* New York: Macmillan Publishing Co., Inc., 1978.

SEBRELL, WILLIAM H., and JAMES J. HAGGERTY. *Food and Nutrition.* New York: Time Incorporated, 1967.

"Stamp Out Nutritional Illiteracy," *Instructor,* Vol. 83, No. 5 (January 1974), pp. 45–54 (series of eight articles).

STEINER, PATRICIA. "Menu Pocket Packs Nutrition Education Wallop," *School Foodservice Journal,* Vol. 27, No. 10 (November-December 1973), pp. 38–45.

TANNAHILL, REAY. *Food in History.* New York: Stein and Day, 1973.

WHITE, PHILLIP L. "New Thoughts on Dietary Practices," *School Food-service Journal,* Vol. 27, No. 9 (October 1973), p. 50.

WILSON, CHARLES C., and ELIZABETH AVERY WILSON. *Healthful School Environment.* Chicago: American Medical Association, 1969.

6

Germs, Pollutions, Degeneration—Disease and Environment

Everyone knows that people live longer these days—that advances in medical technology have greatly extended the average life span. It is indeed true that life expectancy at birth has increased from approximately 49 years in 1900 to 71 years for a child born today, but the factors responsible for these more favorable statistics are often misunderstood. These figures to the average person, immediately evoke thoughts of improvements in the art of keeping old persons alive, of respirators, kidney machines, and heroic surgical procedures that often merely prolong the inevitable. Although the applications of medical advances to the old and critically ill have been widely publicized, the effects on longevity have, as yet, been relatively modest. A 65-year-old person in 1900, for example, could look forward to approximately 12 more years of life on the average, whereas his modern-day counterpart can reasonably expect approximately 15 more years. This is progress, of a sort at least, but certainly nothing spectacular. Actually, it has been the young, not the old, who have benefited most from progress in medicine and public health.

A CENTURY OF PROGRESS

The rapid pace of technological progress throughout this century has produced a mind-boggling array of accomplishments and changes; one of the greatest of these has been the freeing of infants and young people from the ravages of disease. Those who feel that this statement is extreme have probably not considered how conditions were before the advent of modern vaccines, antibiotics, obstetrical techniques, and standards of community

115

sanitation. At the turn of the century a number of infections common to infants were grouped together for statistical purposes as gastroenteritis. This category once constituted the third-ranking cause of death; its mortality rate has since been reduced to a small fraction of its former figure. Diphtheria, which now occurs only as isolated cases of medical neglect, then ranked tenth in mortality, taking approximately 40,000 lives each year, the large majority of whom were children. The influenzas and pneumonias, grouped together as a common category, were the leaders in mortality in 1900 and were indiscriminate in the age of their victims, taking infants, children, and adults of all ages. Since that time this category has managed to stay among the top ten—it is now fifth—mainly by attacking the elderly. It has brought death to those terminally ill with cancer and advanced heart disease so frequently as to earn the title of "the old man's friend." Even syphilis, regarded now as a problem of the young, seems determined to eventually yield to antibiotics, at least as a cause of death, with the mortality rate having been reduced from 5.0 to 0.1 per 100,000 during the period from 1950 to 1974, with reported deaths in 1974 numbering only 250.[1]

The progress against childhood diseases that are primarily cripplers rather than killers has been equally great and only slightly less imporant. Rubella as a producer of congenital defects and measles as a crippler of infants and toddlers are now controllable by means of immunization. Polio was perhaps the last major scourge in America; in epidemic form, it brought widespread anxiety and fear to afflicted communities. It now has gone the way of diphtheria, whooping cough, and other major communicable diseases as merely something "we get immunized for."

A NEW PUBLIC ATTITUDE

One of the cumulative effects of these many advances has been a change in the general public's way of thinking about crippling and life-threatening disease. Illness is now thought of as something that happens to old people. The young have accidents; the old get sick. If one introduces the terms "very sick" or "crippled" into a word association game in these times the responses are likely to be "elderly" or "nursing home." A feverish child may cause parental concern, but this does not now cause the anxiety that such situations evoked in previous generations. Few young people today have had to experience the death of a brother, sister, or playmate because of disease, and few have had to even contemplate such an eventuality. Both the actual fact of this progress against the illness of children and youth and the new "freedom from fear" it has produced are highly worthwhile achievements and ones that have major implications for modern school programs of health education.

[1] Division of Vital Statistics, National Center for Health Statistics.

IMPLICATIONS for SCHOOL HEALTH

AWARENESS THROUGH EDUCATION. Both parents and their children tend to react to the reality of disease far better than to the threat of disease. Few of today's parents have ever seen a case of polio, whooping cough, or diphtheria, and consequently have become careless in carrying out their simple most important responsibility in the prevention of these conditions, namely, obtaining appropriate immunizations for their children.[2] Epidemics of diseases otherwise preventable by immunization periodically return in areas where the general public fails to heed the possible consequences of communicable disease. It is better that this awareness be obtained through education than by actual experience.

CARE FOR THE HANDICAPPED. Despite the tremendous medical progress of this century, children still become seriously ill and permanently disabled. Because of the improved general health of young people, such children have tended to become more isolated than in the past. This effect is now being minimized in many states by new legislation and court decisions requiring schools to provide a suitable educational program regardless of any handicapping disabilities children may have; this has tended in many cases to increase the percentage of handicapped children in many schools. These children have needs that are perhaps even more pressing in these days when the average person is spared much acquaintanceship with death and crippling disease.

CONTINUING THE FIGHT. Although communicable diseases are not the major killers and cripplers they once were, they represent major threats to the quality of one's life. The average schoolchild, for example, loses nearly 5 days of school each year because of upper respiratory infections, to produce a cumulative loss of over 220 millions days per year. At the present time the statistics for syphilis are improving in terms of both numbers of cases and the resulting mortality; however, the incidence of gonorrhea remains high and poses continuing threats of sterility and heart damage, among other complications, if left untreated. A few lethal diseases such as meningococcal meningitis (spinal meningitis) and some forms of encephalitis (brain infections), although low in incidence, still cause old-fashioned tragedies. In general, the virus-caused diseases remain resistant to curative treatment, although many are preventable through immunization and environmental sanitation. The efficient coping with this mixed bag of remaining threats is greatly facilitated by a sound knowledge of disease causation and of the body's resistive mechanism, rather than merely relying on one's parents to see that immunizations are administered when due and then going to the doctor occasionally thereafter when one seems to feel sick

[2] James Brough, "Warning: Epidemics Ahead—Protect Our School Children," *Family Health,* Vol. 4, No. 8 (August 1972), p. 18.

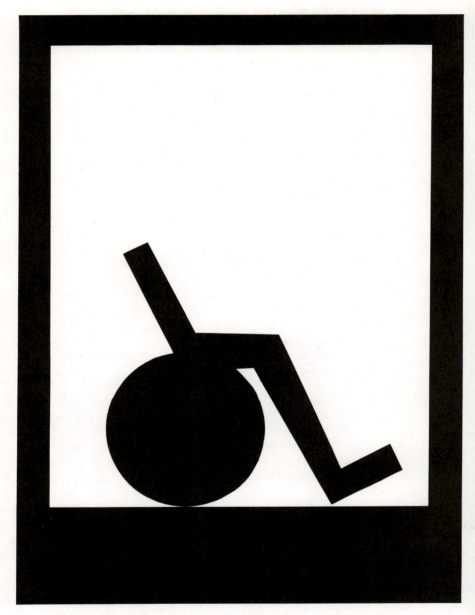

Figure 6.1. Schools Must Provide a Suitable Educational Program Regardless of Any Handicapping Disabilities.

enough. A number of studies of childrens' interests show that they are ready to begin this study in the elementary grades.

MEETING NEW CHALLENGES. Although the public is currently benefiting from a century of fantastic progress against communicable disease, people still succumb eventually to the pain, disability, and death caused by chronic diseases. As long as this situation prevails, which at this point seems to be for an indefinite period, an acceptable level of health for American society appears to remain, in the words of René Dubos, a mirage that keeps moving into the distance as our nation's improvements tend to move us toward it.[3] This is, of course, manifested in the present concern for heart disease, stroke, cancer, and other chronic disorders. The progress against communicable disease must be consolidated; however, it is these chronic conditions that represent the real challenges to physical health in the current century. The battle against these potent adversaries will require changes both in personal health habits and public policies. Although elementary schoolchildren understandably seldom feel threatened by heart disease or stroke, they possess the capacity and the interest to learn about these conditions simply as interesting problems for the human species, and as problems that may affect older persons in their own families.

DISEASE-RELATED PROBLEMS
and INTERESTS OF CHILDREN

The problems and interests of children at particular ages or school levels are regarded as traditional criteria for the selection of content for all phases of the curriculum and particularly for health education with its typical emphasis on immediate, practical outcomes. Health problems in particular also have obvious implications for health services and a healthful environment. Although this type of information is useful, the relationships involved are not as simple as they appear. For example, both dental caries and childhood leukemia are serious problems among elementary pupils, one for its incidence or frequency and the other for its lethal aspects. The implications provided by dental caries are relatively simple. Children can help minimize this problem by their own personal behavior; therefore, the problems may be attacked directly by education. They also need professional care; thus a program of dental screening and referral is logically indicated.

The educational implications are obviously different in the case of leukemia, for the onset or progression of this condition shows little relationship

[3] René Dubos, *Mirage of Health* (Garden City, N.Y.: Anchor Books, Doubleday and Company, 1961).

to the child's behavior. This does not mean, of course, that children do not need to learn about this disease. Cancer is a major national problem worthy of everyone's concern. The fact that the average American tends to avoid the topic and often even hesitates to use the term is indicative of an attitude that also leads to the avoidance of simple precautions such as periodic examinations and the ignoring of symptoms until the disease has advanced beyond control. Also, young people may occasionally come in contact with a seriously ill person and should be able to respond constructively to such a situation.

Health interests likewise provide both opportunities and pitfalls for the selection of health education content. During the heyday of progressive education in the 1930s, interests were regarded by many health educators as direct indicators of health needs. Although this view is still held by many health educators, interests may be regarded as factors to consider rather than principal determiners in the selection of content. Also, a knowledge of children's interests enables a teacher to use them as "motivational hooks" to generate interest in a useful and related topic of which the children may not yet be aware. One hazard in the use of interests is the too-common practice of waiting until the problem is upon the pupil and interest is at its height before presenting the subject. By this time the children have "learned it all" in their peer culture and the educator has little chance to influence attitudes or values. Venereal disease is a case in point. Direct teaching of this topic should probably come not later than the seventh grade; therefore, elementary school pupils need prerequisite learning in the form of general knowledge about bacteria, disease transmission, incubation periods, and so forth if they are to be ready to fully benefit from this later instruction.

DISEASE PROBLEMS

Dental caries constitute the largest disease problem among elementary schoolchildren in terms of prevalence. It is safe to say that the majority of the children in the average elementary school class have teeth that need fillings, or have other uncorrected conditions. At least one study shows that nine out of ten 5-year-olds have never seen a dentist; also, the tendency for neglect on the part of both parents and children continues throughout the cavity-prone years of childhood, with the net result that the average 16-year-old has already lost at least one permanent tooth and has ten untreated decayed teeth.[4]

As noted previously, upper respiratory infections are responsible for the most absences from school among elementary school pupils and, within this

[4] Joanna Jenny and P. Jean Frazier, "Parents' Attitudes About School Dental Services for Children," *Journal of School Health,* Vol. 44, No. 2 (February 1974), p. 86.

group of infections, the common cold is of course the most frequent. Influenza is another fairly common upper respiratory infection that varies greatly both in its severity and infectiousness from year to year as different forms of its viruses become prevelant. Streptococcal infections whether in the form of scarlet fever or a simple "strep throat" are, perhaps, the most serious conditions in this group because of the possible development of rheumatic fever as a sequela to cases that do not receive prompt and adequate treatment.

Among the chronic conditions that afflict children are a variety of heart defects, many of which affect the heart valves to produce a characteristic murmur that can be heard with the aid of a stethoscope. Some of these problems represent inborn birth defects, whereas others occur as a complication of various infections or of rheumatic fever. Many, perhaps most, murmurs are benign and cause no disability, and most others are amenable to corrective surgery; thus they should seldom cause significant handicaps.

Cancer, principally leukemia, is the second leading cause of death among school-aged children, with a mortality rate approximately one-half that of accidents, the leading cause. Although the acute form of leukemia common to children is almost uniformly fatal, treatment often prolongs life for months and sometimes years. Various forms of chemotherapy are the preferred form of treatment and, although relatively severe side effects are common, the child often experiences long periods of relatively good health. A few cases of complete remissions or apparent "cures" have been recorded, and treatment methods are continually improving; therefore, no case should be regarded as hopeless.

Asthma and various allergies are common childhood problems that afflict 10 per cent of the population in their severe forms and another 40 to 50 per cent in milder conditions.[5] These conditions in one sense tend to bridge the gap between communicable and chronic conditions in that they commonly represent malfunctions in the antibody system designed to combat infections. Although seldom life threatening, these conditions can be severely disabling. Severe asthma attacks are frightening and potentially dangerous if not given proper first aid care.

Epilepsy affects a sizeable number of elementary schoolchildren. Close estimates of the actual prevalence are difficult to obtain because of the still-common tendency of parents of epileptic children to keep their child's condition from being known. Some estimates run as high as 2 per cent of the general population, with 75 per cent of these cases developing before the age of 21.[6] Although four out of five persons with epilepsy are likely to have their seizures well controlled with medication, there are occasional slip-ups in the dosage, failure for the medication to be completely effective,

[5] John P. McGovern, "Allergy Problems in School Aged Children," *Journal of School Health,* Vol. 44, No. 5 (May 1974), p. 260.
[6] "The Educator's Role in Epilepsy," *The School Health Review,* Vol. 4, No. 2, (March-April 1973), p. 35.

or occasionally a newly emerging case or some other situation that allows a seizure to take place. Children with epilepsy need understanding from their teachers and help in interpreting the nature of their condition to their classmates.

HEALTH INTERESTS

Children of all ages tend to show a high degree of interest in disease, so much so in fact that teachers sometimes tend to overemphasize this phase of the health curriculum. Although interest is general, particular patterns are apparent at various grade levels; a few examples from the notable study by Ruth Byler and her associates are provided below.[7]

Kindergarten Through Grade Two

• Probably the miracle of teeth is the biggest "production" in these years . . . the first loose ones cause consternation and fear, but this soon turns to joy, as children learn that "more are in the gums" . . . .
• Colds are unwelcome hazards. Some children ask how you get them; some protect themselves loudly against children's coughing and sneezing. The first grader says: "Don't sneeze on me. You give me germs." . . .

Grades Three and Four

• Among illnesses, colds are mentioned most often by third graders . . .
• Children in the fourth grade ask more questions on diseases than about any other topic . . . . Their questions run the gamut of diseases, and about each they want to know its symptoms, causes, cures, and effects, and always, "What's being done to prevent it?"

Grades Five and Six

• Fifth graders name a wide range of diseases about which they want to know causes and cures. There is a technical quality about a few interests, as in the desire "to know about bacteria and fungi."
• Sixth graders ask: What kind of germs does a housefly carry? . . . What else besides smoking causes cancer? . . . How are vaccines made? . . . Why do I get hives when I eat certain things?

ILLUSTRATIVE CONTENT

One of the problems the teacher encounters when planning instruction related to the various diseases that concern man is that there are so many

[7] Ruth Byler, Gertrude Lewis, and Ruth Totman, *Teach Us What We Want to Know* (New York: Mental Health Materials Center, Inc., 1969).

of them. This overwhelming variety when combined with the almost morbid interest that most fourth graders, for example, exhibit toward this topic can easily lead a unit of study into a laundry list rendition of one set of "creepy symptoms and dire consequences" after another. Although a few specific disease conditions should be studied for their particular significance or to illustrate some basic points, the main thrust of the curriculum is better directed toward the pupil's task of developing a valid orientation of disease as general phenomena and valid concepts concerning the general mechanisms of disease and man's natural and technological weapons for its control. This may sound a bit esoteric for the elementary level; however, pupils only need to begin the development of foundations, not complete the whole structure. They have a lifetime to learn about current health problems through the mass media but formal education provides the best opportunity to develop basic tools for attacking these specific and ever-changing problems.

HISTORICAL BACKGROUND

A review of mankind's historical struggle against disease reveals a fascinating and not unexpected kaleidoscope of technological advances and some remarkable consistencies in attitudes, behavior, and public policies. A natural fear of disease and death has been an ever-present phenomenon in the human species as have been the quackery, charlatanism, and desperate behavior it has produced, from the time the first primitive surgeon punched a hole into a hapless patient's skull to the present instances of reliance on spinal adjustments, diet therapy, and copper bracelets to "control" arthritis. Fortunately this dubious behavior has been paralleled by genuine humanitarian efforts beginning long before Hippocrates drafted his oath and extending to the current struggle of American society to bring competent medical care to every citizen as a matter of right.

Within the realm of technology, historical highlights include a blend of ignorant blunders, fortunate or perhaps intuitive guesses, and brilliant discoveries. The Book of Leviticus contains a workable set of directions for the diagnosis and isolation of the victims of leprosy and an equally invalid and impractical explanation of menstruation and related hygenic measures. The "sanitary revolution" that took place in the cities of England during the middle 1800s, with its emphasis on sewer systems and garbage disposal, saved thousands of lives through the reduction of communicable disease several years before Pasteur and Koch identified microorganisms as the basic cause of these maladies. Currently, the research into the causes and the possible methods of controlling the various forms of cancer provides a remarkable example of the bringing together of vast amounts of basic knowledge related to such widely ranging topics as cell structure, antibody responses, mutation, toxins, and many others and applying them to a single

123

task. These various efforts against disease both in the past and in the present may be studied as much for the examples they provide of human ingenuity, persistence, and achievement as for their insights in the understanding of disease itself.

EMOTIONAL ASPECTS

Teachers often lament that young people seem so oblivious to various factors and behavior patterns that threaten their health. However, the other extreme as exemplified by a neurotic concern or hypochrondria is much worse, as the victims must then endure continual emotional stress in addition to whatever physical malfunctions may befall them. Ideally, health-educated persons will incorporate reasonable health precautions into their normal behavior pattern in such a way that they operate in a routine or habitual way and thus expend little emotional energy.

Excessive worry about health is not only a nuisance and, in extreme cases, a disease in its own right, but also very likely is a contributing factor along with other emotional stress to the very physical ills that the worrier fears. In fact, one series of investigations shows a clear relationship between the impact of major changes on one's life, whether they be good or bad, e.g., inheriting wealth or losing it, and the onset of physical disease.[8] On the positive side, every scientific investigator of the efficiency of new drugs is aware of the potency of the "placebo effect," the power of a dummy pill to relieve disease symptoms.[9] And almost every practicing physician puts great store in the value of faith and hope as aids to the healing process.

ENVIRONMENTAL FACTORS

As a topic of study, the environment is perhaps as broad and diverse as it it interesting and valuable. Its many subtopics such as those related to energy supply and agriculture production are perhaps better presented as part of the study of science and social studies. The health aspects of this broad topic center on the more intimate aspects, i.e., the generally unseen world of microorganisms, chemical toxins, and penetrating radiation.

Although Americans receive considerable information concerning disease germs and how to avoid or kill them, there is an almost abysmal ignorance concerning the many harmless and useful microorganisms that form a part of our everyday environment. They not only live in the soil, where they perform the vital function of transforming protein wastes into useful fertilizers in the nitrogen cycle, but also are generally all over and all through

[8] Alvin Toffler, *Future Shock* (New York: Random House, Inc., 1970), p. 281.
[9] Interested teachers will enjoy the brief and readable account on this topic as provided in Berton Roueche, *A Man Named Hoffman* (New York: Berkley Medallion, 1966).

our bodies and interact with us in close relationships. The average person provides a home for perhaps a soup can full of bacteria and other forms of microscopic life, which René Dubos discusses as "the indigenous micro-biota." [10] These tiny residents cause few problems and apparently provide some as yet poorly understood benefits, for laboratory animals raised in germ-free environments do not thrive nearly so well as those raised under more normal conditions. An awareness of the nature and role of these unseen neighbors serves to make one more appreciative of the body's ability to live in harmony with them and of the need to protect these delicate producers of nitrates in the soil, vitamin K in the digestive tract, and carbon dioxide in bread from the onslaught of the same chemical toxins that are threatening the larger members of the living world.

Man has had an opportunity to adapt to microorganisms over several hundred thousand years of cohabitation; however, this is not the case with chemical toxins, many of which are comparative newcomers to the world scene. During the early part of this decade the general public finally became aware of the excessively high levels of carbon monoxide, nitrogen oxides, and other air pollutants, as well as the high levels of mercury that were appearing in ocean fish, DDT and other insecticides in foodstuffs, and various other chemical threats that appear to be permeating all areas of our environment. Some of these pose direct threats to human health, and others threaten to upset certain ecological relationships that are vital to human welfare. The task of cleaning up these environmental insults and preventing their recurrence is both expensive and inconvenient. The maintenance of public support for this task is dependent upon the development of a general understanding of these problems and their remedies.

COMMUNICABLE DISEASE

A wide variety of microorganisms are capable of causing illness in man; the current issue of the American Public Health Association basic handbook on the subject describes 118 such conditions.[11] These tiny offenders include certain varieties of bacteria such as those that cause tuberculosis, protozoa such as malaria parasites, viruses such as those causing the common cold, and a number of others. The process of transmission, infection, and subsequent development of the disease follows a classical pattern including transmission to the host (victim); entrance through a suitable portal of the body such as the nose, mouth, or a break in the skin; and multiplication and overwhelming of the body's resistance. The invading pathogens disrupt the normal functioning of the body with any one or a combination of actions including the production of toxins, the stimulation

---

[10] René Dubos, *Man Adapting* (New Haven: Yale University Press, 1965), pp. 110–146.
[11] Abram S. Benenson, ed., *Control of Communicable Disease in Man* (New York: The American Public Health Association, 1975).

of an excessive reaction of the body's resistive mechanisms, or, less frequently, the physical blockage of various vessels and ducts.

The nature of the organism or organisms that cause a particular disease, the typical mode of transmission of a given disease, and its usual portal of entry into the body dictate different means of control. Some progress is being made, but virus-caused diseases cannot yet be cured by antibiotics or chemical drugs, although many are preventable by immunization. Most diseases caused by bacteria, protozoa, or fungi are susceptible to drug treatment, however. Diseases transmitted via the ingestion of drinking water, milk, or food contaminated by fecal matter are controllable by applying sanitary procedures such as water filtration and chlorination, milk pasteurization, and food sanitation in which handwashing after toilet and before handling food plays an important role.

The spread of respiratory tract diseases such as colds and measles is not subject to effective environmental control, although covering coughs and sneezes may help to some extent. Most respiratory diseases begin to spread from person to person before illness is apparent, or during the prodromal (early) stage, when signs and symptoms are indistinguishable from those of the common cold, so isolation of ill persons is of little value. Active immunization prevents many of these diseases, however, and those caused by bacteria, such as strep throat and meningicoccal meningitis, are treatable by drugs.

Elementary children are subject to a variety of skin diseases, often called nuisance diseases, that are spread either by direct personal contact or by the sharing of personal articles such as caps and combs. These diseases are in part preventable by personal cleanliness and by learning to keep personal things for one's personal use, and most of them are treatable with either over-the-counter or prescription drugs. Insect-spread diseases such as mosquito-borne encephalitis are controllable to some extent at the community level by mosquito control programs. Such programs, unfortunately, disturb ecological balances in the environment. Rocky Mountain spotted fever, which is tick borne, is controllable by avoiding tick-infested areas, using repellants while hiking in wild areas, and removing ticks that do attach themselves by drowning them in oil and gently pulling them off the skin.

Active immunity, or immunity in which persons build their own antibodies against specific microorganisms by exposure to them, can be acquired not only by the injection or ingestion of some killed or weakened varieties of organisms in the form of vaccine but also by natural exposures to them in the course of which the disease a given organism causes may either be acquired or overcome by natural body defenses. Passive immunity, or immunity in which the antibodies are made by another human or some other animal, may be attained through vaccines composed of antibodies. Babies acquire some passive immunities by ingesting the antibodies contained in their mothers' milk. Active artificial immunization has thus far proved to be the most useful means of control of many of the more severe infectious diseases, but it often requires several weeks after active vaccine is given before the body begins to make antibodies. Therefore, passive vaccines are often used to confer quick immunity on persons who have been exposed to a given disease, as in the case of someone exposed to tetanus by a deep, dirty wound. Passive vaccines, however, lose their effectiveness very quickly. Active vaccines provide protection that may last a year or even for life because specialized cells in our bodies "remember" how to make a given antibody once they have done so.

In addition to the antibody response, the body has several features to provide resistance to infections. Certain varieties of white blood cells attack disease germs, usually after their mobility or virulence has been weakened by the antibodies. The skin, with its capacity to let perspiration and certain other secretions out while excluding most foreign material, presents a highly effective mechanical barrier to infection, as do the closely related membranes that line the alimentary canal, respiratory passages, and other body openings. The trachea (windpipe) and the air passages within the lungs are particularly effective, with their lining of countless hairline cilia of microscopic size that provide a continuous sweeping action to remove foreign material from the delicate tissue of the respiratory system. Another mechanical defense is the ability to expel irritating material from the body by vomiting, sneezing, coughing, or the secretion of tears. As a total group, these various resistive mechanisms constitute a highly efficient and flexible system that constantly monitors the external environment of microorganisms and adjusts the body's defenses accordingly. Such general health measures as good nutrition, especially adequate amounts of vitamin C, proper amounts of sleep, and the avoidance of excessive physical or emotional stress are vital to the efficiency of this important system.

CHRONIC DISEASE

The term *chronic disease* tends to be used in different ways and is somewhat difficult to define. Generally, it applies to health impairments that are permanent or may be expected to require a long period of supervision, observation, or care.[12] The various forms of heart disease and cancer merit priority attention because of their high mortality rates; others may be profitably studied by elementary pupils because of their particular significance to children or because of the principles they illustrate.

The allergies merit study on both these latter two accounts. Allergy conditions occur frequently among children, and the study of the underlying dynamics of the condition provides further insights into the working of the antibody mechanism. In making an antibody response to the invasion of disease germs, the body reacts to the alien protein material these germs

[12] Henrik L. Blum and George M. Keranen, *Control of Chronic Disease in Man* (New York: The American Public Health Association, 1966), p. xiii.

contain and produces an army of antibodies to destroy the invader. However, germs are not the only protein material to which this mechanism responds; dog hair, dog dandruff, and pollen are examples of other protein-based materials that in some persons produce a vigorous antibody response that results in the inflammation of the person's own tissue to produce running of the nose, rashes and/or itching of the skin, indigestion, or other manifestations. Treatment of the condition may involve any one or a combination of avoiding the substance that causes the response (the antigen allergen), taking drugs such as antihistamines to suppress the response temporarily or "reeducating" the tissue by giving it frequent and small exposures in a desensitizing process.

The antigen–antibody response also represents an obstacle to the extended use of transplanted organs. Unless the donor has the same type of protein, as in the case of an identical twin serving as a kidney donor, for example, the body will tend to produce antibodies to destroy the presumed invaders in what in this instance becomes the rejection process. Basic strategy for organ transplants involves matching the tissue as closely as possible, then suppressing the recipient's antibody mechanism with drugs until the body comes to accept the new tissue as its own.

This interesting mechanism can also be used as a lead into the study of cancer. It now seems clear the development of cancer involves a failure of the immunity (antibody) mechanism to perform one of its routine tasks. Apparently in the normal process of cell division, which occurs more or less continuously in the body, dangerous mutations occur that produce potentially harmful cells; however, these mutants are normally recognized as different by the immunity system, which immediately generates antibodies to reject this alien tissue just as it would a typhoid germ or a poorly chosen organ transplant. But when this immunity mechanism fails for some reason, then the mutant cells thrive as a newly developing cancer. Sometimes the system can be stimulated, after the fact, as it were, to do its job in a procedure known as immunotherapy; more often, however, the malignant cells must be surgically removed or killed with drugs or radiation.[13]

The study of the effects of cigarette smoking forms a logical part of the overall study of disease. Carbon monoxide and other gases in the smoke tend to paralyze and destroy the delicate cilia that normally sweep the respiratory passages clean, leaving the lung tissue more vulnerable to the irritating tars in other components of the cigarette smoke and to disease germs, dust particles, and other pollutants. As this material accumulates in the mucus lining the respiratory passages it proves irritating and, in the absence of effective action by the cilia, is coughed up. This behavior is known as "smoker's hack," the most prominent symptom of chronic bronchitis. This leaves the smoker more susceptible to colds and other respiratory

[13] For a nontechnical but quite thorough account of the relationship of cancer to the immunity system, see "Toward Cancer Control," *Time*, Vol. 101, No. 12 (March 19, 1973), pp. 64–69.

infections and, as smoking continues, begins to cause physical damage to the tiny air sacs (alveoli) at the end of the air passageways. After some years the suffocating effects of emphysema appear. Among some smokers these tarry deposits somehow stimulate excessive cell growth and cell mutations to produce lung cancer. A few nonsmokers exposed to polluted air also develop this condition.

Thus in many ways lung cancer, although highly publicized because of its mortality rate (95%), is the least of the cigarette smoker's worries. Some degree of bronchitis and increased susceptibility to infections occurs early in the smoker's career. Emphysema is more common than lung cancer; it kills at least as many persons and disables many more. Also among public health officials there is even more concern about the role of cigarettes as a contributor to mortality from heart disease, which takes approximately 700,-000 lives per year, than about its threat as the major cause of perhaps 70,000 lung cancer deaths. Interestingly enough, cigar and pipes appear to have little effect on mortality, with these types of smokers living about as long as nonsmokers.

Most cases of heart disease and stroke result from a basic disease condition called atherosclerosis. In its simplest sense, this condition results from the development of fatty deposits (plaques) on the inner walls of the arteries that eventually leads to the deterioration of the affected blood vessels. This disease may progress slowly and relentlessly to produce many of the symptoms of aging and senility, or, as frequently is the case, a sudden accident may occur as when a major artery supplying the heart muscle is blocked, to cause a heart attack, or one in the brain ruptures to produce a stroke.

Genetic factors appreciably affect the intensity and rate at which atherosclerosis progresses; however, several aspects of health behavior are also strongly related to this condition, which begins in the formative years of childhood. The value of avoiding cigarette smoking has been mentioned; in addition, weight control, reduction of dietary cholesterol and saturated fats, regular exercise, avoidance of excessive emotional stress, and the early treatment of hypertension (high blood pressure) are important factors. In short, the list of measures that can limit the risk of heart disease reads like a standard regimen for good general health and subsequently yields benefits long before the individual reaches the years of high susceptibility to heart disease.

SUGGESTED LEARNING ACTIVITIES

The following suggestions are presented in an effort to demonstrate how the content described in the preceding section might be translated into effective classroom learning activities. They were designed to accommodate a wide variety of classroom groups provided that proper selection and adaptations are made according to the needs, interests, abilities, and maturity level of the particular children involved.

- Take shelf paper or brown butcher paper and make a life line on it from 1900–1978. Block it off in 10-year spans and have the children fill in situations where certain diseases have been controlled, new diseases have been cited, and environmental problems were noted to cause particular problems (e.g., smog–respiratory illnesses) during this life span.

- Many countries (e.g., Russia, Peru) report the life span of many of their people to be over 100 years. Have the children investigate to see if there are any similarities or differences for this longevity in comparison to our life-style (e.g., eating habits) and longevity.

- Have the children make a chart indicating the various diseases for which they have been vaccinated and/or given oral medication. This can be incorporated into their "Life Scrapbook" activity cited in Chapter 4.

- Have the children make a chart of health agencies that provide immunization shots for communicable diseases (e.g., county health department, public health nurses, clinics). Ask representatives from these agencies to speak to the children about their role or arrange to have the children take a field trip to visit their offices. This is a good opportunity to begin developing awareness for future careers.

- Have the school nurse visit your class and show the children how to use and read a thermometer. Have the children practice in small groups.

- Have the children with the aid of the school nurse make a bar graph of the various illnesses that are contracted during the various months of the school year. Have the children watch for time periods and certain illnesses. Discuss control of illnesses that occur at the same time each year.

- While studying American history, have the children consider the various remedies that "medicine men" were advocating and why the people believed they would work. If possible, bring in old medicine bottles and if the labels are still present, read them and determine if they are different or similar from the labels of today.

- Have the children read or listen to stories based on life in colonial and pioneer days involving disease problems. Such simple points as "there were no shots for children to take," "the doctors didn't have very good medicine," and "sometimes the water had germs in it" can give young children an increased awareness of the benefits of modern measures of protection.

- Ask the children to recount episodes when they were sick or hurt and someone helped them. Ask them about their feelings at the time—

Did it hurt very much? Were you scared? When did you feel better? In addition to the development of increased awareness of the ways responsible adults help children, some of the more insightful pupils may come to realize that the attention they received in itself made them feel better.

- Have the children develop an "environmental telephone" service where citizens in their community can call to leave, or have picked up, newspapers, bottles, and cans for recycling.

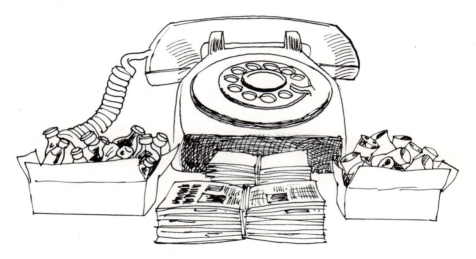

- Have the children build a model of a city in 1800 and a model of a city today. Show how the sanitation practices differed. They can also simulate any air and water pollutants that exist or existed.
- Have the children cut out large letters for the word ENVIRONMENT to be used in a mural for one of the school's corridor walls. Have the students represent in each letter the effects of pollution on people, land, water, etc.

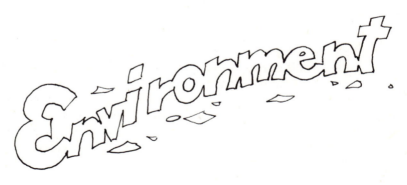

- Have the children draw certain parts of their body (or their whole self) and indicate how these parts can act as pollutants (e.g., dirty hands).

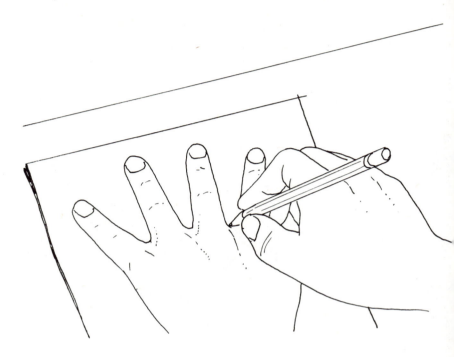

- Ask the children to bring water from a variety of sources, e.g., tap, gutter, pond, and lake. Label each one and observe for clearness and color. Allow to stand overnight. Examine for sediment and any observable organisms. Note: Caution the children to get parental permission and perhaps parental assistance before traveling very far from home for these samples.[14]
- Among upper elementary children, arrange for a small group of volunteers to visit a cooperative auto dealer to examine and discuss auto pollution control devices. The children should ask what pollutants they control, how they work, and how much they add to the cost of the car. Report the findings to the class. This report could be combined with another report from pupils assigned to investigate the dangers of auto pollutants.
- Have the children make posters for environmental week. Have the posters displayed around the various stores in the community.

[14] *Health Education: A Curricular Approach to Optimal Health, Volume I* (Baltimore, Md.: Maryland State Department of Education, 1973), p. 3.

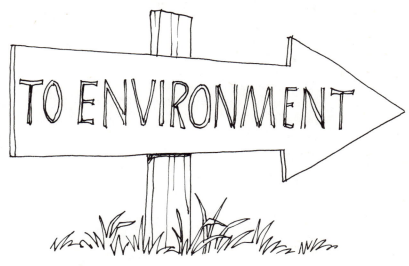

- Construct a "Disease Entrance Wheel." Have the children spin the dial and tell how various diseases can enter the body through the path indicated by the arrow.

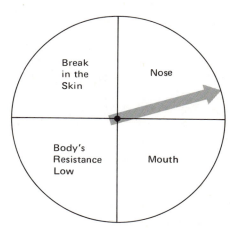

- Have the children draw posters depicting specific ways to combat disease. Poster themes could include getting "shots," getting enough sleep, eating the right foods, staying home when ill, washing hands before meals, and many others.
- Have the school nurse visit the children and bring a stethoscope and a blood pressure kit. Explain to the children what and how these are used and have the children listen to each other's heart beat.

133

- Refer back to the activity in Chapter 4 to show the children what atherosclerosis is (use of toilet tissue rolls and colored clay).
- Rank the following health suggestions as to their importance in maintaining a healthy, long life:
  _____ weight control
  _____ adequate sleep
  _____ proper and regular exercise
  _____ routine medical examinations
- Have the children design a card for their parent (s) and/or legal guardian regarding the good health practices that they should follow according to the message by their son or daughter. Example: on Valentine Day have the children cut out a heart and include in it those risk factors than we can control in protecting our hearts.

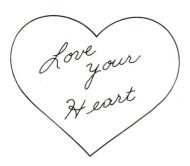

- Ask the children to conduct their own antismoking campaign. One teacher used this general approach and as a culminative activity encouraged the class to write and produce an antismoking play that featured the Flintstones and Snoopy as characters. The total class participated in some way as actors, writers, makers of props, and so forth. In this case the play was aired on local television and was well received.[15]
- Have the children make a banner from different-colored felt pieces to show the ways to limit the risk of heart disease. This banner should be taken home to hang in an appropriate place as a reminder to every member of the family.
  Items that should be included:
  — avoidance of smoking
  — control of weight
  — avoidance of foods high in cholesterol and saturated fats
  — regular exercise
  — avoidance of excessive emotional stress
  — early treatment of hypertension

15 Richard McGuire, "Flintstones and Snoopy Join the Antismoking Campaign," *School Health Review*, Vol. 3, No. 3 (March-April 1972), pp. 10–11.

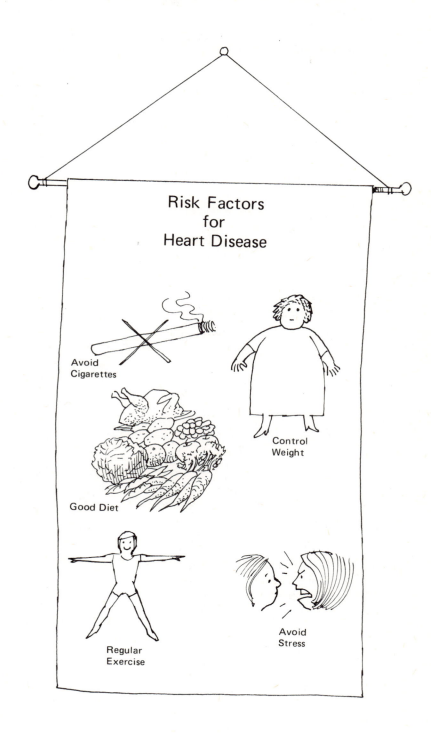

SUGGESTED RESOURCES

The learning resources listed in this section are a selected sample of materials with which the authors are personally familiar. Appropriate grade levels have been included when these were indicated by the source.

BOOKS

McDonald Ecology Pack
McDonald Action Packs
Box 2594
Chicago, Illinois 60698

Noise, Noise, Noise
Scott, Foresman and Co.
Glenview, Illinois 60025

Protecting Our Environment
The Pollution Problem
(by J. Keogh Rash)
Globe Book Co.
175 Fifth Ave.
New York, New York 10010

Wastebasket Full, Wastebasket Empty
Scott, Foresman and Co.
Glenview, Illinois 60025

What Is Air Pollution?
A Story of Air Pollution and Cars
General Motors Corporation
Detroit, Michigan 48202

Who Cares About Pollution
Scott, Foresman and Co.
Glenview, Illinois 60025

FILMSTRIPS

Cities, USA
Guidance Associates
757 Third Ave.
New York, New York 10017

Environment: Changing Man's Values
Grades 5–8
Guidance Associates
757 Third Ave.
New York, New York 10017

Operation Salvage
Guidance Associates
757 Third Ave.
New York, New York 10017

This Earth
Grades 4–6
Guidance Associates
757 Third Ave.
New York, New York 10017

Trees for 2001
Grade 6
Guidance Associates
757 Third Ave.
New York, New York 10017

GAMES AND ACTIVITIES

Energy Activities with Energy Art
Federal Energy Administration
Office of Commissioner and Public Affairs
Washington, D.C. 20461

PAMPHLET
Don't You Dare Breathe That Air!
American Lung Association
Local Chapter

POSTERS

Ecology
Grossman Press
P.O. Box 15246
San Diego, California 15426

137

DISEASE-RELATED CONSIDERATIONS
for the SCHOOL ENVIRONMENT

The great variety of both socioemotional and physical factors in the school environment that have been implicated as either direct or indirect causes of disease form an interlocking network involving virtually every aspect of the school and its activities. Physical factors, such as the sanitation of food, milk and water, have long been recognized, and standards for school practice have been developed that are well accepted. Although the role of stress in disease causation has only recently received commensurate attention, educators have long sought to humanize schools. The state of the art of improving human relations is not so far advanced as that of physical environmental health.

SOCIOEMOTIONAL FACTORS

Horace Mann, the father of American public education, sought to humanize schools by opposing corporal punishment during the mid-nineteenth century. Nearly a century later, John Dewey promoted school humanization by advocating teaching styles centered around the notion that youngsters may better achieve educational goals by selecting and working on projects dictated by their own interest. Although children are still legally spanked in many American schools, and school-prescribed learning activities are still predominant in classrooms, there is less spanking and more concern for individuality than there used to be.

Another stress-reducing trend is the tendency to use test scores more as diagnostic aids and less to label individual pupils as brilliant, ignorant, or lazy. Related innovations include grading systems that include no-fail grading and grading based on individual growth rather than group norms. These reforms are based on observations that pressure to learn more and to learn it faster results in pupils who hate school and who exhibit psychosomatic-related illness such as upset stomachs, virus infections, and headaches. Many teachers have been horrified to learn that some students who receive failing grades also receive beatings from their parents.

Another source of stress, now much less common than it once was, is imposed by the awarding of certificates for perfect attendance. This practice attracts sick children to school, where they may spread infectious diseases to others. It may also encourage parents to send sick youngsters to avoid the loss of a day's work or the expense of a baby-sitter. In most if not all modern schools, teachers who are ill have the benefit of paid sick leave, but many working parents, especially those who work by the day, do not.

Both pupils and teachers are sometimes absent as a result of socioemotional problems. If they do attend school when they are disturbed, they are handicapped in their efforts to learn and teach. Such problems may arise out of family disputes or adverse interpersonal relationships at school or elsewhere. Some persons are able to cope with such problems by themselves. They may do so in ways that are direct, logical, and healthful, or by the use of psychological defense mechanisms, such as blaming their problems on others, that are neither direct nor healthful. Teachers are usually left to their own devices in identifying and using help when they need it. Their sources of help may include friends and relatives or mental health professionals in the community. Most schools provide some sort of help to disturbed pupils. For example, there may be a guidance counselor, school social worker, or psychologist. Recognizing that a disturbed person needs help immediately, not later when a professional may have time available, some schools provide crisis rooms staffed by warm and understanding school staff members to which classroom teachers may refer pupils who are upset themselves or are disturbing to others. Such resources provide immediate help and enable classroom teachers to go about the business of teaching. In many locales, community mental health centers exist that provide both direct help to chronically disturbed pupils and guidance to their teachers and parents.

THE PHYSICAL ENVIRONMENT

Certain factors in the physical environment of the school have significant effects on the spread of infectious diseases. Pollutants may also be present that may cause cancers in later life.

The infectious diseases that are spread by the fecal–oral route are the ones most readily controllable through environmental sanitation. The observable manifestations of these diseases usually include nausea, vomiting, and diarrhea—signs and symptoms that also may be of psychosomatic origin or that may indicate the presence of appendicitis or hunger. Most of these can be effectively controlled by teaching both pupils and adults, especially the food service staff, to wash their hands thoroughly after using the toilet and before eating, and by careful attention to food, milk, and water sanitation. Food must be thoroughly cooked and kept either very hot or very cold until it is served. Dishes and other tableware must be washed in water so hot that they will dry by themselves after washing, or rinsed in a powerful disinfecting solution. Disposable tableware also provides protection. Milk is first protected by pasteurization and then by refrigeration. Leftover food and milk should be discarded. Water is protected by filtration and chlorination and by plumbing that makes it impossible for waste water, such as that in a toilet bowl, to enter and contaminate the drinking water supply pipes. Sanitary drinking fountains are so constructed that the outlet is above the bowl rim and at an angle. This prevents waste water in a clogged bowl from contaminating the outlet, and also prevents contamination by the spittle of users. Pupils can readily observe many of these protective devices as part of their health education.

The most common diseases of childhood—colds and other diseases such as measles, chickenpox, strep throat, and the like—are usually spread either by airborne droplets from coughs or sneezes from the mouth or nose of one person to another, or by contaminated papers or other objects that are touched by fingers that are stuck in mouths. Environmental methods have proven largely ineffective in the control of such diseases; attempts to sanitize the air in school classrooms have proven futile. However, a relative humidity of approximately 30 to 50 per cent both lowers the survival rate of airborne bacteria and increases the resistance to infection of the mucous membranes that line the mouth and throat.[16] This level of humidity also is optimal for comfort at ordinary room temperatures. Proper ventilation (air movement and exchange that is barely perceptible) may also help to dilute and break up contaminated airborne droplets. The idea that chilling and wet feet cause colds is pure hokum, although a room temperature of around 70°F does contribute to comfort and work efficiency. The use of disposable paper tissues to cover coughs and sneezes and to blow noses probably contributes something to the control of airborne diseases.

There is also little that can be done in the way of environmental sanitation to prevent the passage of such personal contact diseases as impetigo, scabies (itch), lice, or fungus infections (ringworm, athlete's foot) in schools. Keeping shower and dressing rooms clean and dry, and providing clean towels to pupils when they shower, probably helps to some extent.

There is little that schools can do to prevent the chemical pollution of air, food, and water. In some schools, policy dictates the suspension of physical activities when air pollution reaches unhealthful levels. In some schools downwind of industries that create chronic pollution problems, windows have been sealed and air-cleansing equipment has been installed in the ventilation system.

Environmental methods of protecting the dental health of school children include the fluoridation of drinking water supplies, preferably at the municipal water plant, or, failing that, in the school buildings themselves. Many schools have taken steps to ban or limit the consumption of sugared sodas, candy, and other such empty-calorie cariogenic items.

DISEASE-RELATED ASPECTS of SCHOOL HEALTH SERVICES

The objectives of the school health service with respect to disease are, first, to prevent disease occurrence to the extent that this is possible; second,

[16] Christopher H. Andrews, "The Viruses of the Common Cold," *Scientific American*, Vol. 203, No. 6 (December 1960), p. 88.

to identify cases of disease that do occur and refer them to community sources for definitive diagnosis and treatment; and, third, to assist school management of pupils handicapped by disease. Teachers and health education as a subject are or should be involved in the attainment of each of these three objectives.

DISEASE PREVENTION SERVICES

The most obvious school health service directed to the prevention of disease is that of involvement in school–community immunization programs. The first step in the development of an effective program is the identification by state and local health authorities of those diseases locally prevalent, or potentially prevalent, for which effective vaccines are available. The second step is to motivate parents, through the enactment of legal requirements, public health education, and outreach programs, to have their children immunized. Although most available vaccines should be administered between infancy and school entrance, laws are most readily enforceable upon school entrance. The third step is to provide immunizations at no charge and at convenient times and places—usually at school during school hours. Finally, the immunization status of the population is periodically assessed and those who should be immunized are notified. In the United States, those adequately immunized upon entrance to kindergarten will generally not need reimmunization until they are of junior or senior high school age. Thus kindergarten teachers are the ones most likely to be involved in gathering immunization histories from parents and in preparing children both through educational procedures and through the necessary paperwork for immunizations. Education is largely a matter of explaining the procedure and its importance so the children will not be frightened.

Crash immunization programs involving the whole school population should not be needed, but occasionally they must be instituted because of poor program planning or execution or when a new vaccine is discovered. Such situations require careful joint planning by public health and school representatives.

Childhood diseases such as chickenpox, mumps, measles, and rubella are generally much more severe in adults than in children. Mumps may cause severe and painful inflammation of the testicles or ovaries, sometimes resulting in sterility when it occurs past puberty. Rubella in a pregnant woman may cause serious defects in her baby. For these reasons, teachers who have not acquired immunity to this disease through prior infection or vaccination should consult their physicians or the school health service about the possibility of immunization. Some school health services provide immunizations against influenza and other diseases to adult school members.

Another major disease prevention program provided by school health services is preventive dentistry. In communities where the water supply is

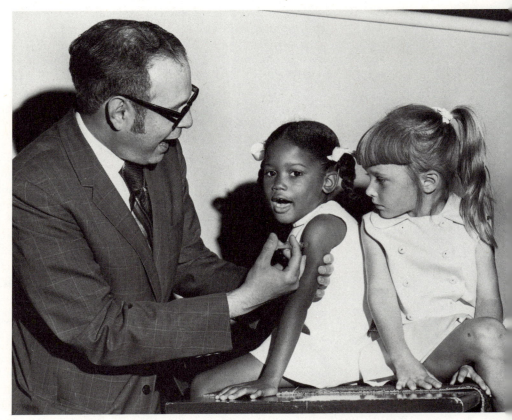

Figure 6.2. Immunization: A Little Pain Now Can Prevent a Big Problem Later. (Philadelphia Health Department)

not fluoridated, dental hygienists may apply fluoride or decay-preventive plastic sealants to children's teeth, or fluoride tablets or mouthwashes may be administered to children. Dental hygienists may also clean and scale children's teeth, a procedure important in the prevention of gum disease. These procedures require parental permission and acceptance by the children, both of which are best obtained as a result of health education as to the nature and purpose of the procedures.

EARLY IDENTIFICATION and REFERRAL

Most children benefit from the early diagnosis and treatment of both infectious and chronic diseases. A conspicuous exception is the common cold, for which no effective treatment is yet available. Strep throat infections, which often mimic colds at onset, are curable, and treatment helps prevent rheumatic fever and rheumatic heart damage. Children with such diseases as epilepsy and diabetes also benefit from the medical control of their conditions.

In most states and local school systems, children are required to undergo medical health examinations upon school entrance and periodically thereafter in the hope of discovering health problems early. As a guide to the examiner, parents are usually asked to fill out a questionnaire about the child's disease and immunization history prior to the examination. The examinations may be conducted in school by school physicians or nurse practitioners at the school's expense, or by private practitioners in their offices at the expense of the parents. Studies indicate that school entrance examinations are productive and useful but that periodic reexaminations result in the identification of few new problems not otherwise discoverable through the screening tests and teacher observation of children. As a result, many authorities believe that reexamination should be limited to those children suspected of having acquired a new health problem, including those recently seriously ill or injured.

Teachers are more likely to discover incipient infectious diseases and mental health problems through observation than physicians and nurses are through periodic examinations. Teachers see their pupils daily in all kinds of activity and for extended periods, whereas examiners see them rarely and for only a few minutes at a time. Most communicable diseases begin with such observable signs as headache, nausea, lethargy, fever or chills, pallor, skin rashes, redness of the eyes, or signs of a cold. The routine procedure in most schools in the presence of such indications is referral to the school nurse for further evaluation and decision as to the appropriate disposition of the case. Mental health problems of a serious nature usually result in inappropriate or markedly changed behavior: failure to play with other children, extreme changes in academic achievement in relation to ability, socially unacceptable behavior, or behavior too good to be true. Here, the appropriate procedure in most schools is initial referral to the counselor or other school mental health professional. In some schools, nurses also receive mental health referrals.

Dental health examinations or inspections by a dentist or school dental hygienist are also routine in many schools. Almost all children have existing dental problems in need of correction, so identification of problems is a bit like trying to find hay in a haystack. The real hope is that all children will be seen by a dentist twice a year for preventive treatments, but this hope is somewhat unrealistic because of the expense to poor parents and the lack of dental services in many communities. In-school examinations and inspections are worth more in terms of their educational value and the preventive services that may be applied along with them than for their case-finding value. It is also useful, however, to assess the dental health

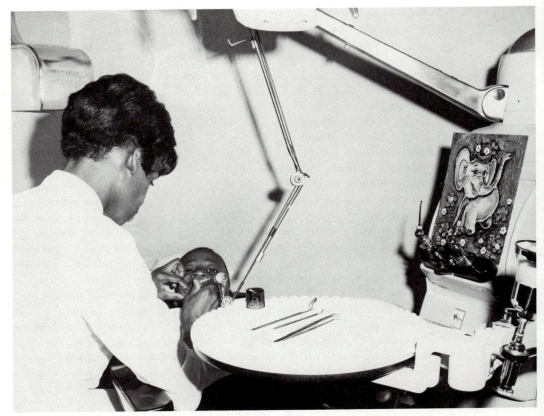

Figure 6.3. Regular Dental Care Is Important. (Philadelphia Health Department)

status of the child population from time to time to provide data for program planning and evaluation.

Screening tests to detect vision and hearing problems and obesity have been discussed. In some localities, particularly those in which the disease is still a threat, both pupils and teachers are screened periodically for tuberculosis infections. The usual procedure is a skin test, which, if positive, is followed by a chest X-ray. A positive skin test is readily apparent to any intelligent person well before it is read as such by the nurse or physician and can therefore be extremely anxiety producing. Education stressing the fact that a positive test indicates prior exposure to tuberculosis, not necessarily active disease, is therefore an essential component of the program. Tuberculosis is now treatable with drugs and no longer requires prolonged hospitalization. Another screening test used in schools to detect scalp ringworm, a fungus disease, is the examination of the scalp under an ultraviolet (Woods) light in rooms in which a case has occurred. Infected hairs glow under the light. The test is usually performed by the school nurse, and the disease, although unsightly, is not serious and is curable.

Appropriate referral patterns vary with both the nature of the disease and the family situation of the pupil involved. Although most infectious diseases have already been spread about the classroom by the time they are discovered, some control value may be gained by excluding those with certain diseases from school until recovery occurs or effective treatment has been given. The control value of exclusion is generally low for virus diseases such as colds and measles. There is also little to be gained by referring youngsters with these diseases to a physician; only symptomatic treatments are available. For lice and scabies, some over-the-counter drugstore remedies are as efficacious as those that can be bought only on prescription. Most bacterial diseases, on the other hand, respond to medical treatment and their communicability is controlled by treatment as well. Children with serious noncommunicable disorders such as epilepsy or diabetes belong under medical care, despite the incurability of the disease. Given the information that their child may have a medical or dental defect that requires diagnosis and, if indicated, treatment; most affluent and well-educated parents will respond quickly and appropriately. Those who are less well-off financially or less well informed may be enabled or motivated to act only after counseling, including referral to a specific community agency, by the school nurse.

To many persons, a referral to a source of help for socioemotional problems is seen as a disgraceful indication of personal weakness or incompetence as a parent. Such referrals, like those for costly medical or dental problems with which parents need help, are therefore best made by a skilled professional in a face-to-face conference. In such instances, the nurse or other counselor tries to keep the conversation focused on the child's problem and on developing ways of solving it. When a source of help is agreed upon, the professional may make the actual appointment for the parent and child.

SCHOOL MANAGEMENT

Many ill children require some adjustment in their school routine to enable them to attend school and learn and to comply with medical orders. These adjustments range from providing emergency care for those who become acutely ill at school to placement in special education classes or the provision of visits by a special teacher for children confined in hospitals or at home for extended periods of time. They also include the commonsense and kindly things many teachers do to make life easier for children handicapped by illness, such as providing opportunities to make up missed work and sending get-well cards. The nature and scope of the kinds of adjustments that may be helpful vary considerably, both with the problem and with the individual child.

ACUTE ILLNESSES

Children who become acutely ill at school must be cared for until they can be returned to the care of their parents. If a communicable infection is suspected, they should be isolated from others. Such care is usually provided by the nurse, whose responsibilities may also include notifying the parents, advising them as to whatever or whether medical care is indicated, and helping them arrange transportation. Legal restrictions exist in most places that prevent the nurse from administering medication without medical advice (aspirin is sometimes excepted) or from obtaining medical care without the express knowledge and consent of the parents. The nurse's task is made more difficult by the fact that in most modern families both parents work outside the home and are not easy to reach.

Most acutely ill children recover rather quickly and return to school in a few days. They will need an opportunity to make up missed work. Some will return too soon, and have to stay home again for a day or two. Most will return during convalescence and before recovery is complete, and may therefore not be able to participate fully in all activities. They may be better off at rest while the others engage in physical play.

CHRONIC ILLNESSES

Parents and teachers alike tend to pamper children with severe illnesses, and to be alarmed at the prospect of having to deal with the recurrent medical emergencies that accompany some of them. Pampering or allowing such children to opt out of important school activities does not help these children prepare for a productive life in the real world. The medical emergencies that occur may be dramatic, but their appropriate management is, in fact, quite simple. Appropriate management varies with each case and is usually best planned individually in case conferences involving the school nurse, teacher, and parent.

ASTHMA. Asthma is a serious form of respiratory tract allergy. Attacks may or may not be seasonal, depending on the allergies, and they may be precipitated by socioemotional stress as well as by the presence of the substance to which the pupil is allergic. It is important to try to identify such precipitating stresses and avoid them if possible. It is equally important that asthmatic youngsters participate as fully as possible in physical exercise and all other common school activities.

Attacks are marked by wheezing, choking, and gasping that persists until the plug of mucus that blocks the respiratory tract is expelled. Most asthmatic youngsters carry medication, often in the form of an inhaler, that helps them through an attack. During an attack, the child should be

146

placed in a sitting position. Most victims need to rest after an attack, and some may need to be taken home.

DIABETES MELLITUS. Diabetes in childhood is a much more severe form of the disorder than that which begins in adult life. All diabetic children need insulin injections to stay alive, and are much more likely than adults to experience emergencies. Young diabetics benefit from vigorous exercise, including participation in athletics. The only caveat is that adequate feeding should precede exercise to prevent insulin reactions. The extent to which an individual is subject to attacks must be considered in determining the appropriateness of specific activities, such as climbing ropes.

Insulin reaction, which results from some combination of too little food, too big an insulin dose, and/or too much exercise, is the most common emergency. Experienced diabetics learn to feel a reaction coming on and act to prevent it by consuming sugar in some form—a candy bar or sugared soda, for example. Signs of insulin reaction are its sudden onset, usually following exercise, and include a pale, ashen complexion and moist, clammy skin. As long as the person is conscious and able to swallow, the attack can be aborted within 10 to 15 minutes following ingestion of sugar in any available form. If the person is unconscious, granulated sugar can be placed under the tongue. If the person does not respond to sugar, he or she should be sent to a hospital emergency ward.

Acidosis, which results physically from lack of insulin, is gradual in onset. The complexion of the person is flushed, the skin is dry, and the odor of acetone (like cheap wine) is obvious on the breath. Cases of acidosis do *not* respond to first aid treatment. The victim should be sent to a hospital emergency ward for treatment, together with the information that he or she has diabetes.

In either event, the pupil's parents and physician should be notified of the occurrence.

EPILEPSY. Epilepsy is a brain disorder manifested by several forms of convulsions or lapse of consciousness. In children, nonepileptic convulsions sometimes occur as a result of infections, hyperventilation (prolonged periods of rapid breathing), or other causes. Epileptic convulsions can be adequately or completely controlled by medication in about four out of five cases. Modern electrosurgical techniques offer the possibility of cure for a least some victims. The two most common forms of epileptic seizure are *grand mal* and *petit mal,* the latter being more common among children than in adults.

Grand mal seizures are usually preceded by an aura, a sensation that informs the victim that a seizure is about to occur. Those with reliable auras can thus remove themselves from hazardous situations (such as swimming pools) before they lose consciousness. Falling, convulsive muscular spasms,

147

foaming at the mouth, vomiting, and bladder and bowel evacuation may accompany an attack. Attacks usually last only a few minutes, and their first aid management is simple. The first and most important rule is to keep composed, and to help the other children do so. Help the victim lie down on the floor and move funiture away to prevent injury. The first aid person may place the victim on his or her side to prevent choking on mucus or vomit. If clothing is tight around the neck, loosen it. *Do not put anything hard in the victim's mouth.* To do so may cause the victim to choke, or result in broken teeth. A rolled soft cloth may be inserted between the side teeth. Most attacks end by themselves in a few minutes. After an attack, the victim will probably appreciate a drink of water and a chance to rest and go home to change soiled clothing. Effusive expressions of sympathy are likely to prove embarrassing and unwelcome. Attacks from other dramatically convulsive forms of epilepsy should be treated in the same manner. One such form is *focal* epilepsy, in which convulsions usually start at one extremity and become generalized.

In petit mal epilepsy, signs are not at all dramatic: the victim does not fall or lose full consciousness. There may be a failure to respond to questions, and minor convulsive movements such as a rapid blinking of the eyes. Recovery usually occurs in a few seconds or minutes. Teachers need only be aware of the problem so that the pupil is not blamed for lapses.

Most epileptic students remain free from seizures and perform as well as others in school. No modification of the elementary school program is usually needed. Some may need to take medication while in school. If so, special arrangements for safekeeping and administration of the drug must be worked out in accordance with school policy by the nurse, parent, and the child's physician. A convulsion at school may be the first one, and follow-up by the nurse is then needed to make sure appropriate medical care is obtained. Teachers should be informed of known cases and their individual peculiarities by the nurse. Because of the social stigma attached to epilepsy, there is some question as to whether classmates should be informed prior to occurrence of a seizure in school. Doing so in a calm way does, however, help prevent panic. Once a seizure does occur in school, children should be told of its cause and nature and given an explanation of first aid procedures.

CANCER. At this writing a diagnosis of leukemia still means, in the average case, that the child can look forward to long courses of medication, often with severe side effects, periods of hospitalization, and death sometime between 6 months and 3 years. However, it also means that there will be months of relatively symptom-free life and at least a glimmer of hope for a complete remission of the disease. The occurrence of this condition is surely a tragedy. Unfortunately, this tragedy may be compounded by the emotional and sometimes physical abandonment of the affected child by his or her family, friends, and the school. With continual improvements

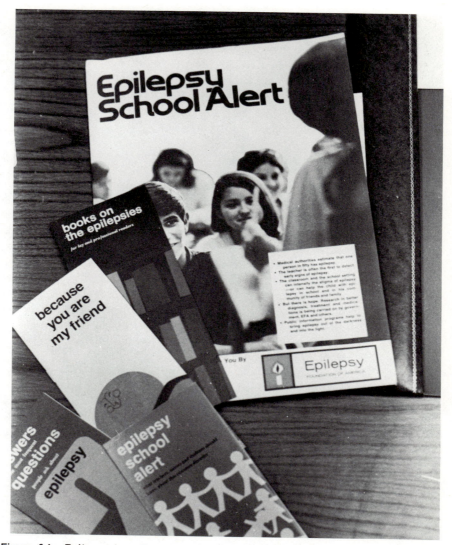

Figure 6.4. Epilepsy Is a Common Disorder Which Should Carry No Social Stigma. (Carol Ashton)

occurring in treatment methods, it is becoming more often advisable and feasible for the leukemic child to return to school.

This situation presents, of course, a severe challenge to the resourcefulness and leadership ability of the teacher. Generally, the ill child's situation needs to be discussed with the class, as the gossip is often more morbid than the reality. Although the life-threatening aspects should not be evaded, the hopeful aspects should be emphasized in most cases. Beyond this, the ill child needs the same feeling of acceptance and concern from his or her

149

teacher and classmates that every child needs. Singling out the child for special attention obviously cannot fill this need; the seriously ill child needs most to be part of a classroom where good morale and interpersonal relationships are the rule. The presence of a seriously ill child merely illustrates something that we all know but sometimes forget. Life does not go on forever and the way we treat each other each moment of each day matters.[17]

REFERENCES

BENENSON, ABRAM S. *Control of Communicable Disease in Man.* New York: The American Public Health Association, 1975.

DUBOS, RENÉ. *Man Adapting.* New Haven: Yale University Press, 1965.

———. *Mirage of Health.* Garden City, N.Y.: Anchor Books, Doubleday and Company, 1961.

FOX, JOHN P., CARRIE E. HALL, and LILA R. ELVEBACK. *Epidemiology.* New York: Macmillan Publishing Co., Inc., 1970.

FRIEDMAN, LAWRENCE A. "Impact of Teacher-Student Dental Health Education," *Journal of School Health,* Vol. 44, No. 3 (March 1974), pp. 140–143.

HENDERSON, JOHN. *Emergency Medical Guide.* New York: McGraw-Hill Book Company, 1973.

HIATT, JANE, and DARLENE STEWART. "Is a Child in Your Class 'Always' Ill?" *Instructor,* Vol. 83, No. 6 (February 1974), pp. 92–93.

JENNE, FRANK H., and WALTER H. GREENE. *Turner's School Health and Health Education.* St. Louis: C. V. Mosby Company, 1976.

JENNY, JOANNA, and JEAN FRAZIER. "Parents' Attitudes About School Dental Services for Children," *Journal of School Health,* Vol. 44, No. 2 (February 1974), pp. 86–91.

KAPLAN, DAVID, AARON SMITH, and ROSE GRABSTEIN. "School Management of the Seriously Ill Child," *Journal of School Health,* Vol. 44, No. 5, (May 1974), pp. 250–254.

McGOVERN, JOHN P. "Allergy Problems in School-Aged Children," *Journal of School Health,* Vol. 44, No. 5 (May 1974), pp. 260–264.

READ, DONALD A., and WALTER H. GREENE. *Creative Teaching in Health.* New York: Macmillan Publishing Co., Inc., 1975.

ROSNER, ARIA C. "Modifying Attitudes of Upper Elementary Students Towards Smoking," *Journal of School Health,* Vol. 44, No. 2 (February 1974), pp. 97–98.

ROUECHE, BERTON. *A Man Named Hoffman.* New York: Berkley Medallion, 1966.

---

[17] For a sensitive discussion of this problem complete with specific case histories, see David M. Kaplan et al., "School Management of the Seriously Ill Child," *Journal of School Health,* 44, No. 5 (May 1974), pp. 250–254.

TERHUNE, JAMES A. "Developing Positive Dental Health Practices," *Health Education*, Vol. 6, No. 1 (January-February 1975), pp. 23–26.

TERRY, POLLY. "Is There an Epileptic in Your Class?," *Instructor*, Vol. 73, No. 6 (February 1974), pp. 82–84.

WALKER, JAMES E. "What the School Health Team Should Know About Sickle Cell Anemia," *Journal of School Health*, Vol. 45, No. 3 (March 1975), pp. 149–154.

WILSON, CHARLES C., and ELIZABETH AVERY WILSON. *Healthful School Environment*. Washington, D.C.: National Education Association, 1969.

Courage? Carelessness? Caution?—Safety

Most people in our society are aware of the seriousness of accidents as a cause of death and disability and of the particular vulnerability of school-age children to these hazards. Public concern for the accident problem has resulted in both direct efforts at prevention in the form of more intelligent and cautious behavior of individuals and indirect efforts in the form of public pressure for legislation prescribing tighter safety standards for almost all aspects of human endeavor. For example, the laws for the electrical wiring of homes have been tightened, hard hats and protective goggles are frequent industrial requirements, clothing often must be flame resistant, child-proof caps have appeared on most medicine bottles, and a host of safety improvements have been prescribed for the automobile and traffic safety in general. Improvements have also been made in emergency care within most communities so that accident victims are more likely to receive better treatment than in past years.

APPROACHES to CONTROL

Public safety organizations, out of a natural fear of engendering public complacency, have been reluctant to publicize the success of these many efforts. Consequently, the considerable progress that has been made in the reduction of accident risk and the mitigation of the consequences of accidents is less well known than are the remaining problems. At the turn of the century, for example, over 70 of every 100,000 Americans were killed in accidents in any given year. Since that time exposure to accident hazards has most likely increased because of increased mechanization and mobility; however, the mortality rate for accidents has declined to approximately 55 deaths per 100,000 population. There is even some room for optimism for

152

automobile deaths, perhaps the most difficult problem. Although deaths have increased since the early decades of the century, the rate per million passenger miles has declined from approximately 20 per 100 million passenger miles to less than 5 today; thus the increase in traffic deaths is almost purely the result of more travel rather than increased hazards per trip.

One important generalization may be derived from this brief historical sketch: safety precautions "work"—they save life and limb—the effort is worthwhile. There is a tendency for many persons to throw up their hands in despair as they hear the latest holiday death toll, but this reaction is inappropriate. The average American is living in a safer world (at least, with respect to accidents) than he or she did 50 or even 10 years ago, not because of fate or chance or unknown factors, but because of deliberate human efforts to reduce accident risk. This reassuring conclusion must be immediately tempered by some sobering facts: first, the large majority of the more than 100,000 accidental deaths that do occur represent needless tragedies that could have been prevented; second, these deaths occur far more frequently among young people who otherwise could have expected many years of life; and, finally, despite the progress in prevention during this century, accidents have increased in rank from seventh to fourth place as a cause of death because of the greater progress made in other areas, particularly among the communicable diseases.

SAFETY in the SCHOOLS

Accident prevention and injury control are especially important within the elementary school. As with other health concerns, this problem area provides implications for health education, health services, and the school environment. This can be illustrated by the following hypothetical situation:

Mary was the most shy and insecure child in her fourth grade classroom. Mr. Kraft, the teacher, decided to try to build up her self-esteem by asking her to stay late at school to help prepare a bulletin board, a task that Mary enjoyed. After the last picture had been pinned in place, Mr. Kraft left Mary in the lobby of the school building after being assured that she had arranged to have her mother pick her up at school for a ride home. The weather had been unusually cold and a snowfall had started earlier that afternoon. Mr. Kraft was reluctant to leave Mary under such circumstances, but he was anxious to get home and, consequently, went on his way after reminding Mary that Mrs. Benett, the principal, was still available in her office in case a problem arose. As soon as Mr. Kraft left, Mary began to worry. Outside it was dark and gloomy; the snow that evoked feelings of pleasant excitement earlier that afternoon now took on a menacing appearance. Inside, the school was silent and deserted. The fact that Mrs. Benett was still there was not that reassuring as Mary had always been somewhat afraid of her.

As the minutes dragged on Mary became concerned that her mother might have forgotten her. They had made the arrangements the night before but, in her hurry to get off to school, she had not reminded her mother that morning. "She forgot me once before and left me stranded at the YWCA pool last summer," Mary thought to herself. The sound of a few footsteps and a door closing came from the distant reaches of the building as the custodian left for home. Mary wondered if it might have been Mrs. Benett and if she might be completely alone. Just then she saw what appeared to be her mother's car go slowly past the entrance to the school's access road. "She's not stopping!" thought Mary in a moment of panic. "She thinks I rode home with someone else." Mary ran out the door and down the sidewalk to wave; she stepped on an icy patch; she landed on her back; her head snapped back sharply and hit the concrete.

Mrs. Benett reached her first and rather excitedly pulled Mary to her feet. Although a bit dazed she didn't appear to be badly hurt. Mary's mother arrived a few moments later and, after chastising her for running on icy sidewalks, took her home.

ANALYSIS OF CAUSES. Mary's fall was "a sudden, unplanned event that carried the potential for producing injury or damage" and thus conforms to the classical definition of an accident.[1] In terms of causes, an analysis of this incident reveals a typical pattern of interacting factors that tended to form a chain of events leading to the occurrence itself. To say simply that a little girl ran on an icy sidewalk and fell down is an appealing conclusion but one that ignores a host of useful items of information and overlooks a number of useful possibilities for prevention.

- *Personality Factors.* It is true, but somewhat irrelevant, that if Mary had been less insecure the teacher might not have asked her to help with the bulletin board, but more to the point is the fact that this insecurity left her vulnerable to the type of emotional tension that contributed to her reckless dash out the door. Earlier efforts on the part of both parents and school personnel to increase Mary's sense of security and confidence as a person might have reduced her accident proneness as well as yielding all the more direct benefits of such a personality change.
- *Situational Factors.* A number of factors related to both the physical and the emotional setting were important contributions to Mary's fall. The ice on the sidewalk is, of course, most obvious, but the snow and the late afternoon darkness added to the emotional tension. Had the hour been earlier or the day sunnier, the accident might not have occurred. If she had not been alone she probably would not have been

[1] Kenneth F. Licht, "Safety and Accidents—A Brief Conceptual Analysis, and Point of View," *Journal of School Health*, Vol. 45, No. 9 (November 1975), pp. 530–534.

so upset, as would have been the case if a classmate or Mr. Kraft had been with her. Also, she would have been under far less pressure if her mother's past behavior in such situations had provided her with more reassurance that she would indeed come for her.

- *Triggering Event.* The most visible component of any accident situation is the often random factor that causes all the preceding factors to culminate in a single event. In this case it was the passing car that was similar to that of Mary's mother. In other cases it might be a child's grabbing of a pot handle, a playmate's call from across the street, or the drifting of a bright water toy into the deep area of the pool.

MODES OF PREVENTION. This incident also illustrates a number of specific points regarding the school's direct responsibilities for accident prevention and injury control. If Mary had been more thoroughly aware of (1) the dangers of slipping on icy surfaces and (2) the special need for caution when emotionally upset, she might have been able to act more prudently despite the hazards and pressures of the situation. In terms of a healthful school environment, it seems clear that the ice should have been removed and the sidewalk salted or sanded for better footing. Also, there appears to have been a need for better school policies concerning the supervision of children after the regular school hours. There appears to have been a need for the principal to have become better acquainted and more friendly with the children so that she might more often represent a source of support rather than an added emotional burden. Finally, the principal and all other school personnel should know at least the rudiments of first aid. The hauling of this dazed child to her feet could have produced permanent disability or death had her neck been injured in the fall. Also, any blow to the head strong enough to produce unconsciousness or a dazed condition should always receive medical attention to preclude the possibility of danger from hemorrhaging within the skull.

TEACHING APPROACH

Several sets of long-range goals for safety education have been developed for various state and district curricula. Although these efforts encompass a wide variety of expectations, they can generally be reduced to two prime considerations: (1) producing favorable changes in the behavior of children with respect to current hazards in their environment, and (2) helping them develop the type of attitudes and understandings that equip them to cope with hazards of future situations. Specific examples of learning experience within the first category include those related to pedestrian and playground safety. The second category includes those related to more general concepts such as the role of emotional stress, fatigue, and personality factors in accident causation. Although this latter category may seem advanced for the elementary level, the specific points can be put in very simple terms. Primary children have no difficulty understanding that "people have more accidents when they get excited," for example, or that "some people seem to take chances more than others."

HERE and NOW SITUATIONS

Fortunately, these two general goals are extremely compatible with one another. The best way for children to build good safety habits and concepts for the future is to learn to cope successfully with the present-day hazards. (In fact, if they do not accomplish this, they might not have any future.) Conversely, the development of general concepts for future situations tends to reinforce and make more meaningful the specific warnings related to current problems. This latter point also provides a key to the most useful general teaching approach in regard to the organization and presentation of content in safety instruction. In reference to this area of study, Alton L. Thygerson states:

> It is becoming increasingly clear that the way to influence a person's behavior is to help him develop clear concepts of the objects and events which make up his world.[2]

In simpler terms this means that the teacher should place emphasis on the task of helping children understand the reasons why accidents happen, and the reasons why various precautions serve to minimize their frequency or consequences. Because Thygerson utilized Asahel D. Woodruff's [3] definition of a concept, one can assume that this concept development process also includes the attachment of the proper affective components in the form of values or attitudes to these cognitive understandings. An example of one form this approach could take at the classroom level would be a learning activity in which the children studied the accidents or the accident potential of a particular locale, such as the school cafeteria, for example, identified the hazardous factors, and developed rules or procedures for offsetting these hazards. Any shortcomings could be corrected with judicious teacher guidance; the children would gain experience in analyzing and identifying accident potential and the rules they developed would be likely to have more impact on behavior than those imposed by others.

[2] Alton L. Thygerson, "Safety in Health Education: Some Precautions," *Journal of School Health*, Vol. 44, No. 9 (November 1974), pp. 508–510.
[3] Asahel D. Woodruff, "The Use of Concepts in Teaching and Learning," *Journal of Teacher Education* (March 1964), pp. 81–89.

OVERUSED DEVICES

Thygerson contrasts this approach with three other devices that he feels are generally overused by teachers. These are statistics, scare techniques, and the use of rules. All of these have occasional value, but their abuse can quickly undermine the effectiveness of any attempt to provide safety instruction.

STATISTICS Although statistics are not so often abused at the elementary level, teachers should still beware of the tendency to overwhelm children with numbers in an effort to impress them with the seriousness of some particular accident risk. Few adults, much less children, have a clear concept of what 100,000 or a million really means, and the various "rates" can become even more obscure than the crude totals. Obviously, some statistics merit use, but they should be used sparingly and translated into terms the children can understand. For example, rather than tell the children that 115,000 accidental deaths occur each year in the United States, say that, on the average, one person dies from an accident every 5 minutes.[4]

SCARE TECHNIQUES Threatening stories and gory movies are a traditional favorite of many nonprofessional and quasi-professional health teachers. As one enthusiast explained, "I like to hit them right between the eyes," presumably with the hope that if the impression is strong enough the children will avoid the related accident situation for the rest of their lives. Unfortunately, or perhaps fortunately, the human brain in most cases responds to this treatment by forgetting the whole distasteful experience as soon as possible. The children are far more likely to avoid safety lessons than accident situations in future years. There is a place for a realistic presentation of the consequences of accidents, including the negative emotional tones; however, emotion-laden material should be offered within the context of creating a balanced picture of reality, not as an isolated attempt to play on the emotions.

USE OF RULES Of these three overused devices, safety rules probably have the most legitimate use, particularly in the elementary school program. Often, to save time and circumvent complexities, it becomes necessary to simply establish rules to protect children from serious hazards. Also, elementary schoolchildren tend to accept this approach better than adolescents or adults. Problems soon arise, however, when the program of safety education fails to supplement these rules with learning experiences designed to show the reasons for their use. Rules should be presented both as quick protection and as the first step toward a full understanding of the situations to which they apply.

4 Thygerson, op. cit., p. 508.

CHILDREN'S HEALTH INTERESTS as RELATED to SAFETY

In their comprehensive study of children's health interests, Ruth Byler and her associates reported comparatively few comments on safety and first aid from children at the lower grade levels; however, what comments were offered were often presented with considerable urgency. Children at the fifth and sixth grade levels frequently expressed a need for first aid instruction. A few representative comments are included in this section.[5]

Kindergarten Through Grade Two

• They take great pride in fulfilling these duties well [hygiene and safety]; their concern, if any, is to please the teacher and gain her recognition and praise.

A teacher reproved a kindergarten child for ignoring an important safety rule. The child had run out onto the street without looking. Ann: "I didn't mean to do it. Frank was chasing me and I ran into the street." Frank: "But I didn't run into the street. I'm not supposed to." Ann: "A car might come along and he'll end up in the hospital."

Grades Three and Four

• Third graders do not mention these areas.
• Fourth graders say: If you fall and you think you are hurt, what should you do? What do you do for frostbite? A burn, a snakebite, a bee sting, animal bites, if there is no doctor around?

Grades Five and Six

• Fifth and Sixth graders say: We need first aid in case of accidents. . . . And the requests are accompanied by horror incidents.

CONTENT OVERVIEW

There are a number of schemes for organizing the content of safety instruction into logical subcategories; however, one of the most logical and direct ones is the use of various locales or living environments as the organizing centers. This practice yields such unit titles as "Safety at Home," "Safety

[5] Ruth Byler, Gertrude Lewis, and Ruth Totman, *Teach Us What We Want to Know* (New York: Mental Health Materials Center, Inc., 1969).

at Play," and "Safety at School." This is perhaps less sophisticated than a principles approach, which might be organized into units on "Causation," "Consequences," and "Prevention," for example, but is also more effective for achieving the vital short-term goals of safety instruction. Within this section the priority areas of content most closely related to these goals will be discussed.

SAFETY at HOME

As Marland K. Strasser and his associates remind us, "The traditional concept of *your home is your castle* connotes a sense of security NOT borne out by accident facts." [6] In support of this contention they explain that the home is the site of more accidental injuries than any other locale and that it ranks second only to automobiles in the number of accidental deaths. Moreover, young children are common victims in a wide variety of home accident categories. Approximately 10,000 people die each year as the result of falls within the home, with the very young and the very old most frequently affected. Poorly anchored rugs, objects left on stairs, and improper supervision of toddlers with respect to stairs and ladders are among the more frequent causes.

Suffocation can result from a variety of situations in the home and is particularly threatening because of its quick and deadly results. Blockage of the windpipe following the ingesting of buttons, small components of toys, and poorly chewed food items is one cause of these tragedies; plastic bags and abandoned refrigerators are other common culprits. The closely related category of accidental drowning is another significant cause of mortality, with home swimming pools a frequent site.

Burns caused by fire or hot liquids pose a particular threat to young children, as do the suffocating smoke and poisonous fumes that accompany most house fires. Although the main burden of responsibility for prevention rests on the adult members of the household, they can often be encouraged to take more thorough precautions by children who have learned to inquire about escape plans, smoke alarms, and the safe disposal of cigarettes.

Aspirin tablets and other forms of medicine, both prescription and over-the-counter items, cause the majority of the 2,000 to 3,000 deaths by poisoning in American homes each year. Alcohol, pesticides, and cleaning agents such as ammonia are significant contributors to this category. Poisonous fumes such as carbon monoxide and natural gas are less frequent but nonetheless important threats in this general category.

No inventory of home hazards is complete without the mention of fire-

---

[6] Marland K. Strasser et al., *Fundamentals of Safety Education* (New York: Macmillan Publishing Co., Inc., 1973), p. 269.

arms. As one would suspect, males are the more frequent victims. A particular problem is caused by adults who purchase hand guns for home protection. These fascinating objects are frequently stored in places accessible to children and thus constitute an attractive and serious hazard. The victims of these "protective" devices are more frequently friends and loved ones than criminal intruders.

SAFETY at PLAY

Although serious accidents can occur on occasion even in the better-designed and -supervised parks and playgrounds, they more frequently occur when children venture into areas not intended for play or recreation. Construction sites, for example, provide a vicious combination of interesting and dangerous objects and situations, as do many deserted or abandoned buildings. Old cisterns and cesspools are other sources of trouble, as are railroad sidings and warehouses. Parents have an obvious but too frequently neglected responsibility to inspect their children's neighborhood play areas and see that their children stay within designated limits. Appropriate safety instruction can complement the efforts of conscientious parents and compensate to some degree for the neglectful ones.

Another common threat to children at play is posed by child molesters and, less frequently, by kidnappers. The majority of children tend to look to adults as sources of help and support, as they appropriately should; therefore, a strong educational effort is needed if they are to protect themselves from the occasional deranged adult they may encounter.

TRAFFIC SAFETY

Parents too often seem to place their faith in strict laws and the judgment of automobile drivers rather than in the education and training of their children as a means of protecting them from traffic accidents. This policy is obviously unwise in view of the large amount of evidence that many drivers are habitually careless, that careful drivers are not always at their best, and that there are definite limits to the degree to which a careful driver can compensate for a careless child. Pedestrian safety and bicycle safety merit emphasis at both the primary and intermediate levels. Although many elementary schools prohibit the use of bicycles as a means of transportation to and from school or restrict it to the upper grade levels, the parents of many young cyclists permit them to venture into the streets as early as 5 or 6 years of age.

As with most other areas of safety instruction, children have a need for firm and definite rules of conduct in regard to traffic situations, closely followed by teaching activities designed to develop an understanding of the need for these rules. As two elementary school teachers with special competencies in bicycle instruction state:

> The best programs *teach* bike safety; they don't just *preach* it. Since a part of safe riding rests on an understanding of how a bicycle works and the laws governing its use, start with these points.[7]

This same approach, which rests on an understanding of how accidents occur and the rules and laws that tend to prevent them, can be applied to pedestrian safety.

SAFETY at SCHOOL

As noted in the preceding section, the school is a relatively safe environment for children in comparison with other common areas they frequent. This fact carries two general implications for the school safety instruction program: First, despite the careful engineering of the physical plant, the careful development of safety rules and procedures, and the careful adult supervision a good school provides, the children must do their part if the program is to succeed. There are never enough playground supervisors to enforce the rules, for example, if the majority of the children do not really accept these constraints. This degree of acceptance requires more than a mere awareness of their existence; a thorough understanding of their protective qualities and, ideally, a role in their development are also needed.

The second implication pertains to the use of a safe school as a model to be applied to other areas of the child's life space. A school is in many ways a home, a play area, and part of the traffic network of its community, at least in regard to its sidewalks, parking lots, and access roads. Consequently, it is useful for the children to question that if a school has an evacuation plan for fire, should not a home also have such a plan? If school personnel keep flammable liquids and poisonous chemicals under lock and key, should not parents do the same at home? If school crossing guards enforce traffic rules, should not the same rules be followed on the streets near home? The parallels are virtually endless and provide experience in the important skills of identifying common elements of different locations and applying these to a variety of situations.

---

[7] William Truesdell and Carol Wicks, "Bike Ed. for Teachers and Kids," *Instructor*, Vol. 86, No. 1 (August/September 1976), pp. 68–69.

INJURY CONTROL

Children as well as teachers have a role to play in assisting those who have been injured. At school and occasionally at home or at play, a child may have to take primary responsibility for obtaining help. Strangely enough, even among adults, one of the greatest threats to the injured persons is a well-meaning but poorly trained first-aider. The literature of emergency care contains many stories of damaged spinal cords resulting from the improper moving of victims, crushed arteries caused by unneeded tourniquets, and even deaths from massive doses of table salt given to induce the vomiting of substances thought to be poisonous.

Because the relative inexperience and immaturity of children increases the likelihood of such paradoxical results, the emphasis in first aid instruction at the elementary school level is placed on training children to seek outside help as the first consideration in an injury situation. They will tend to do this far more readily if they are taught that speed is seldom important in the case of injuries, and that it is seldom necessary to move an injured person prior to the arrival of expert assistance. With the increasing number of single-parent families or families with two parents working outside the home, it becomes even more essential that children of all grade levels learn to use the telephone to secure help in an emergency. Here, the main task is to stress the importance of knowing one's address and being sure to clearly present this vital item of information to the party on the opposite end of the line.

SUGGESTED LEARNING ACTIVITIES

The following suggestions are presented in an effort to demonstrate how the content described in the preceding section might be translated into effective classroom learning activities. They were designed to accommodate a wide variety of classroom groups provided that proper selection and adaptations are made according to the needs, interests, abilities, and maturity level of the particular children involved.

- In small groups have your students complete the following statements:
  — You wake up and your room is full of smoke_____
  — Items in the mouth other than food_____
  — Plastic bags_____
  — Riding my bicycle alone at night_____
  — Swimming alone_____
  — Matches should_____
- During "Fire Prevention Week" in October, have your students design posters and display them around the community or have them paint murals of safety rules on store windows.

- Select one month and designate it "Safety Month." Have your students keep track of the number and types of accidents that occur and graph their results. When they have compiled their results, have them discuss how the various types of accidents could have been prevented. Have them submit their results to the local safety council or newspaper.

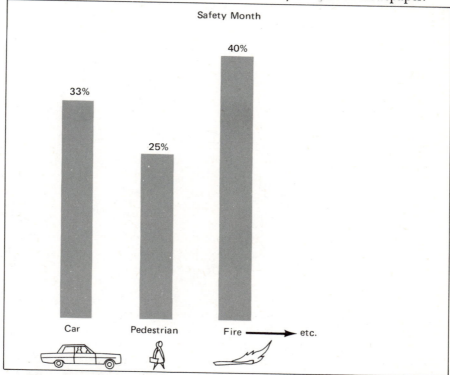

Safety Month

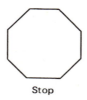

- Have the children study the various road signs that are seen every day and then select various areas around the school and design rules for that area. Place the appropriate rules on one of the signs and place the signs at these places. Possible areas for selection include stairwells, drinking fountains, and playground.

Crossing Danger Stop Yield

• Using colored construction paper, have your students construct blocks (4 by 4 inches). On each block they are to describe pictorially those rules that develop good safety habits. Display the blocks in the library on top of one of the book shelves.

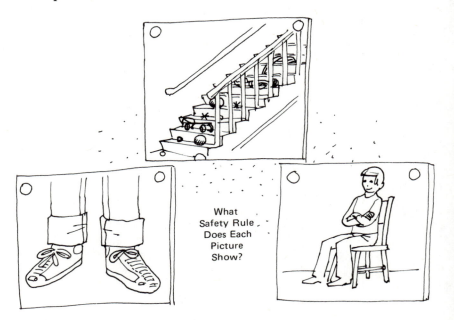

What Safety Rule Does Each Picture Show?

• From different colored pieces of construction paper, have the class cut out footprints approximately 12 inches long. Have them develop those safety rules that they feel are necessary while eating in the school cafeteria. On each foot, either in printed words or pictures, place a rule (one foot for each rule developed). When they have completed their rules have them display the footprints on the cafeteria walls.

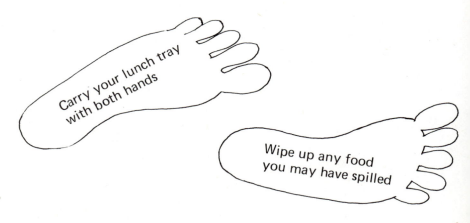

Carry your lunch tray with both hands

Wipe up any food you may have spilled

• Have the class design a house of their choice. When the house is complete, divide the class into groups and have one member from each group draw from an envelope a slip of paper with the name of a room on it that would be found in the house. Have them then design all the rules for safety in that room. Each rule will be placed on a flag and attached to the room for which they were responsible.

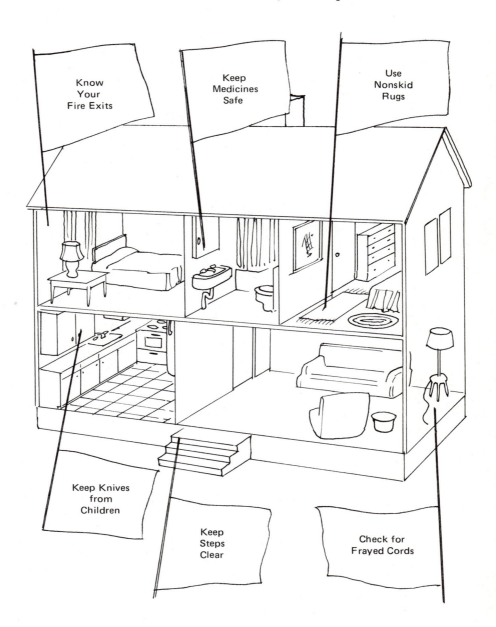

• Select various holidays during the year and have the children create rules of safety for that holiday and/or season. Place them on a "seasonal wheel of safety rules" and when the holiday appears, have the children refer to the chart as a reminder.

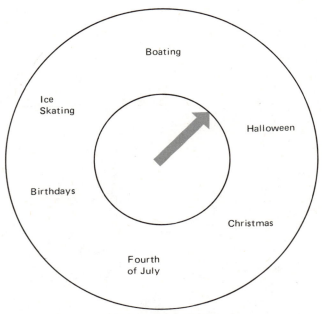

• Arrange your class in pairs and have each dyad select three occupations and investigate the various pieces of protective clothing associated with them. Have the students find out what purpose each item has and report their findings back to the class (e.g., hard hats for construction workers).

• Have the students design an emergency chart of phone numbers for their community. When it is completed and they have discussed the purpose of each number and how to reach it, have them take the charts home to be displayed in an appropriate place. (Numbers to include: police, fire, doctor, hospital, emergency squad, poison control center, etc.)

• Have the students draw a picture of a swimming pool, lake, pond, river, or ocean depending upon which is most appropriate for your geographical location. Around the picture, write in safety tips on water safety.

• Divide your class into small groups to discuss why accidents occur when people get excited or fatigued. When they have compiled their lists, have them cut out two life-sized torsos of human beings. On one torso list or draw those reasons for accidents when you get excited and on the other those caused by fatigue. Display the torsos in an appropriate area of the school.

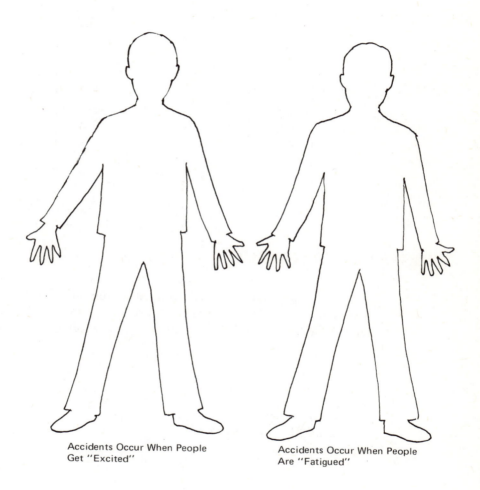

Accidents Occur When People
Get "Excited"

Accidents Occur When People
Are "Fatigued"

• Have the students design rules for pedestrian, bicycle, and skateboard safety.

• Have the students design cartoon characters depicting safety while camping.

• Have the children design and stock their own first aid kit.

- During "Fire Prevention Week," have the students design a calendar of rules for that week showing the community how they can keep their homes safe from fire. Ask your local newspaper to run this calendar during the appropriate week.

Fire Prevention Week

Sun.	Mon.	Tues.	Wed.	Thurs.	Fri.	Sat.
Furnace filters changed	Check electrical cords for frayed wiring and for over loaded circuits	Cleaning substances are in appropriate containers and labeled	Number of electrical items used in the bathroom	Old oily, rags and paint cans are thrown away	Matches are properly stored	S A F E H O M E

SUGGESTED RESOURCES

The learning resources listed in this section are a selected sample of materials with which the authors are personally familiar. Appropriate grade levels have been included when these were indicated by the source.

BOOKS

Bicycle Safety
Aetna Life and Casualty
151 Farmington Ave.
Hartford, Connecticut 06115

Bicycle Safety
American Automobile Association
Consult your local office.

Dennis the Menace Takes a Poke at Poison
U.S. Consumer Product Safety Commission
Washington, D.C. 20207

FILMSTRIP

Smokey the Bear and Little Marcy
Fire Safety
Grades K–6
Singer Educational Filmstrips
1345 Deversey Parkway
Chicago, Illinois 60614

GAMES/ACTIVITIES

Health and Safety Course for Primary Grades
Packet of Activities and Posters
Teacher's Guide
Youth Division
American Red Cross
Local Chapter

PAMPHLET

Bicyle Blue Book
Public Relations Department
Goodyear Tire and Rubber Company
Akron, Ohio 44316

THE SCHOOL ACCIDENT CONTROL PROGRAM

The basis of an ideal school accident control program is a data-collecting system that requires that injuries resulting from accidents be reported by teachers and/or nurses, coupled with formal periodic safety inspections of school buildings and grounds. The most important purpose of such reports and surveys is to identify those locations, activities, and equipment most commonly involved so that a program can be designed to reduce the number of injuries that occur. The second most important purpose of reports and surveys is to provide data for evaluating the effectiveness of the program; if accidents decrease, the program can be assumed to be effective. An effective program requires that a trained person assume responsibility for coordinating and directing it, and that all those concerned—teachers, pupils, parents, and police, for example—be involved in planning and carrying out the program. This is often accomplished through permanent school safety councils or committees at either the building or systemwide level, or both.

169

An injury-reporting system requires the selection or local development of a form that elicits information on the circumstances, nature and severity, and probable cause or causes of the injury. Many school systems use the form developed by the National Safety Council, which lends itself nicely to either hand sorting and tabulation, or to coding and keypunching reports for computer analysis. Some states and local school systems have developed safety inspection forms for buildings and grounds that are helpful in locating hazards and that may be used either by adult professionals or by committees.

Almost all schools involve older pupils in the safety program by participation in the school safety patrol. Standards for this program have been developed with the cooperation of national organizations of parents, teachers, police, and safety organizations and are published by the National Safety Council.[8] The local program ideally is planned by local counterparts following national guidelines. Patrol members assist adult crossing guards in directing pupils as they cross streets near the school. They are not legally authorized to direct vehicular traffic. They may serve on school buses and on playgrounds to help maintain order and thus promote safety. They play an important part in safety education. Responsibility for organizing, training, and supervising patrol members is often delegated to a teacher.

School fire safety is so important that standards are often written into state law and enforced by state or local fire marshals. These officers periodically inspect schools for fire hazards such as chained exit doors, electrical dangers, and dangerous accumulations of combustible material. The standards, which vary from state to state, also require a certain number of fire drills per year. Most fire deaths are caused by toxic fumes rather than heat. Pupils and staff should therefore acquire and maintain the ability to empty the school in the few minutes before fires spread. In a desirable program, fire drills are unannounced, a different exit is blocked on each occasion as would be the case in a real fire, and pupils leave without their coats and books.

Most injuries in elementary schools occur on playgrounds and in gymnasiums. Injuries are most likely to occur during the unorganized and unsupervised play that is sometimes permitted before and after school and at noon. Many such injuries result in part from broken play equipment or from debris such as broken glass or sharp stones. Play areas should therefore be supervised by an adult—either a teacher or a trained aide—at all times, and play areas should be inspected frequently to discover and correct hazards.

Injuries can and will occur despite the best of preventive programs. Provision for the first aid care of injuries is therefore part of the responsibility of every school health service program. The nature and extent of care

[8] Current editions of *Policies and Practices for School Safety Patrols, Accident Facts,* and other useful materials may be purchased from the National Safety Council, 425 N. Michigan Avenue, Chicago, Illinois 60611.

provided vary, depending in part on school laws and policies and in part on the community resources available for the transportation and definitive care of injured persons. In some districts, the first aid providers include teachers whose roles are often limited to providing minor first aid and whose class-rooms are often equipped with first aid cabinets containing appropriate supplies. Such a plan usually envisions the school nurse and/or other trained and designated persons as providing care in cases of more severe injury. The nurse may train selected pupils to serve as first aid assistants to their teachers and to keep the room first aid cabinet clean and filled with supplies. This is a sensible plan because almost all school injuries are minor cuts, scrapes, and bruises that require little care and necessitate no absence from the classroom. It also helps the children acquire basic first aid skills and frees the nurse for more important work.

ENVIRONMENTAL CONSIDERATIONS

A safe school environment depends on good architectural design and good maintenance of building and grounds. Some safety features that should be planned into every new or renovated school include drinking fountains recessed into walls, exit doors that are equipped with panic hardware (bars that open the door when pressed), doors that swing outward in case of fire, non-skid floor coverings, and separate appropriately equipped playgrounds for younger and older pupils. Good maintenance for safety includes the daily removal of inflammable trash, immediate mopping up of spilled liquids, maintenance of resilient surfaces under play equipment from which children might fall, and immediate repairs or removal of worn or broken playground equipment. Good school housekeeping requires the cooperation of teachers and students; school custodians can clean up the building and grounds but they cannot keep them clean without help.

Hazards exist within the classroom, although serious injuries rarely occur there. Injuries sometimes occur as a result of unsafe use of paper cutters, scissors, staplers, and similar equipment. Such accidents can be reduced in numbers and severity by teaching students how to use the equipment safely and by supervising its use. Climbing on chairs results in falls. When pupils need to climb, as when they are placing decorations on the walls, a step-ladder should be provided. Other falls may result from tripping over items carelessly left on the floor; these accidents can be prevented by picking up things such as building blocks when they are not in use. Broken furniture may also present a hazard and should be taken out of use and perhaps stored in a corner until it is repaired or replaced. Some cuts can be pre-vented by using plastic containers instead of glass ones as vases for flowers or other objects. Young children are sometimes shocked when they insert metal objects in electrical outlets out of curiosity. Therefore, outlets should

171

be replaced with safety fixtures or equipped with childproof plugs. Modern crayons and other art material specifically designed for child use are composed of nonpoisonous materials. Care should be taken to avoid the introduction of hazardous art materials, such as organic solvents, that children might inhale or ingest.

HEALTH SERVICE CONSIDERATIONS

Regardless of whether teachers are officially given primary responsibility for first aid to injured pupils, it is desirable that all of them receive some training in first aid because the designated first aid persons in a school might not be present when an injury occurs. Such training is available through Red Cross chapters. It may be provided as part of the school's own program of in-service education. Many colleges and universities also offer courses in first aid and safety.

First aid is the care given at the outset to an acutely ill or injured person. It includes calming and reassuring the person and summoning any needed assistance, as well as providing physical care. In many instances, this is the only type of care needed. In other cases, it is necessary to preserve life, prevent further injury and prepare the person for transportation to a hospital or other source of expert care.

In cases where the victim is exposed to danger, removal of either the victim or the danger is the first step. For example, connection of a person with a live electrical wire must be broken by use of a nonconducting tool such as a dry wooden pole. If multiple injuries are present, those that are most life threatening—suspended respiration or heart beat, severe bleeding, or ingested poison—must be attended to first.

In general, however, an injured person should not be moved until the extent of injury has been determined; victims with possible neck, spine, or head injuries, or broken bones should not be moved. Immediate care for life-threatening injuries can usually be given on the spot, and the victim kept warm by blankets or coats until persons trained and equipped to provide transportation to a source of medical care arrive.

BLEEDING

Uncontrolled and copious bleeding is a problem that demands immediate attention. In most cases, bleeding can be stopped if direct pressure is applied and the part is elevated; a protective clot will form. If pressure points (places where main arteries lie close to the skin and just over bone) are known, pressure may be applied to the supplying artery. Tourniquets are dangerous and should be used only as a last resort. Excessive pressure should *not* be applied to bleeding head wounds because the skull may be fractured. No pressure at all should be used on a bleeding eye. Such wounds, and all large, deep, or dirty wounds, require medical care. Some of these require stitches, others require expert cleansing, and many victims will require reimmunization against tetanus. Therefore, no attempt should be made to remove the pressure bandage or a blood clot or to clean such wounds. Foreign bodies should be left in place. The victim should be transported to a hospital emergency ward or other source of medical care and turned over to parental supervision.

Small cuts and scrapes, on the other hand, usually require no more than first aid care. The first aiders' hands should first be washed thoroughly. Then superficial splinters or other objects can be removed with tweezers. Other loose dirt or foreign matter can usually be washed out with clean tap water. Some recommend the use of soap, others the use of plain tap water only for cleansing wounds. After the wound has been blotted dry with a sterile bandage, a dry bandage should be applied and fixed in place with tape or a roller bandage. The parents should be instructed to seek medical care if signs of infection (inflammation, pus formation) appear.

SUSPENDED RESPIRATION

If no signs of breathing can be seen or heard, and no exhalations are felt from the mouth or nose, immediate attempts to restore breathing are required. The art of mouth-to-mouth resuscitation is best learned in a first aid course in which demonstration and supervised practice are possible. The victim's head should be tilted back as far as possible to clear the airway and kept in that position with firm pressure from one hand on the forehead. The thumb and forefinger of the same hand can be used to pinch the nostrils closed. In small children, the rescuer's mouth may cover both the child's nose and mouth. The rescuer's lips are then sealed about the victim's mouth or mouth and nose, after inhaling deeply. The air is then blown into the victim's lungs until they are felt to expand. The rescuer's mouth is then removed to permit exhalation, and the process is repeated at 5-second intervals.

Children and adults sometimes choke when they try to swallow large chunks of food, or when they play while carrying objects in their mouths. Persons who are still able to breathe despite the obstruction may be able to remove the object themselves by reflex coughing. Rescuers are sometimes able to remove offending objects with their fingers, but such attempts should be limited because the object may be driven further into the throat. Whacking the victim repeatedly and firmly on the back between the shoulder blades may also dislodge the object. The Heimlich maneuver involves strong thrusts against the center of the abdomen below the rib cage that cause air to be expelled and the object with it. The thrusts may be applied from a standing position behind a victim who is standing or seated on a chair, or from the front when the victim is lying down. The thrust should be directed upward as well as inward. The maneuver should only be attempted after other means fail.

FRACTURES

Some fractures are apparent; others can only be suspected. Whenever a fracture is suspected or known, an ambulance should be called. No attempt should be made by unskilled persons to move the victim without first immobilizing the affected part. Open fractures in which the skin is broken should be covered with a sterile bandage. Pressure may be applied to control bleeding, if necessary.

BRUISES, SPRAINS, and STRAINS

Bruises and sprains (injuries to the soft tissues around joints) may be relieved by applying cold, wet compresses—never initially by heat. If such injuries do not improve in 24 hours, a physician should be consulted. Strains (pulled muscles), on the other hand, respond best to rest and applications of heat.

SHOCK

Severe injury of any kind can result in shock, the indications of which include a pale or bluish skin that is cold or moist and clammy to touch and a rapid pulse. Breathing is usually rapid. There may be nausea. To prevent and minimize the effects of shock until medical help arrives, victims of severe injuries should generally be kept lying down and body heat conserved by use of blankets or coats, avoiding overheating.

POISONING

Poisoning should rarely occur in school. If a pupil ingests something suspected of being poisonous, specific information as to its toxicity and what to do about it should be obtained by calling the Poison Information Center, whose number is listed in the emergency section of the telephone book. It helps to dilute any ingested poison with water or milk. Vomiting should be induced except for petroleum products or strong acids or strong alkaline substances, as indicated by the container label, a breath odor of gasoline or kerosene, or burns around the mouth. Vomiting can be induced by the

174

administration of ipecac or using a finger to tickle the back of the throat. *Never* give salt water to dilute a poison or induce vomiting.

EYE INJURIES

Students often complain of having something in an eye. The something is sometimes a sty—a pimple on the eyelid that touches and irritates the eye. Styes usually burst and heal by themselves in a day or two; if too uncomfortable, they can be treated by a physician. Commonly, the irritation is caused by a foreign object that the nurse may be able to remove if it is located on the inner surface of the eyelid. If not, it may be washed out by tears or by flushing the eye with clean tap water. If this fails, or if the object is embedded in the eye surface, medical help is indicated. The student should be kept from rubbing the eye, and may be more comfortable if the eye is kept still and closed and is covered lightly with a sterile bandage. "Black eyes" are bruises around the eye, and should be treated with cold applications.

Medical treatment is indicated for any injury that results in visible bleeding from the eye or under the eye surface, loss of vision, double vision, or complaint that vision is partially blocked by a "curtain" in the eye. Some specialists feel that anyone with a black eye should have medical attention. Chemicals in the eye should be flushed with tap water for 15 minutes before the victim is taken to a hospital.

HEAD, NECK, and BACK INJURIES

Any head, neck, or back injury is potentially serious. Pupils with such injuries should be kept where they are until the nurse or other trained person can evaluate the case. Cut scalps tend to bleed profusely. Such cuts should not be cleaned by amateurs, however, and excessive pressure on them should be avoided because of the possibility of a skull fracture. A sterile bandage may be placed snugly on the wound and moderate pressure applied to control bleeding.

FROSTBITE

Frostbite is characterized by lightened color and glossiness of exposed skin. It may or may not be accompanied by pain. Severe frostbite may cause impaired breathing and impaired mental functioning and result in shock. The frozen part should be warmed quickly, using *warm* (102°F to 105°F) water. The part should *not* be rubbed. Blankets are useful in rewarming the whole body. A dressing may be applied while the victim is transported to a source of medical care.

175

BURNS

Burns should rarely occur in elementary school settings, and most that do will be of a minor nature. Recommended first aid for minor burns consists of immersing the part in cold water, or cold water applications. No medication or ointment should be applied. No attempt should be made to cleanse a burn, but a sterile bandage may be applied loosely to protect it. Severe cases should be transported to a hospital, and steps should be taken to prevent shock and treat it if it occurs.

DENTAL INJURIES

Teeth are sometimes broken or knocked out as a result of fights or accidents. Such injuries are always dental emergencies, and dentists will make room in their appointment schedules to provide immediate care. If the tooth is knocked out, the dentist may be able to reimplant it, so the tooth should be taken with the child to the dentist.

FOLLOW-UP

Injuries severe enough to require medical attention or ones that result in school absence should be followed by at least a telephone call from school. One reason is that some parents may need the nurse's assistance in securing necessary medical help. Some schools offer accident insurance to pupils, which encourages needed medical care, and parents may have questions about how they can file their claim. Children who miss much school may be helped by giving them their assignments and arranging for a parent to pick up books and work sheets. Expression of sympathetic interest by the teacher or nurse may also serve to discourage a damage suit.

DEFUSING the RISK of DAMAGE SUITS

Teachers and other school employees are sometimes sued for damages to children that result from accidents under school jurisdiction. Certain legal principles help protect teachers against unjust decisions in such cases. More important, there are a number of things teachers can do to reduce the likelihood of being sued or of being required to pay damages as a result of suit.

To sue a teacher successfully for injury to a child, a plaintiff must prove that the child was actually injured as a result of either the teacher's failure to act as a prudent teacher would have acted or the commission of an imprudent act. For example, a teacher might have failed to foresee that a child might try to use a broken swing and be injured as a result. On another occasion, a teacher might slap a pupil in anger, causing a hearing loss. In either case, the plaintiff would have to prove that the teacher's inaction or action was the direct and immediate (or proximate) cause of the child's injury. The teacher, on the other hand, might mount a successful legal defense in several ways. It might be shown, for example, that a student was injured as the result of some force beyond the control of the teacher, such as a sudden thunderstorm. It might also be shown that a student voluntarily assumed the risk that resulted in the injury: that he or she played on a broken swing despite the teacher's warning, for example. Another possible defense would be to show that the injured student's own negligent behavior contributed to the injury. The usefulness of these last two defenses depends on whether the student's actions would be considered negligent in light of his or her maturity and ability.[9]

Some of the actions teachers can take to protect themselves follow from the law. The law, for example, holds that teachers serve in place of the children's parents during school hours. *Good* teachers therefore treat and care for their students as *good* parents would. Prudent teachers constantly observe the school environment for safety hazards and then neutralize the hazards observed or at least warn students of them. Good teachers seek to identify the risks inherent in school activities and reduce them through safety instruction and supervision. For example, they will not only teach youngsters how to use staplers and paper cutters safely, but observe and stop their unsafe use as well. When accidental injuries occur, teachers have a legal obligation to see to it that appropriate first aid is immediately provided.

Other protective actions go beyond legal requirements. Teachers can protect themselves against much of the cost and worry that arise out of school-related liability suits by obtaining the professional liability insurance available to them through their unions or school districts. They can improve their competence in safety and first aid by taking courses, and they may reduce the likelihood of being sued by making phone calls or home visits and sending get-well cards to seriously injured students.

REFERENCES

AARON, JAMES E., A. FRANK BRIDGES, and DALE O. RITZEL. *First Aid and Emergency Care.* New York: Macmillan Publishing Co., Inc., 1972.

THE AMERICAN RED CROSS. *Cardiopulmonary Resuscitation.* Washington, D.C.: The Red Cross, 1974.

[9] The principles cited were adapted from Dean F. Miller, *School Health Programs: Their Basis in Law* (Cranbury, N.J.: A. S. Barnes and Co., 1972), pp. 66–71.

————. *First Aid for Foreign Body Obstruction of the Airway.* Washington, D.C.: The Red Cross, undated.

————. *Standard First Aid and Personal Safety.* Garden City, N.Y.: Doubleday and Company, 1973.

HENDERSON, JOHN. *Emergency Medical Guide.* New York: McGraw-Hill Book Company, 1973.

LICHT, KENNETH F. "Safety and Accidents—A Brief Conceptual Analysis, and Point of View," *Journal of School Health,* Vol. 45, No. 9 (November 1975).

STRASSER, MARLAND K., and others. *Fundamentals of Safety Education.* New York: Macmillan Publishing Co., Inc., 1973.

THYGERSON, ALTON L. "Safety in Health Education: Some Precautions," *Journal of School Health,* Vol. 44, No. 9 (November 1974).

————. *Safety: Principles, Instruction, and Readings.* Englewood Cliffs, N.J.: Prentice-Hall, Inc., 1972.

TRUESDELL, WILLIAM, and CAROL WICKS. "Bike Ed. for Teachers and Kids," *Instructor,* Vol. 86, No. 1 (August/September 1976).

WOODRUFF, ASAHEL D. "The Use of Concepts in Teaching and Learning," *Journal of Teacher Education* (March 1964).

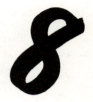

Medicine and Medicine Men—Health Care

A famous professor of medicine once assessed the state of medical care at the turn of the century in a widely quoted statement to the effect that the average patient, with the average complaint, when visiting the average physician had a 50 per cent chance of benefiting from the encounter. Although perhaps a bit harsh, this assessment was not far from the mark because physicians then could offer no penicillin for those with infection, no insulin for the diabetic, no Rh test for the expectant mother, and little hope of surgical intervention for congenital defects or most other heart impairments.

Although American medicine still does not lack for criticism, the most valid complaints are usually directed at the political and economic rather than the technological aspects. Most Americans will generally ignore advice that they secure routine medical examinations, and that they control their weight, exercise appropriately, get enough sleep, and follow other health suggestions. But when obviously sick or injured they are quite willing to put themselves in the hands of a physician, not as a last resort, but with genuine hope and faith that they will receive the needed help. Mistakes and failures are widely publicized, but do not discount the fact that many of the life-threatening problems of the past such as appendicitis and tuberculosis are handled routinely, and the scope of those cases considered hopeless grows narrower day by day. However, this increasing efficiency has been accompanied by major problems and complexities.

In the past many persons could buy the best care available for the price of a two-dollar office visit even for something serious because the physician had little to offer. Now the physicians may be able to work veritable miracles for their patients, but these patients must often thread their way through a complex maze of general practitioners, specialists, and subspecialists to find their miracle workers and somehow arrange for financing their treatment, operation, or whatever once the helpful persons are found. In other words, the practice of medicine has become very complicated. As John Knowles said at the beginning of this decade:

> What used to be a one patient one doctor relationship is now one patient to one doctor to another doctor to fifteen to twenty people standing behind each doctor in the hospital and in other institutions related to health. . . .[1]

Each year new types of supportive personnel develop. Some of these are specialized technicians needed to operate the ever-growing array of electronic equipment that is crowding its way into consultation rooms and hospital facilities; others, such as the various forms of physician associates and nurse practioners, represent entirely new roles designed to help in the tasks of dispensing care to the patient. In this latter regard the changes extend beyond the individual role and into the structure of the medical care system itself. Although many persons still rely on a "family doctor" who refers them to specialists or arranges hospital care as needed, others are provided for by alternate patterns of care. Some choose internists to care for adults and pediatricians to care for children, for example. Others join Health Maintenance Organizations (HMO), where a single monthly fee guarantees full service, or enroll in government-subsidized neighborhood health centers managed by the local public health department; still others living in communities with few doctors and no public clinics rely on the emergency room of the local hospital for all their medical needs. And, regardless of who dispenses the care or who pays for it, the general trend is for sharply rising costs and continual controversy as to how these costs should be met. Care for some poor families is provided through the federal–state Medicaid program, but the care thus provided ranges from poor to excellent, and the system often permits providers of care to cheat the government.

Somehow, this huge and ever-changing system, or nonsystem as some prefer, provides quite good care for many persons, and somehow the bills get paid. At this point, however, it appears that a period of ferment will prevail for several years as the search for better modes of delivery and better methods of financing medical care continues. The current quality of care is better than it has ever been; it seems to be improving, but it is too often not at its best. It is frequently insensitive or simply not as good as it could be. As long as one person dies or suffers unnecessarily because of poor care or lack of access to needed care, efforts at improvement must continue.

All of these developments tend to increase the burden of decision making for the average consumer. Each person may have to choose between a

---

[1] John Knowles, "Where Doctors Fail," *Saturday Review* (August 22, 1970), p. 21.

personal physician or affiliation with a private or public clinic or health maintenance organization. Consumers who rely on a personal physician must take care of their own medical insurance needs, which may or may not be available on a group basis at their place of employment. Those who select an individual insurance plan must be sure of the adequacy of their coverage and how to file their claims. If they do not like the choices available, they must be prepared to seek additional alternatives through the political process.

Once good health care becomes available and is securely financed, the consumer must be astute enough to use it properly, a process that requires both good understanding and a constructive attitude. Modern physicians are aided in their diagnoses by modern tests and other diagnostic techniques that may include computer analysis. However, no test or technique is of any value until the patient makes the decision to seek treatment; once this step is taken, the physician's diagnostic skill may be wasted if the patient refuses to take the prescribed medication, or to authorize proposed surgery. It is the patient who decides how thoroughly the treatment will be carried out: if the full course of antibiotics is completed, if a child is brought back for the next series of immunization shots, if psychotherapy will continue. The growing realization of these facts has led to the view that the patient is one of the most important members of the therapeutic team as well as the recipient of the therapy, and this role, like the other health care roles, is destined to get more demanding year by year.

The process of becoming an intelligent and enlightened consumer of health products and services begins in early childhood with the first experiences with doctors, nurses, and dentists and their work. Later, children may encounter the dental hygienist, the lab technician, and the pharmacist. Attitudes begin to form as children develop impressions of these helpers and of their differing roles. Classroom experiences can condition these experiences; they can moderate extreme viewpoints, reducing unreasonable fears and building up the trust that comes from a real understanding of the various health professionals.

A television commercial for vitamin pills or pain relievers may represent a child's first exposure to the world of health products. Here, of course, the main educational task is to help children develop the proper degree of skepticism and objectivity necessary to counteract the Madison Avenue puffery that they will encounter in advertising. This task consists of more than casting all TV ads in a bad light. Many advertisements present a mixture of truthful statements and sound advice, together with exaggerated claims of the special merits of their products. Toothpaste companies represent a case in point; there is nothing wrong with brushing twice a day or visiting the dentist twice a year, it's just that many brands of toothpaste do their job equally well. Thus in the case of attitudes toward legitimate health personnel it is probably best that the children develop faith and trust but stop short of blind faith. And with regard to over-the-counter health products it seems best if they develop a critical attitude that falls short of blanket rejection.

Most beginning teachers, who, as young adults, may visit physicians infrequently, may forget the prominent part that medical care plays in the lives of children. Many parents, although careless of their own medical needs, are reasonably conscientious regarding their children's needs for periodic checkups, vaccines, and so forth. Because children have not yet built up resistances to many common disease germs, they are frequently hauled off to the physician with high fevers and runny noses. Then, too, there is the inevitable tonsillectomy, which usually makes a lasting impression on young patients. Consequently, most elementary schoolchildren are ready to study consumer health topics with more than average interest. Here are some illustrative responses from the study of Ruth Byler and her associates.[2]

Kindergarten Through Grade Two

- The familiarity which children have with hospitals and the faith they have in them is a tribute to services hospitals and doctors are giving.
- Hospitals are where they help you. They make you all well again. Dentists help you, too. They clean off the dirt and fill up the cavities.

Grades Three and Four

- Practical situations. Medicine, needles, stitches, casts—all inspire curiosity. How the doctor knows what is wrong and what to do stimulates wonder.
- Why doesn't the nurse give shots in school? What would she do if you needed stitches?

This study did not report specific findings on these topics as applied to fifth or sixth grade pupils. However, many curriculum guides suggest ambitious plans for those grade levels, and emphasis is often on analyzing advertisements in the mass media.

AN OVERVIEW OF CONTENT in CONSUMER HEALTH

The study of consumer health may be logically divided into two basic subdivisions—health services and health products. Within each area, the specific task of consumer selection is the most widely publicized aspect and the one

[2] Ruth Byler, Gertrude Lewis, and Ruth Totman, *Teach Us What We Want to Know* (New York: The Mental Health Materials Center, 1969).

that perhaps merits the most emphasis at the elementary school level. This involves the development of a basic familiarization with the various functions of health practitioners and of the purposes of various drug categories, together with an examination of sound criteria for selection within each category. A second major aspect that applies to both health services and products is public policies in the forms of laws, regulations, subsidies for professional training, and so forth. These matters are generally related to the task of ensuring the quality of services and products and their availability, in terms of both an adequate supply and a reasonable price. Although heavy emphasis in this latter area of consumer activism is perhaps more appropriate at the secondary level, it is not too early to acquaint children with their coming opportunities and responsibilities regarding direct participation in this area of citizenship.

PROFESSIONAL HEALTH CARE

Although the health care needs of increasing numbers of children are being met in more impersonal clinical settings, the majority of children still have their first experiences with family physicians and dentists. However, many innovations and variations are developing within the context of these conventional patterns; changes are occurring both in the types of doctors and dentists who serve families and in the manner in which they conduct their practice.

MEDICAL CARE. Few factors can be more important to the welfare of a family than the services of a competent physician who is trusted and who responds with a genuine concern for the health of family members. At least four different types of physicians have the training that normally equips them to serve in this role:

- *The general practitioner* often provides routine care in all areas except obstetrics and surgery, and, in localities not served by specialists, these services may be provided as well. Because of the wide scope of their practice and their still-large numbers (despite the recent trend toward specialization), the quality of their performance perhaps varies more widely from physician to physician than in the more tightly controlled specialities. In many instances the "G.P.'s" combine good training with old-fashioned dedication to the practice of medicine and the welfare of their patients.
- *The pediatrician* is a physician specialist in child health care. His or her responsibility may begin at the child's birth and continue into the child's adolescence.
- *The family specialist* is a member of a relatively new medical speciality created in 1969 that generally combines the features of obstetrics, pediatrics, and general practice. Somewhat unique to this speciality is a

quite rigorous policy of reexamination every 6 years to ensure that these physicians have kept up with recent advances and have otherwise maintained their qualifications.

- *The osteopath,* once on the fringe of professional respectability, has recently emerged as a thoroughly acceptable choice for family medical needs because of his/her improved standards of training. Except in a few states where they have been absorbed by the state medical associations, osteopaths represent an independent alternative for one's choice as a physician who is not an M.D. but who is fully licensed by the state for the practice of medicine.

Regardless of the type of physician who is primarily responsible for the child's care the child will usually encounter some of the physician's supporting personnel.

- *Nurses* have enjoyed traditional acceptance as persons qualified to carry out the instructions of the physician. They often take medical histories, conduct some phases of the examination such as measurement of height and weight, determination of blood pressure, and so forth, and may do routine procedures such as administering immunizations.
- *Medical technicians* such as X-ray technicians are trained to carry out certain tests and laboratory procedures such as those for glucose level, hemoglobin, blood cell counts, and so forth.
- *Nurse practitioners* are more highly trained than the regular registered nurse and thus are able to diagnose and treat minor ailments and provide counsel and advice on routine health problems. In some rural areas where physicians are scarce, these "supernurses" function quite independently and refer only the more serious conditions to the nearest physician who may be many miles away.
- *Physician's associates* represent another effort to free the physician from routine tasks. Many P.A.'s gain their basic experience in the military service, then obtain supplementary training to equip them to function much like the nurse practitioner.[3]

Children generally receive care within the context of one of a number of medical practices or organizations. *Solo* practice, a single physician working out of his office, is the traditional pattern but is dropping increasingly out of favor as pressures encourage various *group* practice arrangements. These arrangements often reduce the financial overhead of each physician because supportive personnel and equipment can be more efficiently utilized. The patient may benefit because more efficient back-up service is provided, together with a more complete pattern of auxiliary service, X-ray, lab work, and so forth. Physicians who associate with one another in group practice

[3] John A. Brown et al., "The Physician's Associate—A Task Analysis," *Journal of the American Public Health Association,* Vol. 63, No. 12 (December 1973), pp. 1024–1028.

are occasionally of similar specialities (a group of obstetricians or pediatricians), but the present trend is toward a balanced group of physicians who organize a private clinic and offer a comprehensive pattern of services to patients who wish to enroll. When such organizations are large enough to offer hospital services, they take on the status of a health maintenance organization that provides total care to its members. Many inner city areas and some rural areas where private physicians are particularly scarce are serviced by comprehensive clinics managed by the local health department. Although these clinics are normally tax supported in part, nominal fees are usually charged to all patients except those who cannot pay or who are covered by Medicaid.

DENTAL CARE

The new developments in dental care are generally proceeding along the same lines as those for medical care, with group practice arrangements becoming more common, with more aggressive use being made of support personnel, and with new financial arrangements such as dental insurance becoming available. These are personnel the child may commonly encounter.

- The *dentist* does diagnosis and drilling, provides other more complex treatment services; even though today he or she is getting more and more help from support personnel.
- *Dental hygienists* may be familiar to both teachers and pupils because of the dental screening and education services they provide as employees of the school district. In private practice the hygienists often associate with a dentist or, more often, with a group of dentists, and normally do all the cleaning and X-raying of teeth.
- The *chair-side assistant* normally receives less training than the hygienist and works directly under the supervision of the dentist. Some are trained to place fillings in cavities after the dentist has drilled.
- The *pedodontist,* a specialist in children's dentistry, and the *orthodontist,* who specializes in straightening teeth and correcting malocclusion or improper bite, are two specialized dentists that children may encounter.

EYE CARE

All children should receive at least one thorough examination from an eye specialist, or at least a screening test offered to preschoolers in many communities, by the age of four years. However, many parents do not seek such an examination unless their child shows signs of eye strain or vision problems. Thus in contrast to an almost universal experience with doctors and a familiarity with dentists, many pupils have no experience with eye care other than that provided by the school screening procedures. The following personnel may be encountered in the field of eye care and vision correction:

- The *ophthalmologist* is a physician who specializes in eye care; although much of his or her time is normally spent in the diagnosis of simple refractive problems and the subsequent prescribing of glasses, the ophthalmologist's medical training also qualifies him or her to prescribe drugs and to do surgery to correct eye defects.
- The *optometrist* is a nonmedical eye specialist whose practice is generally restricted to the correction of refractive errors by use of glasses. Although not permitted to perform surgery, optometrists are now legally permitted to use drugs in some states.
- The *optician* grinds lenses and fills the prescriptions as provided by the ophthalmologist or optometrist.

PARENTAL RESPONSIBILITIES

One of the more general goals of the study of health services is the development of a proper degree of trust and appreciation regarding the various health practitioners. This goal can be met in large part by providing learning opportunities that enable the pupils to become familiar with the specific work that these helping people perform. Within almost all school districts there are parents who flagrantly disregard their responsibility to obtain needed professional health care for their children despite the often heroic efforts by nurses and administrators to prod them into action. There are also parents who are simply unable to afford decent health care for their children or, more rarely, whom physicians and dentists refuse to treat because of their skin color. The pupil of today is the parent and community citizen of tomorrow; it is not too early to begin the development of a knowledgeable and a positive orientation within these future parents.

Most health care activities can be divided into (1) the treatment of existing impairments or illnesses and (2) the prevention of the future occurrence of such conditions. Although prevention is seldom as glamorous, the teacher should not neglect any opportunity to allow childen to develop insights into the special value of prevention. Generally people do not need to be told to seek help when they are ill or injured, certainly not to the degree that they need to be encouraged to take preventive measures.

HOSPITAL CARE

Because of their lower resistance to communicable disease and consequently greater likelihood of being carriers of infections, children are commonly not allowed to visit hospitals. Also, the greater vulnerability of preschoolers

186

to the emotional trauma of separation and to the risk of postoperative complications often causes physicians to delay recommendations of elective surgery until after a child has reached school age. As a result, most first graders will have had little experience with hospitals other than their non-rememberable stay following their birth; or treatment of injuries in emergency wards. However, many of them may soon require tonsillectomies or surgical correction of minor impairments. In addition to the immediate emotional and physical significance, these upcoming hospitalizations will influence lifelong attitudes toward this phenomenon.

VALUE OF UNDERSTANDING. Children, like adults, tend to fear the unknown. Therefore, by providing the opportunity to learn about hospital procedures, teachers can do much to affect the child's reaction to any forthcoming hospital experience and to a lesser extent to affect the opinions and interpretations of children who have already been to the hospital. These latter, of course, represent valuable teaching resources as they relate their experiences and impressions. Teachers, through appropriate use of discussion leadership, can lead the class toward valid assessments of this first-hand information. Although the modern hospital is an immensely complex organization, it is relatively easy to highlight the major activities. As one 6-year-old child observed upon his hospitalization,

"The important thing about this hospital is ME." [4]

HISTORICAL DEVELOPMENT. Although the history of the hospital as an institution can be traced to a number of precursors such as the pagan temple of healing in the ancient world, the modern hospital evolved most directly from the early Christian period when houses were established where weary travelers could obtain food, lodging, and nursing care. Except for the destitute, who, like the travelers, relied on the hospital when they were ill, the crude medical care of the day was commonly dispensed in the patient's home. These early hospitals were houses of despair for the sick, poor, and homeless travelers, and persisted in large part until the early part of the present century. [5] However, since the advent of anesthesia, modern surgical techniques, antiseptic procedures, and antibiotics to prevent the spread of infections among patients, hospitals have become, in general, highly efficient centers of health care.

HOSPITAL ACTIVITIES. A child entering the hospital will probably stop first at the admissions office. Hospitals, like schools, try to keep careful records of the people they serve. Hospital stays are becoming shorter because

[4] "Red Is the Color of Hurting," *Public Health Service Publication No. 1583* (Bethesda, Md.: National Institute of Health, 1965), p. 1.
[5] John H. Knowles, "The Hospital," *Scientific American*, Vol. 229, No. 3 (September 1973), p. 128.

care is improving, and rising costs create pressures for the removal of long-term patients to nursing homes and similar facilities. Therefore, hospitals are serving more and more people for acute conditions involving short stays, and the admissions office is likely to be a busy place. In past generations most people paid their own hospital bills or were served on a charitable basis if they could not pay. Now most hospital stays are financed by a "third party" such as an insurance company, or the federal government as in the Medicare and Medicaid programs. Most of these arrangements are complicated by payment limits for certain operations or other procedures and by co-pay features where the insured person pays a portion of the bill. These factors also contribute to the hospital's burden of record keeping and paperwork.

Patients often go directly from the admissions office to their room or ward. Although some people are still willing to pay the high cost of a private room, most persons choose to stay either in a semiprivate room with one or two other patients or in wards where several patients share the same large room. Adults are commonly assigned to wards on the basis of their sex and the general nature of their illness or injury. Expectant mothers are assigned to obstetrical wards, people with broken bones go to orthopedic wards, people needing surgery are assigned to surgical wards, and so forth. Children are usually grouped together in pediatric wards so that they can provide companionship to one another, so that play space and toys can be made available, and so that other arrangements including special education can be made for their particular needs.

Patients are often taken to special rooms within the hospital for X-rays and other tests. In most modern hospitals first-time patients are impressed by the mazelike complexity of the hospital building. A tour would reveal the hospital as a city within itself, with up to 50 different kinds of staff members, a huge kitchen that prepares dozens of special diets, its own coffee shop for visitors and some ambulatory patients, its own laundry, and provisions for its own emergency power supply in the event of a power failure.

Patients scheduled for surgery are usually denied solid food for several hours before their operation to prevent vomiting during anesthesia. The night before the operation the patient is often given a sleeping pill, and a tranquilizer injection is usually given before the patient leaves the ward. If the operation involves an incision, the patient's first stop after leaving the ward may be a preparation room, where the incision site will be shaved and scrubbed with detergents and antiseptics.

Once in the operating room the patient may feel threatened by the generally cold atmosphere of tile floors and walls, trays of gleaming instruments, and electronic apparatus. The nurses, who will probably arrive before the surgeon, may speak in friendly and reassuring tones, but their smiles will be hidden by face masks. However, the patient's preparation in terms of a general knowledge of the nature of the operation, together with the effects of the drugs he or she has received, usually prevents undue concern. An anesthetist or an anesthesiologist (a physician specializing in this procedure) will put the patient to sleep with a gas or with a liquid dripped into the vein of the arm. After one drug has been used to put the patient to sleep, other drugs may be administered to block pain, relax muscles, or prevent certain reflex actions that might interfere with the surgery.

The patient's next sensation may be one of waking in a somewhat confused state in a strange new room. One will also sense that "something is different about my body"; the feeling may not be specific or painful, and it may not even center on the site of the operation, but it will usually be very apparent. The recovery room nurse will appear and provide reassurance that everything is fine and the worst is over. He or she will keep close check on the recovering patient's respiration, pulse rate, blood pressure, and other vital signs for a few hours until the effects of the anesthesia and any postoperative shock have subsided. The patient will then be returned to the ward for a period of convalescence before going home.

On the day of discharge the business office may provide a copy of the bill even though an insurance company may be paying most of it. It may be quite long, with an entry for each medication or service as well as the daily charge for the room and the fees associated with the operating room. A few days after the patient arrives home, the surgeon's bill may arrive, illustrating this contract is with the patient rather than with the hospital.

Although one is usually happy to be coming home, this feeling is often mixed with at least a little sadness. Even a short stay at the hospital is usually sufficient for making some genuine friends among the staff members and other patients. Even though there may have been some unpleasant instances, the general impression one carries away from the experience is that these people were good at their job and "they seemed to care about me."

HEALTH PRODUCTS

The factors that affect one's health status are so broad and diverse as to almost defy definition. This applies to the realm of health products just as surely as it does to behavior patterns and environmental factors. Two categories appear as logical inclusions, namely over-the-counter drugs sold on the open market without a physician's prescription and ethical drugs that by law require a prescription for their purchase. Beyond these two relatively distinct groups lies a huge conglomeration of food products sold on the basis of exaggerated nutritional claims, exercise devices of dubious value, household cleaners and disinfectants purchased in the false hope of preventing disease, and many other items that by claim or implication offer health advantages. One source estimates the annual national expenditure for health products at $37 billion. Although such figures carry little meaning to most persons, it makes the motives for the vigorous and often diabolically clever advertising efforts in this field a bit easier to understand.

189

ETHICAL DRUGS. A drug, by definition, is a substance that alters the functioning of the body. Many drugs that may alleviate noxious symptoms or effect a cure at the proper or effective dose level become extremely dangerous and in many cases lethal at higher levels. In fact, no drug that is effective can be said to be completely safe. The safer drugs have a lethal dose level that is many times higher than their effective level. Aspirin represents perhaps a borderline case in drug safety, although it normally takes several times the recommended dose to kill, it is one of the leading causes of accidental death due to poisoning. Death, of course, is not the only risk associated with patent drugs; some may cause harmful or disabling side effects, and others possess addictive or habit-forming qualities. For these reasons the more potent drugs are restricted to a prescription-only basis.

The relatively effective federal laws that govern the development, testing, and marketing of ethical drugs represent in large part a response to the inadequacies and tragic episodes of the past. One of the more infamous of these involved the release of a sulfanilamide compound in 1937. Although the main ingredient had apparently undergone some preliminary testing, the form that went on the market included a dangerous and untested chemical (diethylene glycol) as a vehicle or solvent for the sulfa compound. This caused over 100 deaths from kidney damage before the mistake could be corrected.

Another public shock occurred in 1961 when the United States was spared the ravages of thalidomide, the notorious cause of birth defects, not by the systematic operation of legal regulation, but only by the intuitive judgment of Dr. Frances Kelsey, a Food and Drug Administration officer who deliberately pigeonholed the authorization papers for United States sales until the tragedy broke in Europe. These and similar influences have resulted in relatively strict laws that are enforced by the Food and Drug Administration and that provide for (1) laboratory analysis, (2) animal testing, and (3) field testing with human volunteers under medical supervision. Although application of these laws causes considerable delay between the development of a new drug and its availability to the sick whom it will benefit and adds considerably to its price, it provides a high degree of protection to American consumers. Therefore, a fine balance in these factors is needed if the public is to be served in the optimal manner.

After a drug company has incurred the costs of developing and testing a new drug, it usually obtains a patent and the drug is marketed for several years under a brand name to recover its development costs and take full advantage of its temporary monopoly on the drug's sale. During this period other companies may purchase the right to market the same drug under their own different brand names and after the patent has expired these brands may sell at a premium because of the confidence that has been established with physicians and because of advertising pressure. Drugs in these situations, however, are often marketed by other companies under their commonly accepted descriptive title or generic name. Because the purity and potency of all drugs must meet standards established by law, generic brands usually combine lower costs with a level of effectiveness equal to that of brand-name drugs.

OVER-THE-COUNTER DRUGS.   In recent years public opinion regarding over-the-counter drugs has often tended toward extreme positions. Some, who for religious motives or in reaction to the recent upsurge of drug abuse, tend to avoid any drug use, particularly by self-administration, feel that all drugs should be banned to the general public. Others, with their *Merck Manual* or *Physician's Desk Reference* (diagnosis and dosage handbooks) in hand, call for the right to purchase any drug available and attack the physician–pharmacy arrangement as a monopolistic "rip-off" of the public. Somehow, public policy has managed to steer a middle course, and thus average citizens can purchase such items as aspirin tablets, cough syrup, and decongestants on their own; these compounds often bring noticeable relief from minor symptoms and irritations. However, the same laws that make a few useful items conveniently available have opened a veritable Pandora's box of generally useless and sometimes dangerous attractively packaged and highly advertised items.

Among the most serious problems associated with OTC items is the out-

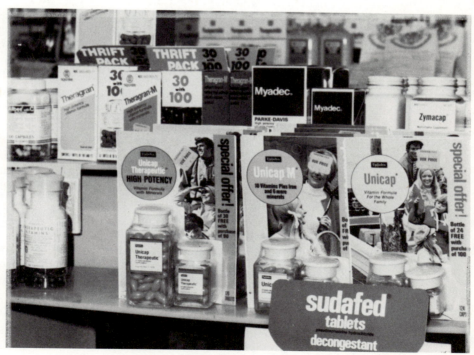

Figure 8.1. Health Products: How Do I Choose? (Carol Ashton)

191

right harm that is often caused by overdosage or other misuse. Aspirin poisoning, particularly among children, is the classic example within this category, but other examples occur such as the occasional auto or industrial accident attributed to the doziness that antihistamines can produce or the aggravation of acute appendicitis with a strong laxative compound. A second type of risk occurs when OTC drugs provide symptomatic relief of serious conditions and thus delay the time when the needed medical attention is obtained. Consequently, we find occasional cases of rectal cancer being treated with hemorrhoid compounds, stomach ulcers being treated with antacids, and active tuberculosis being treated with cough syrup. Finally, even in the absence of harmful outcomes, there is the awesome siphoning off of literally millions of dollars from the public in return for unneeded or worthless items. The uneducated poor are among the hardest hit by this practice, which must be considered criminal in an absolute if not in a legal sense.

Efforts directed at the control of these problems are currently proceeding on two main fronts: (1) federal laws and regulations as spearheaded by the Food and Drug Administration and the Federal Trade Commission and (2) consumer education as to both appropriate sources of help for various health complaints and the ability to properly evaluate various advertising appeals. The current thrust of the FTC is being directed toward the prevention of outright fraud and deception in advertising and the development of stricter standards of proof for advertising claims. The FDA is evaluating the effectiveness of OTC drugs and is removing useless and dangerous ones from the market. On the educational front the more promising efforts seem to resemble a "Vance Packard know-your-enemy" approach in which pupils analyze the various psychological appeals that have been incorporated into specific ads. Also, of course, the straightforward testing or trying out of products in efforts to objectively assess the validity of advertising claims is an equally promising approach.

OTHER HEALTH PRODUCTS. Cosmetics and exercise aids are two other major categories of products related to health that are subject to abuse in the market place. Although there are some real differences in the quality of different brands of cosmetics, one often pays more for the attractive containers and the advertising behind the cleansing cream, lipstick, or other product than for the item itself. Also, the consumer is often tricked into relying on the purported effects of cosmetics to the neglect of good health care. A good night's sleep is often the best remedy for dark circles under the eyes, regular bathing controls body odor quite effectively in the absence of special soaps or deodorants, and regular exercise often helps the complexion.

In the areas of exercise and weight reduction, the key point is that there is no easy way. Exercise programs or apparatus that demand little in the way of effort will return equally little in the way of benefits regardless of how elaborate the equipment or how high the cost. For general health, endurance exercises that tax the cardiovascular system are the most valuable. Therefore, stationary bicycles with friction devices and rowing machines may have some value, but little can be said in defense of pedaling devices that offer no resistance or that come equipped with their own power supply. The various jiggling belts and powered rollers sold for reductions of fatty trouble spots constitute enduring monuments to the powers of hope and self-deception. Although some improvement in tone may result from efforts to maintain one's balance, all available scientific evidence supports the conclusion that body fat is retained until energy consumption exceeds food intake regardless of how vigorously the body is stroked, shook, pounded, or steamed. For elementary-age children vigorous play is the best reducing agent.

SUGGESTED LEARNING ACTIVITIES

The following suggestions are presented in an effort to demonstrate how the content described in the preceding section might be translated into effective classroom learning activities. They were designed to accommodate a wide variety of classroom groups provided that proper selection and adaptations are made according to the needs, interests, abilities, and maturity level of the particular children involved.

- *Crystal Ball of Health Professionals.*

  Write on slips of paper the names of various health professionals that your children encounter at some point in their lives. Have them select a slip of paper from the cyrstal ball (a fish bowl or other appropriate container) and explain to the class the role that each of these individuals plays (e.g., general practitioner, nurse, dentist, dental hygienist, optician).

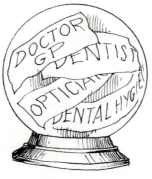

Crystal Ball
of
Professionals

- Have the children rank the following health examination that they feel is most important to them and explain why.
  - eye exam
  - dental exam
  - medical exam

  Step 1 is the most important, step 3 the least.

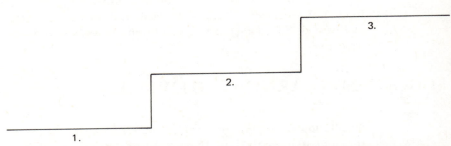

- Have the children write and present a play regarding good oral hygiene for "Dental Health Week" in February. Some of the cast of characters (puppets could be used) might include Timothy Tooth, Betsy Brush, and Dr. Dan.

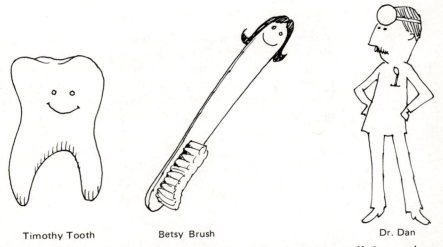

Timothy Tooth   Betsy Brush   Dr. Dan

- Have the children make a poster for their classroom wall from pieces of felt indicating all the ways we need to protect our teeth in addition to brushing and regular checkups with the dentist. Example: when taking a drink of water at the fountain, don't shove and push, because you may cause someone to chip a tooth. Have the children think of other ways teeth can be chipped. What are some of the other ways that we need to protect our teeth? For example, wear your mouth guard when playing football.

• During Halloween, have the children start a campaign to encourage parents and other people who give out treats to make the treats orally healthy rather than orally hazardous. Encourage local businesses and papers to participate. You can have the children write letters to the editor so that the whole community can become involved.

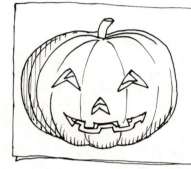

ORALLY SAFE TREATS
for
HALLOWEEN

Examples: fruits
sugarless gum
small packages of potato chips
toothbrushes (donated by the
American Dental Association
of your community)

• Divide the class into small groups and have them make a list (with brand names) of the following products found in their homes. If they do not have one of the items, have them leave it blank.

    Items: 1. dishwashing soap
          2. bread
          3. aspirin
          4. toilet tissue
          5. vitamins
          6. cereal
          7. soft drink beverage

After they have made their list with the brand names, have them discuss the reason that brand name product is in their home (e.g., influenced by ads from TV). Ask them to see if there were any similarities in products and the reason for them.

• After instructing the children in the proper method of brushing and flossing their teeth, have them brush and floss as a group after lunch each day. A peg board can be used to store labeled tooth brushes. To check progress, distribute disclosing tablets. Have the children keep a record of their progress and reduction of dental caries in their "Life Scrapbook" (see suggested activity in Chapter 4).

• To have the children appreciate the importance of their eyes, have them blindfold themselves for an hour (or any other designated period of time) and have them go about their regular activities. Assign a guide and have the students record their feelings while participating in this experience.

• Ask your local Blind Association to bring in books written in braille and show the children how they are used. Have them learn to read some braille regarding a story that they have already read in class and that they would be familiar with.

- Many children may have unwarranted fears regarding the doctor's or dentist's office or hospital. Arrange a field trip to these places or have someone from them come and speak to the children and discuss what happens at each place. They may show some of the equipment and instruments that they use.

- Have the children visit their local pharmacist to ask about drugs. Some of their questions might be: Which ones need a prescription? What can be sold over the counter? What does "generic name" mean? What is the difference among brands, for example, of aspirin? What kinds of records does a pharmacist have to keep of his sales of drugs? [6]

- In at least one city arrangements were made to have all first graders visit a hospital. This occurred when the public relations director of the Rochester, Minnesota, Methodist Hospital made the opportunity available to the city's schools.[7] This visit was recommended as the culminating activity of a one-week unit on the hospital. Children's stories were reviewed, with emphasis on such titles as *Curious George Goes to the Hospital,* and *How Hospitals Help Us.* Two nurses were regularly assigned to work with the children to provide orientation including such experiences as getting into an adjustable hospital bed, taking routine tests, role-playing the taking of anesthesia, and other such experiences. Although few school districts have this opportunity, the apparent success of this particular program suggests that more indirect methods of instruction such as films and classroom role playing would be highly effective with this age group.

- Fifth and sixth grade pupils will often respond well to "Hospital Miracles" as a unit theme, with each pupil assigned the task of finding one dramatic hospital achievement as reported in the newspapers or in some recent magazine, such as the successful treatment of a badly burned or severely injured person, the successful transplant of some organ, or the development of some new artificial device for a damaged part of the body. Ask the children to bring in magazine pictures to illustrate their report and to use in a bulletin board display. As the unit develops, shift the class's attention to the more normal everyday work of the hospital to convey the idea that when you are the patient even the routine procedures are little miracles in themselves.

- Children are prime targets for many TV advertisements and are relatively easy to involve in learning activities focused on this phenomenon. One approach is to first ask each member of the class to carefully note

[6] *Yellow Pages of Learning Resources* (Cambridge, Mass.: MIT Press, 1972), p. 60.
[7] Warren W. Zimmerman, "A Hospital Visit for First Graders,' *School Health Review,* Vol. 4, No. 2 (March-April 1973), pp. 19–21.

the contents of one health-related TV commercial in terms of (1) the claims or hinted benefits (implications) and (2) the method used to appeal to the viewers' interests or readiness to believe the claims. Discuss these in class, with the purpose of selecting the interesting examples for further study by a group of volunteers. This investigation can take the form of obtaining the product and reading the label carefully, talking to someone who has actually used it, reviewing the results of independent tests by consumer organizations, or possibly writing the manufacturer for further information on their advertising claims.[8]

• Have the children design a calendar for one month and relate it to some health topic.

Example:

MARCH — BEAUTY AIDS FOR COMPLEXION

S	M	T	W	T	F	S
		1 Regular cleansing	2	3	4	5
6	7	8	9	10 Exercise	11	12
13	14	15 Sleep	16	17	18	19
20	21	22	23	24 Good Diet	25	26
27	28	29	30	31		

[8] For a detailed account of a similar technique, see Michael W. Radis, "Consumerism Belongs in the Classroom Too," *Grade Teacher*, Vol. 90, No. 9 (May-June 1973), pp. 54–56.

Have the children draw pictures or write in words for the various days as a reminder for beauty tips. Also, they can make a calendar for the entire year and give it as a present for an appropriate holiday.

SUGGESTED RESOURCES

The learning resources listed in this section are a selected sample of materials with which the authors are personally familiar. Appropriate grade levels have been included when these were indicated by the source.

FILMS

American Society of Dentistry for Children
Catalog of films
211 East Chicago Avenue
Chicago, Illinois

Toothkeeper
Programmed Unit
American Society of Preventative Dentistry
435 North Michigan Avenue
Chicago, Illinois 60611

FILMSTRIPS

Goodlandlord and Your Teeth
Grades K–2
Colgate Palmolive Company

The Mouth I Live In
Grades K–2
Colgate Palmolive Company
740 North Rush Street
Chicago, Illinois 60611

KITS

Colgate Professional Services Department
Colgate Palmolive Company
740 North Rush Street
Chicago, Illinois 60611

Toothbrush/Plaque Control Kits:
(available free to third grade classes)
1. John O. Butler Co.
   540 N. Lake Shore Drive
   Chicago, Illinois 60611

2. Oral B Company
   Fairfield Road
   Wayne, New Jersey 07470

3. Crest Kits
   Procter and Gamble Company
   Professional Services Division
   P.O. Box 171
   Cincinnatti, Ohio 45201

Toothtown
Programmed Unit
111 North Canal Street
National Dairy Council
Chicago, Illinois 60606

PAMPHLET

National Foundation for the Prevention of Oral Disease
1804 East Indian School Road
Suite No. 4
Phoenix, Arizona 85016

POSTERS

American Dental Association
Catalog of posters, materials, etc.
Bureau of Dental Health Education
211 East Chicago Avenue
Chicago, Illinois 60611

Florida Citrus Association
Posters on Dental Health and Nutrition
P.O. Box 148
Lakeland, Florida 33802

HEALTH SERVICE ASPECTS of CONSUMERISM

The school's health service staff can contribute to consumer health education not only by serving as resource persons in health education but also by giving individual consumer advice and guidance to parents and pupils as part of the process of referral and follow-up of those with suspected health problems. School nurses, for example, are expected to know the health service resources available in the community, to assist parents in selecting an appropriate source of care, and to find ways of overcoming intervening economic and social barriers to care. For example, the nurse may assist a poor parent through the maze of red tape that stands in the way of getting a Medicaid card in many states. The nurse should know that Medicaid children are eligible for a valuable service called the Early and Periodic Screening, Diagnosis, and Treatment Program (EPSDT), and should refer poor parents to an agency that provides this service if one is locally available.

In addition, the specialized knowledge of the nurse and dental hygienist enables them to teach parents and children about referral for such potentially frightening services as neurological diagnosis and treatment of suspected epilepsy, or orthodontia, and thus to remove fear as a barrier to successful follow-up and also enable them to judge the adequacy of the service received.

School nurses also often act as liaison persons between the school and outside sources of health care. The information nurses can provide to physicians about screening test results and health observations of children is often useful in establishing diagnosis. The information provided by a physician to the school nurse about a given child's health problem often results in better management of the child within the school setting.

School health service workers are also often able to give helpful advice in the selection and use of safe, effective, and appropriate health products. They are, for example, well informed about items that should be included in a home first aid kit and which over-the-counter materials are useful in treating head lice or other nuisance diseases. They may know of an agency through which a temporarily crippled pupil can borrow rather than buy needed and expensive orthopedic equipment.

Teachers and parents, however, are sometimes disappointed when a health professional refuses to recommend a specific medical specialist or product by name, or to contact a physician directly about a pupil's problem. To do any of these things may be a violation of the nurse's perception of professional ethics. For example, a nurse could tell a parent how to go about selecting a pediatrician, but the nurse could recommend Dr. Mary Smith only if she were the only pediatrician in the community. A dental hygienist might recommend fluoride tooth paste, but not a specific brand. And Dr.

Smith might refuse to discuss her patient's case with the school nurse without first obtaining a signed release statement from the child's parent.

REFERENCES

KNOWLES, JOHN H. "The Hospital," *Scientific American,* Vol. 229, No. 3 (September 1973), pp. 128–137.

————. "Where Doctors Fail," *Saturday Review,* August 22, 1970, p. 21.

LAMBERG, LYNNE. "Patient Help Thyself," *Family Health,* Vol. 7, No. 1 (January 1975), pp. 35–38.

LEE, RUSSEL V., and SAREL EIMERL. *The Physician.* New York: Time Incorporated, 1969.

The Medicine Show. Mount Vernon, N.Y.: Consumers Union, 1975.

MODELL, WALTER, and ALFRED LANSING. *Drugs.* New York: Time Incorporated, 1969.

RADIS, MICHAEL W. "Consumerism Belongs in the Classroom Too," *Grade Teacher,* Vol. 90, No. 9 (May-June 1973), pp. 54–56.

Red Is the Color of Hurting (Public Health Service Publication No. 1583). Bethesda, Md.: National Institutes of Health, 1965.

SEHNERT, KEITH W. "But Has Medicine Forgotten the Patient?" *Family Health,* Vol. 7, No. 11 (November 1975), pp. 41, 60–62.

VACALIS, T. DEMETRI. "Determination of Vital Areas of Knowledge Needed for Wise Consumer Use of Health Care Services," *Journal of School Health,* Vol. 44, No. 7 (September 1974), pp. 390–394.

ZIMMERMAN, WARREN W. "A Hospital Visit for First Graders," *School Health Review,* Vol. 4, No. 2 (March-April 1973), pp. 19–21.

9

Families Big and Small— Living Groups

Human infants are among the most helpless of the world's living creatures; they must have years of care before they can maintain an independent existence. And, in comparison with other of the world's species, a relatively high percentage of human babies receive this care and reach maturity, a point at which there would presumably be a fair chance of surviving on their own even in a primitive environment. Of course, few people choose to live this way. One of the most distinguishing features of human beings of all cultures is their universal desire to experience close, affectionate interpersonal relationships. Various social scientists disagree as to the origin of this characteristic, with some maintaining that people learn to value people during their long years of dependence when their very lives depended upon the behavior of someone else, and others maintaining that a need for affectionate relationships is as instinctive to humans as nest building is to birds.

TRADITIONAL VALUES VERSUS MODERN PRESSURES

The issue concerning the origin of this quality appears to have little practical significance to most human affairs, for when virtually every person manifests a need for affection it must be dealt with whether it is instinctive or is a product of some near-universal human learning experience. Within Western culture the family based on monogamous marriage has endured as the main social institution designed as a setting within which affectional needs could be met. The current family model within the United States is the small, nuclear family that, according to the current ideal, consists of a man, a woman, and two children.

202

INFLEXIBLE SCENARIO

It would seem that there is no responsible alternative to this normative family pattern. The committed bachelor or spinster is commonly regarded with various combinations of pity and condemnation depending on whether the individual appears as lonely and unwanted or as simply unwilling to assume "normal" adult responsibility. The childless marriage is commonly termed "empty" or "barren," and is pitied or condemned according to whether the couple is regarded infertile or as simply selfish and unwilling to assume the personal and financial burden of child rearing. Another invalid stereotype is the "only" child, who is foredoomed to become a neurotic brat who will never learn the joy of sharing. Therefore, there must be one brother or sister, but certainly no more than one if the parents are not to commit the worst sin of all, contributing to the population crisis.

Surely someday this scenario will yield somewhat to the forces of reason and respect for the other human qualities of individuality and integrity; however, it seems clear that the very factors that have figuratively painted the American family into a corner will continue to have their effects on this very important and sometimes very troubled social institution. This process appeared to begin with the many scientific and industrial advances of the nineteenth century that provided the basis for the industrial revolution and the consequent shift from a rural to an urban society. The old-time extended family with its aunts and uncles, cousins, and grandparents all living under one roof worked well on the farm but proved inappropriate and unwieldy in the town and the city. From an economic standpoint the family fortunes became focused on the husband's job rather than on a plot of ground, and these jobs often proved to be more temporary than enduring as work either dried up or as more attractive opportunities developed elsewhere. Families began to move more frequently, thus rendering the extended family even more impractical. With the more peripheral members trimmed away, the erosive forces of economics began to reduce the number of children as additional offspring shifted from being useful rural farmhands to becoming urban liabilities.

PERIOD of TRANSITION

Previously, in the agrarian family the most important part of the child's education was provided by the parents as boys learned to till the soil and care for the animals and girls learned cooking and housekeeping for large families in the absence of electrical appliances and convenience foods. As modern technology continued to accelerate, the ability to read, once looked upon as a tool for Bible study, now became a requirement for economic success, as did arithmetic, which now had use extending far beyond activities at the general store. The three R's were obviously a mere starting point,

203

as the need for more sophisticated levels of education began to place a strain on taxpayers in general and the parents of college-bound youth in particular. The increased need for education was only one aspect of the demands for an increasingly higher standard of living. The doctors of the horse-and-buggy era dispensed many of their services right in the farmhouse rather than at any hospital, and were often paid with jars of pickles or a sumptuous evening meal. Considering the qualities of their services, they often received the better part of the deal. Their modern counterparts, by comparison, are efficient and expensive, another good reason to keep families small.

Reductions in the basic responsibilities of the family as a social institution have roughly paralleled the reduction in size. The elderly and the infirm have been left behind, often to the care of government facilities or commercially operated nursing homes. The major portion of the educational task has been, out of necessity, given over to professional educators. The availability of the automobile and other forms of transportation and the expansion of commercial entertainment have taken many recreational functions out of the family context except for the passive watching of television. Finally, the family has surrendered its role as the primary source of economic support for women; both the technological advances that reduced the need for muscle power and the political advances that are placing women on an increasingly equal footing with men have produced a situation where the modern woman is under less pressure to marry or to stay in an unsatisfying marriage for economic reasons. Thus the American family entered the decade of the 1970s vastly reduced in size and shorn of many of its traditional functions except those of providing a source of affection and companionship, a socially endorsed context for the rearing of children, and a socially acceptable pattern for satisfying sexual needs. However, the most severe challenges are yet to come.

The traditional efforts of society to restrict sexual activities to the confines of a proper marriage have never been more than partially successful. Even in Victorian days most people advocated premarital chastity while knowing in their own minds that the majority of young men were destined to gain their experience from "loose women" long before marriage and that many men of means and discretion were often able to maintain a mistress without placing undue strain on their marriage. Kinsey marks the year 1900 as a turning point in women's acceptance of this blatantly unfair double standard. He found that "Among the females in the sample who were born before 1900, less than half as many had had pre-marital coitus as among the females born in any subsequent decade." [1] Although many women who have come to maturity since the early part of this century showed an increasing willingness to participate in premarital sex, they steadfastly expressed support for the ideal of sex only after marriage during

[1] Alfred C. Kinsey et al., *Sexual Behavior in the Human Female* (New York: Pocket Books, Inc., 1965, p. 298). Reprint of W. B. Saunders edition (Philadelphia, 1953).

the 1930s, 1940s, and 1950s. More recently, however, there has been a tendency to bring professed standards more in line with the realities of actual behavior. Robert C. Sorensen's more recent study, for example, showed that "Two-thirds of all adolescents agree that if two people love each other and are living together, getting married is just a legal technicality which they should not be required to comply with." [2] Clearly, sexual gratification outside of marriage is becoming not only more frequent but also more acceptable.

Although the trend toward increasing degrees of sexual freedom is complex and lends itself to different interpretations, it represents in one sense part of the general effort on the part of women to achieve equality in all respects with men. This effort took its most visible form, of course, with the "Women's Lib" movement that came to national attention in the 1960s. However, as a general trend, it extends historically back to the sufferage movement of World War I. It was reflected in the social changes of the "Roaring Twenties" and in the new vocational opportunities typified by "Rosie the Riveter" during World War II, as well as in the formally organized movements of recent years. The trend toward equality of the sexes within present-day society also extends well beyond its formal organization to change the lives of even those women who do not particularly like the ideas associated with the movement. The most profound of these changes are those related to the women's traditional responsibilities for the care and raising of children. Child-rearing chores are increasingly viewed as obstacles to the higher goal of vocational fulfillment and thus the demand has developed for more day-care centers, for early childhood education, for school breakfast programs, and for similar developments motivated wholly or in part by a desire to shift a significant part of the childrearing burden to persons and agencies outside the family. Closely related are trends toward the delay of having children until later in the marriage, having fewer children, and the increasing acceptance of childless marriages.

Just as it would be unwise to underestimate the many factors that are placing heavy stress on the modern family, it would be even more ill-advised to conclude that this social institution is about to drop from the scene. Its roots extend back beyond the dawn of history and in a contemporary sense permeate our social, religious, and legal traditions. Even among Sorensen's modern-day teenagers, "85% of all boys and 92% of all girls . . . expect someday to marry and have children." [3] Although many of its traditional functions have been usurped by other social institutions, the ideal of establishing a loving, enduring, monogamous relationship with the eventual prospects of raising children is still supported by the overwhelming majority of young people. Other possibilities exist such as the communal movements and various forms of single life-styles, but for most these repre-

[2] Robert C. Sorensen, *Adolescent Sexuality in Contemporary America* (New York: World Publishing, 1972), p. 358.
[3] Ibid.

sent untested alternatives. The conventional marriage with its prospect of a satisfying family life is still the normative mode of meeting these human needs.

Like virtually every other human organization, the family has had to change in the process of adapting itself to its dynamic environment; and, as the case of other organizations, these changes sometimes lead to success and improvements and sometimes leave the original problems unchanged or exacerbated. Both the successful changes and the continuing problems of the family carry important implications for elementary teachers both in their roles as surrogate parents in the classroom and for their responsibilities as teachers of health education. Some of the most important characteristics, changes, and problems of the modern family will be discussed as potential content for family life education; however, first a sampling of children's interest patterns within this topic will be presented.

CHILDREN'S INTERESTS as RELATED to the STUDY of FAMILY LIVING

The landmark study of children's health interests as conducted by Ruth Byler and her associates yielded evidence that led the investigators to conclude that children are receptive to the study of content related to parents and family at all grade levels, with particularly high levels of interest occurring at grades six through nine.[4] A few sample responses and findings are as follows:

Kindergarten Through Grade Two

- He [my dad] plays ball with me—swims with me—reads to me.
- My mom gets us new babies; she feeds us—picks me up when I fall down—cleans me off.
- My mudder always hollers at me—she just likes to play with the baby.
- A little girl who missed her recently divorced father and was concerned over the possibility of her mother's remarriage confided to her teacher: I don't think I have enough love for two fathers.

Grades Three and Four

- My brother picks on me—my sister bugs me—I hate my sister. She gets me in trouble. I don't know why you can't hit girls. I'd sure like to hit her.
- I get mad at my mother when I have to go to the tutor.

[4] Ruth Byler, Gertrude M. Lewis, and Ruth J. Totman, *Teach Us What We Want to Know* (New York: Mental Health Materials Center, Inc., 1969), p. 169.

• My mother and father don't love each other any more. Which one shall I love?

• Why do I get so lonely?

Grades Five and Six

• Why does my mother get mad at me when I try to do something right? My mother spends more time with my sister.

• Why do people fight between each other if they were born within the same family?

• My father never spends much time with me. When he comes home from work, he is so utterly exhausted and in a terrible mood. What should I do?

• Why do people get married if they don't love each other?

AN OVERVIEW of CONTENT
for FAMILY LIFE EDUCATION

The factor of major importance in the formation of children's concepts of the family, its basic value, the appropriate behavior of its various members, and how it should generally function is their real-life experience within their own family. This influence is crucial regardless of whether the reactions are those of enthusiastic endorsement of the "way we did things" or of vehement rejection as with those who say "I'll never do that to my kids." Teachers cannot and should not hope to superimpose some ideal concept of family life over this potent program of natural education; however, they can help children respond more constructively to their ongoing experiences within the family. Through study of what happens generally in families, they more clearly determine whether or not their particular problems or strengths are unique; their study of the motives of parents and siblings can make them more empathetic and analytical and less prone to overly harsh judgments. This is by no means easy, but few tasks are more worthwhile, for poorly functioning families probably account for more maimed and disfigured personalities than any other single phenomenon. The school, through its educational program, represents perhaps society's best means of systematically improving this highly important and greatly troubled component of society.

FAMILY PATTERNS

The modern nuclear family with husband, wife, and two or more children is, as noted, still the national norm. Recently it has become so popular among educators to debunk the idea that all children come from intact homes that it is sometimes overlooked that the majority of elementary children in the average classroom are still from nuclear families, although the exceptions are indeed sizable. Moreover, the prospects of someday following this American ideal in a family of their own formation still remains a firm if somewhat distant goal for most children. The variations from this norm, however, are becoming both more frequent and, perhaps most important, more acceptable as viable alternatives.

Perhaps the most workable of these alternatives is the family formed by a second marriage of one or both partners that includes various combinations of stepchildren, step-siblings, and/or half-siblings in a "yours, mine, and ours" type of arrangement. The emotional dynamics operating within these families can be highly complex and can contribute to intense conflicts between or among the children. The fact that the children in conflict may

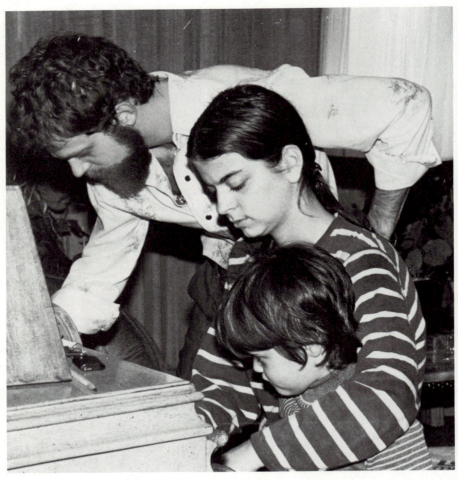

Figure 9.1A. Most Common, Everyday Activities Are Important to Family Unity. (Sheila Bernstein)

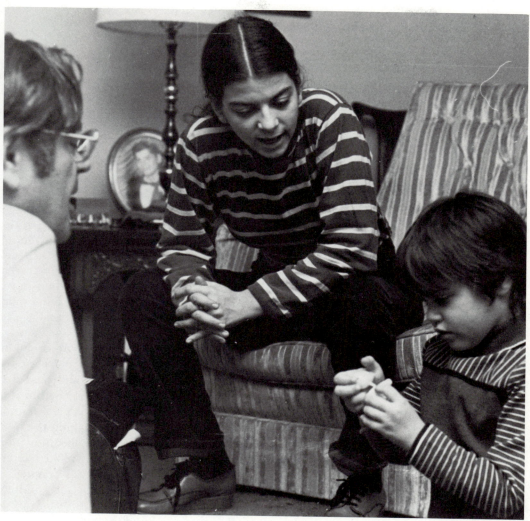

Figure 9.1B. Even the Simplest Family Interaction Carries Some Degree of Emotional Significance. (Sheila Bernstein)

be stepbrothers, for example, is often seized upon as a convenient explanation for a problem. In actual fact the family of a second marriage may have fewer rather than more such conflicts because of the unique assets such families possess. Although divorce may involve considerable trauma, it dispels many romantic fallacies and often contributes to the maturity of the participants; consequently, second marriages are often more firmly grounded in maturity and realism. Also, skills in personal relationships may be more assiduously applied to a second marriage because of the obvious challenge of the new situation and a mutual awareness that a good marriage relationship requires care and attention rather than passive dependence upon tradition. This approach is, of course, precisely what is needed for the long-term health and survival of any marriage.

The single-parent family, which in its most common form consists of a divorced or separated woman and one or more children, is one with more significant but not overwhelming liabilities. Freudian-based psychologists, in particular, argue with considerable merit that normal personality development requires that children experience close interpersonal relationship with both a male and a female model during their preschool careers. According to this theory young children need a same-sex model for the development of appropriate sex-role behavior and a cross-sex model if they are to learn to act appropriately toward the opposite sex; the crucial aspect of this dual learning process is held to be the affective or emotional response rather than any superficial training in social customs or etiquette. Although this point of view has its critics, both research evidence in its favor and its commonsense basis provide considerable credibility.[5] However, it should be noted that the intact family produces its share of warped personalities also, particularly when there are serious and prolonged conflicts between the parents. Also, parents are not the only role models the children have. Consequently, the old-time virtue of holding a hopelessly unsatisfying marriage together "for the good of the children" has justifiably become the object of near-universal disfavor.

Many variations of the single-parent family are becoming more common as various forms of hypocrisy are dropped in favor of openness and honesty. Examples are the unmarried mother who has chosen to keep and raise her child, the mother who is struggling on her own, or, particularly within the black ghetto, the mother who is living with her own parent or parents in a vertically extended family. In some cases these mothers are making the best of a difficult situation, but frequently they chose this pattern because they were more interested in parenthood than in marriage. A closely related variation that is growing in acceptance is the single person who has adopted a child. Because of abortion and the shortage of white infants, the children involved are usually nonwhite or multiracial in background. This arrangement has its liabilities but appears as a much better alternative than permanent institutionalization of otherwise unwanted children.

Another type of family that is subject to special problems despite the recent progress in racial tolerance is the multiracial family. Although still quite rare, there is every indication that such families are increasing in number. The 1960 census showed that there were 51,400 black–white married couples in the United States as compared with recent estimates which run

---

[5] For supportive evidence together with an interesting review of this point of view, see E. Mavis Hetherington, "Girls Without Fathers," *Psychology Today*, Vol. 6, No. 9 (February 1973), pp. 46–52.

as high as 1 million such couples.[6] Such marriages tend to be more unstable than intraracial marriages; however, it is difficult to determine how much of this instability results from cultural differences between the partners and how much results from the added pressures produced by society's unwarranted hostility toward such couples.

Perhaps the most important concept related to family patterns is that the quality of the personal interaction that transpires between the members of a family is far more important than the particular configuration of its structure.

FAMILY FUNCTIONS

People in general and children in particular tend to view families as things that simply exist and to give little thought to the possible reasons for this existence. Sociologists, however, see the family as representing a social unit that serves certain functions related to important human needs. They realize that it is not permanent, that it can and no doubt will change just as it has when viewed in historical or cultural perspective. Probably of more importance to the average person are some insights into its present functions as a cooperative venture where the members put something in, pay their dues, so to speak, and get service in return. This is a somewhat cold-blooded view, perhaps, of what many regard as a sacred institution, but this objective understanding can lay the groundwork for the more secure basis of mutual appreciation, concern, and love.

The love relationships within a family unit are regarded by most persons as of primary importance, but more clearly understandable to the child are the more prosaic functions related to living arrangements. If life is to proceed with any degree of comfort and civility, beds must be made, laundry must be done, meals must be prepared, lawns must be mowed, and garbage must be emptied. Despite modern conveniences, considerable work is required if the average home is not to degenerate into a modern hovel. Somewhat less visible to the child is the work required to keep water flowing through the faucets and power from the outlets, to keep food in the pantry and freezer, and to keep the title or lease to the home or apartment. Any communal living organization functions much more smoothly in all respects when responsibility for these day-to-day tasks is well defined and effectively carried out, and the family is no exception.

The child who learns to understand and accept the need for each person in a living group to carry his or her share of these household burdens will have acquired an attractive personality trait. The behavior that naturally follows this attitude and understanding is related, not merely to some sense

[6] Ernest Porterfield, "Mixed Marriage," *Psychology Today*, Vol. 6, No. 8 (January 1973), pp. 71–78.

of industry or desire to be a hard worker, but to the basic concept of treating other persons with fairness and empathy rather than as objects to be manipulated in the service of one's own personal desires. As this quality develops as part of the total process of social maturity it will serve children well, both in the family of their parents and in their future interpersonal relationships, whether these occur in a military academy, a Walden Two commune, or in some future version of an equalitarian marriage.

As children are encouraged to take a relatively objective look at the appropriate contributions of each member to these many and varied tasks, they become consciously aware of a fact that many psychologists feel they already know intuitively, namely, that they are rather completely dependent upon the adult members of the household. The adults obviously provide the money that maintains the household, they take steps to protect their children from injuries and death by accidents, they seek to promote positive health by encouraging the child to eat proper foods, get proper rest, and so forth, and they provide home care or obtain professional care for their children in times of illness.

Children during their developing years need to learn about the burdens and reponsibilities of parenthood as part of the long task of preparing themselves for both the adult decision as to whether to have children and the adult task of caring for children should they become parents themselves. Some appreciation of the effort their own parents are making in their behalf is, of course, appropriate, but children's attitudes toward their parents will probably be improved not so much by belaboring their indebtedness as by making them aware of what they as children are contributing and can contribute to the total welfare of their family. Haim Ginott describes the emotional dynamics that support this approach:

> Parents ask why children are not our friends after all that we do for them. The answer is: They are dependent on us, and dependency breeds hostility. It follows, then, that by diminishing dependency, we can make friends of our children.[7]

The children of two or three generations ago who were raised on the farm before its rather complete mechanization could look forward to the time when the daily chores they performed made a positive contribution to the overall family enterprise. In contrast, modern suburban or urban children may be asked to fold clothes or mow the lawn, chores that appear far less important. "Slopping the hogs" may be mean, dirty work, but to an 11-year-old boy it must seem far closer to "a man's job" than trimming the hedge or weeding the flower bed.

Perhaps the primary function of a family lies in the opportunity it provides for the interchange of love and affection among its members. Here the children are in a somewhat better position to give as well as to receive

[7] Haim Ginott, "Driving Children Sane," *Today's Education* (November–December 1973), p. 22.

212

and thus satisfy in part their need for self-esteem as well as their need for affection. The popular literature leads one to believe that every child represents either an accidental pregnancy or the decision of some culturally brainwashed soul who seeks parenthood as a badge of normality rather than for any intrinsic value it may offer. However, many persons reach a stage in their development where they want and perhaps need the affectional relationship provided by parenthood. Indeed, single persons may defy society's norms as they consciously seek parenthood for the stated purpose of obtaining something of their own they can love and trust. Unfortunately, the success rate for these love affairs appears to be no greater for these parents, married or not, than are the affairs between adults, although the need that motivated them is nonetheless real. Love in any of its forms tends to defy logical analysis or explanation; however, Erik Erikson and many other psychologists believe that expressions of parental love satisfy intrinsic needs for both adult and child.[8]

The key to the success of this important aspect of the parent–child relationship is of course the emotional maturity of the parents, who must provide the setting for this normal growth of their children's personalities and their subsequent abilities to reciprocate appropriately at each stage of development, from their spongelike dependence as infants through their equal partnership of adulthood to their eventual dominance as caretaker, in an emotional sense at least, of their aging parents.

FAMILY SUCCESS and FAMILY PROBLEMS

The practices of entering marriage to resolve the situation created by an unplanned pregnancy, to satisfy the social strivings of one's parents, or simply to meet the social norm that dictates marriage for everyone are fortunately occurring less frequently than in the past. Consequently, there are fewer reasons to establish a family on any other basis than mutual affection and love. Experience has shown, however, that certain rather clearly defined factors serve to determine or strongly influence the future quality and survival of a marriage and family relationship.

Sexual compatibility is often viewed as a factor that determines to a large degree whether a marriage will endure. In specific cases, particularly where there are serious inadequacies or emotional conflicts that are not treated constructively and compassionately, sexual problems can place a severe strain on a marriage. It appears, however, that sexual dissatisfaction more often represents a symptom related to other problems of the relationship rather than a direct cause.

Part of the attraction that leads to the emotional involvement and eventual marriage of two people is the discovery that they value many of the same things, that their important goals are either similar or mutually

8 Erik H. Erikson, *Childhood and Society* (New York: W. W. Norton and Co., Inc., 1963), pp. 266–267.

compatible. Both partners may have important goals related to their work, whether it be "blue collar," professional, or in some commercial field. Each may have definite ideas as to priorities in the allocation of money for home, travel, and savings. When children are involved, each parent may have definite ideas as to the approach toward discipline and the importance of good school performance as opposed to music, athletics, and social development. Religious values in many families can exert strong effects on the relationships among family members. Through time, as financial fortunes improve or erode, as children arrive and develop, a family's values and goals can change considerably. According to the dynamics operating in specific situations and the ability of family members to communicate, these changes can be toward increased agreement and harmony, or toward divergence and conflict.

However, divergence does not have to lead to conflict if another factor important to family unity prevails, specifically, a mutual respect for the integrity of each family member. This means that the uniqueness and individuality of each person are allowed reasonable expression, that both adults and children are allowed to grow and develop along lines of their own choosing. Mother might wish to return to school on a part-time basis; father might choose to take a new job in another city to further his career or to decline a promotion and higher pay because of the nature of the new responsibilities involved; daughter might want to drop piano lessons and join a local swim team; her brother may wish to drop little league baseball and spend more time making model ships and airplanes.

Respecting personal integrity means more than merely granting each person license to "do their own thing." Mother's plans to return to school may place a heavy burden on the older daughter who must now assume many new household duties; conversely, a daughter's new mania for competitive swimming might convert one parent into a perpetual chauffeur. Many other examples could be drawn to illustrate that the family represents human ecology in its most intimate form. Each person's growth or change must be accommodated with this semi-closed system, and accommodation requires, among other things, another major factor, good communication.

The ability to communicate, like most other factors important to human relationships, looks deceptively simply, but deficiency in this skill is a common cause of family disorganization and failure. Too often members of a family operate with their "transmitter on full power" and their "receivers" virtually turned off. They speak in words and phrases that are perfectly clear to themselves, but the person spoken to, assuming he's listening at all, tends to hear what he wants or expects to hear. The problem extends well beyond the realm of semantics or an effort to pay more attention, because good communication requires that feelings be communicated as well as mere ideas. The young mother who exclaims to her husband, "those kids are driving me out of my mind," may be releasing a little tension after a very normal day with a couple of preschoolers, or may be headed for actual suicide or emotional illness; the husband in this instance has the greater responsibility for the accuracy of this exchange because he is more detached from the specific situation. If his wife is indeed close to emotional collapse, she cannot be expected to be as lucid or persistent in her efforts to convey her feelings. Likewise, where children are involved, more mature persons have a greater responsibility to work at the communication process. Children are notorious for expressing ideas that are important to them in language that could appear frivolous to an adult. One cannot, of course, respond to all of a 6-year-old's chatter with great seriousness, but it is necessary to remain alert to notes of urgency and concern, and then listen, watch, and probe until the ideas and feelings have been perceived.

The greater power and influence of adults make it exceedingly difficult for children to take corrective action when patterns of abuse and injustice prevail within their families; however, just as families seldom meet the ideal of agreed-upon goals, well-defined roles, good communication, and mutual respect for each member, they are seldom complete failures. Children who have learned the basic principles of family dynamics in their own terms will be in a better position to contribute to the positive aspects of their families and compensate in part at least for family weaknesses. The child who comes to understand the difficulties involved in true communication can work harder to get through to the parents and may not make so many assumptions that they already know his or her feelings. Children who learn that adults also have dreams and goals toward which they are still striving may be able to better accept the inconveniences these strivings may produce for them. Education cannot solve family problems but it can exert a positive effect on the child's current efforts to function as a junior family member. Where a family education curriculum spans grades K–12, children should be better equipped to someday live in healthy families of their own formation.

SUGGESTED LEARNING ACTIVITIES

The following suggestions are presented in an effort to demonstrate how the content described in the preceding section might be translated into effective classroom learning activities. They were designed to accommodate a wide variety of classroom groups provided that proper selection and adaptations are made according to the needs, interests, abilities, and maturity level of the particular children involved.

- Take pieces of rugs or felt and make a placemat on which the children can sit. Attach the words "The World Around Me." In order to promote positive feelings, ask those children who wish to volunteer to sit for a few moments on the mat and share with the class a person in their life who makes them feel loved and wanted.

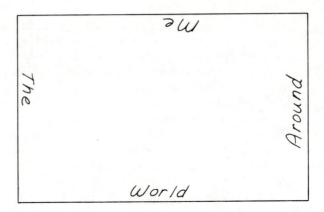

- Inflate different-colored balloons and have the children paint pictures on each balloon representing those people they are most closely associated with (e.g., mother, father, grandparent). If they feel strongly about a pet, they can include it. They may use as many balloons as they need. When they are finished, they should tie their balloons together with yarn or ribbon as a display of those who influence them the most in their lives. Following the activity, have the children share with the other members of the class why they chose the people that they did.

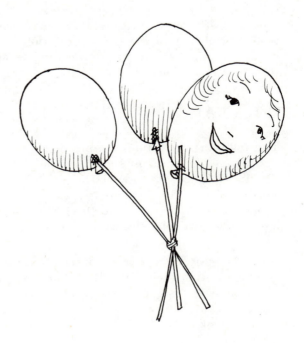

• Have the children make a tree from pipe cleaners and secure it to a stand (e.g., piece of wood, clay). Have them bring in pictures of each member of their family (pets can be included). On the back of the pictures or on a piece of paper hanging from each picture, have the children complete the following phrase for each person they selected for their tree: "I feel good when my_____."

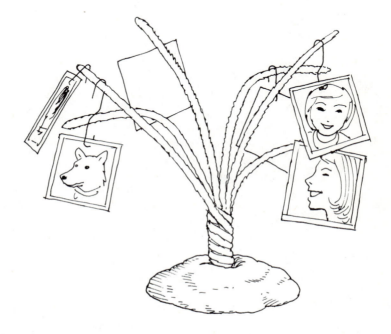

• As the children are studying the various cultures of countries around the world, have them look at family patterns as they existed many years ago and how they may be different or similar today. Example: families in the early 1900s in the United States as compared with today's families.

• Divide the class into four or five groups with each group having only members of one sex. Give each group a piece of newsprint, opaque paper, or shelf paper and crayons or magic markers. Have the groups of boys make a list of all the roles (jobs, sports, etc.) girls should be allowed to be involved in today. Have the girls do the roles for boys. When they are finished, have the students hang their lists up around the room and have all the children look at the other lists. When they are finished doing this, have them discuss how they feel about the lists and ask them if they agree or disagree, and why?

• Ask the children to list the family chores they do each week. Share these lists in a class discussion.

217

• Ask the children to think about "how my family makes me feel"; prepare a work sheet as shown and give the following directions: "In each of the ovals, draw your face when one of your family members tells you the following situation will occur."

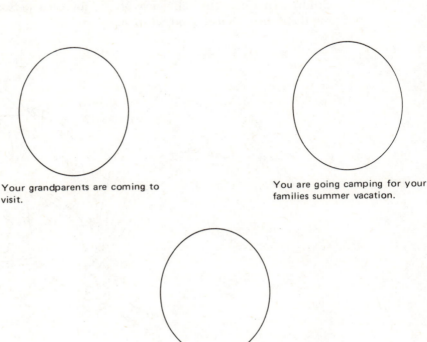

Your grandparents are coming to visit.

You are going camping for your families summer vacation.

Your room needs cleaning

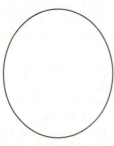

Your pet needs feeding.

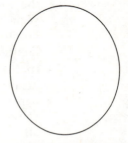

Your mother and father are going away for the weekend and you can't go with them.

• Have the children draw a picture of their father and one of their mother on separate sheets of paper. When they are finished, have the children list on the reverse side those responsibilities that each parent

218

has. (If there are single-parent children, have them draw the one parent or select another relative.) Have the children discuss their pictures with the class and then take the pictures home and discuss them with their parents. On the reverse side of the picture when they have finished discussing the roles, have them complete the following sentence: "I discovered that my father_____."

- Have the children form two circles, one facing in and the other facing out so they have someone standing directly in front of them. Ask the person in the inner circle to tell the classmate facing him or her "one thing that makes me feel good about my family." When the child in the inner circle finishes, have the child in the outer circle make a similar statement. When both are finished, have the child in the inner circle move one person to his or her left. This will continue until all the children in the inner circle have been all the way around.

- Have the children get into groups of four or five. Give each group a piece of newsprint and crayons. As a group, ask them to design the car that will be driven in the year 2000. While designing their auto, they may not communicate verbally with each other, they can make no more than two lines at a time, they cannot make a line again until someone else in the group does, and they must use a different-colored crayon. Allow 10–15 minutes for the activity. Following the activity, have each group tell how and what went on with the group during the activity.

- Ask primary children to draw a "family portrait" with a stick figure or a more elaborate figure for each member of their family. On a new piece of paper, ask them to draw a similar picture of another family with which they're acquainted that they would like to spend a day with in some pleasant activity or activities. After the pictures have been completed, ask for volunteers to describe their own family and tell what they like about the other family of their selection.

- Have the children make a paper chain of different-colored links. On each link have them name the various responsibilities that are needed to make a home run smoothly. When they have completed their chains, have them discuss what would happen if one of the links were to break.

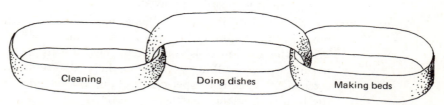

- Have the children make measuring cups from construction paper and then indicate how much time they spend with the following activities:

219

— eating with their parents
— watching TV
— doing homework
— doing chores around the house
— exercising

After making their cups and measuring the amount of time they spend a day on each activity, have them see if there is any portion in one of the cups that they feel should be changed and have them explain why.

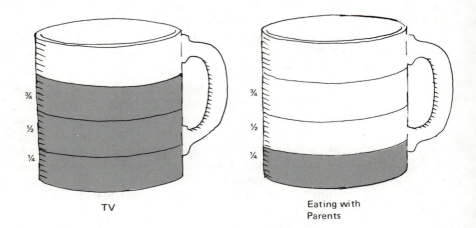

TV   Eating with
                                       Parents

- Ask upper elementary children to pretend that a new national law has been passed that requires all children to be raised in comfortable and well-managed boarding schools whose rules would allow them to see their parents only one day each month on a visit home. Then ask them to write an essay or story telling (1) what things about their home life they would miss most, (2) what things they do with their parents that the parents would miss most, and (3) the way in which they would want to spend their time on their one-day visit. During the ensuing discussion ask the class members to express their feelings about the idea of parent-child separation and why it would be good or bad for the people involved.

- Put the children into triads. Have one member of the group take 2 minutes to tell another member about his or her favorite TV program. When the 2 minutes is completed, have the listener feedback to the person who was talking what he or she said. The third student acts as a recorder to see if the person listening was listening accurately. After the feedback, change partners (roles). If tape recorders are available, tape the sessions to give even more accurate feedback.

SCHOOL HEALTH SERVICE
RELATED to LIVING GROUPS

When the family runs smoothly, a number of important and complex health needs are routinely satisfied; this is a major accomplishment, somewhat of a daily miracle. Unfortunately, most families suffer periods when their functioning is anything but smooth because of serious conflicts between adult partners or between adults and children. These may be mild, brief, and self-healing or severe, protracted, and fatal to the ability of the family to endure or to function in a satisfactory manner. It may be less harmful when an apparently satisfactory family disintegrates suddenly over a period of several weeks because of the discovery of an adulterous relationship or some sudden onset of emotional illness or instability on the part of one of the partners. More commonly, however, troubled marriages "die hard," and endure extended periods of conflict and physical and/or emotional estrangement before the end finally comes.

Where human relationships are involved, the only safe generalization is that "anything can happen." Undoubtedly, some strife-ridden marriage has yielded mature and compassionate children who have benefited from this bizarre nurturing context, but, more often, emotionally vulnerable children in these situations suffer severe and often permanent personality damage. This is often manifested in various symptoms of emotional distress that interfere with academic progress or produce behavioral problems that eventually require professional counseling and/or treatment. As part of the routine procedure in helping the emotionally disturbed children, strong efforts are made to involve the parents in the counseling process; consequently, the underlying marriage problem often comes to light, with the result that marriage counseling is obtained by or for the parents. This additional help will not guarantee success but it may improve the chances for saving the marriage and minimize the harm done to family members. This general situation will be discussed further in Chapter 10 on mental health.

Children are emotionally vulnerable; however, they also are adaptable and possess coping devices to protect themselves to some degree from the malevolent forces of a poor family situation. Any symptoms such children may exhibit as a result of what they are enduring may not be severe enough to justify referral; in some cases, they may even take the form of over-achievement in school tasks. The implications for the teacher here are quite complex and do not lend themselves to any easy formula. The school's primary responsibility is to the child; its relationship to the family, although very real, is nonetheless indirect. Perhaps the most appropriate behavior for teachers is to remain alert to comments and other signs that particular children are enduring troubles at home and provide them emotional support by leaving the way open for them to seek sympathetic understanding in their own way. Human beings are prone to serious problems, and when they happen to be children they may have few people to whom they can turn. One of these persons is their teacher.

One type of case that demands decisive action on the teacher's part is that of the battered child, the child who has been brutally and sometimes seriously injured by his parents. Although infrequent, these cases unfortunately are not rare. As one concerned psychologist writes: "About 40,000 cases of serious injury to children inflicted by parents or their caretakers are recorded annually. Researchers in the field assume this is merely the tip of a iceberg." [9] It has been estimated that about 2,000 American children are murdered by their parents each year—more than the number killed by leukemia or other cancers.

The chain of events and the emotions that result in parental abuse of children are complex and form the object of much study by behavioral scientists. Such research reveals that practically all abusive parents were themselves abused as children, and that most abused children were unwanted by their parents. This suggests that much child abuse can be prevented by encouraging contraception, and by breaking the vicious circle created by societal acceptance of the physical punishment of children as appropriate adult behavior—a potent argument for the absolute prohibition of corporal punishment in schools.

Abused children typically try to hide their injuries and to accept their injuries as justified punishment. Likewise, a nonabusive spouse tends to protect the abuser. The parents tend to take their injured children to a different hospital or physician on each occasion and to claim that the injuries were the result of accidents. Abuse occurs among families of all ethnic groups and all social classes. Careful observation of all children by their teachers for signs of abuse is therefore essential to its detection, and detection is essential to prevent the maiming and murdering of these children. Signs of abuse include withdrawn behavior on the part of a child as well as such obvious indications as the constant wearing of attire that hides arms and legs, bandaged or unbandaged cuts, welts, burns, and bruises.

State laws now generally require both school and health care professionals to report suspected child abuse cases to an agency designated by state law. The law also protects those who report these cases against damage suits should a reported case be found not to be a case of abuse. Most schools have established procedures for reporting; the school nurse is the person usually designated to receive reports from teachers and other adults in the school. Some states like Pennsylvania have established statewide hot lines that may be used to report cases to the authorities.

The objective of most modern abuse laws is the rehabilitation rather than the punishment of offenders. It is recognized that abusive parents,

[9] Arlene S. Kolnick, "Families Can Be Unhealthy for Children and Other Living Things," *Psychology Today*, Vol. 5, No. 3 (August 1971), p. 106.

like alcoholics, need help in controlling their behavior. An organization patterned after Alcoholics Anonymous exists to provide such help. Professional psychological help is also available. If necessary for their protection, abused children can be taken from their families and placed in institutions or foster homes. There should thus be no reluctance on the part of anyone to report suspected cases.

REFERENCES

CRAWFORD, CHARLES O. (ed.) *Health and the Family*. New York: Macmillan Publishing Co., Inc., 1971.

ERIKSON, ERIK H. *Childhood and Society*. New York: W. W. Norton and Co., Inc., 1963.

GINOTT, HAIM. "Driving Children Sane," *Today's Education* (November-December 1973), p. 22.

HENKE, LORRAINE J. "A Health Educator's Role in the Problem of Child Abuse," *Health Education*, Vol. 6, No. 3 (May-June 1975), pp. 15–18.

HETHERINGTON, E. MAVIS. "Girls Without Fathers," *Psychology Today*, Vol. 6, No. 9 (February 1973), pp. 46–52.

KILMAN, ANN. "Children in Crises," *Instructor*, Vol. 84, No. 8 (April 1975), pp. 51–58.

KILWEIN, JOHN H. "Social Class Differences in Family Attitudes," *Journal of School Health*, Vol. 45, No. 1 (January 1975), pp. 27–29.

KOLNICK, ARLENE S. "Families Can Be Unhealthy for Children and Other Living Things," *Psychology Today*, Vol. 5, No. 3 (August 1971), pp. 18–22, 104.

PORTERFIELD, ERNEST. "Mixed Marriage," *Psychology Today*, Vol. 6, No. 8 (January 1973), pp. 71–78.

RAMOTH, JANIS. "A Plea for Aging Education," *Health Education*, Vol. 6, No. 4 (July-August 1975), pp. 4–5.

SORENSON, ROBERT C. *Adolescent Sexuality in Contemporary America*. New York: World Publishing, 1972.

Feelings and Emotions—
Mental Health

10

Few things are more important in the care and education of children than fostering wholesome personality growth. In simple terms this task consists of helping children to feel good about themselves and to get along with other people or, more precisely, encouraging each child to develop (1) a positive self-concept and (2) skills in interpersonal relationships. Those children who are fortunate enough to acquire these qualities have thus managed to avoid what appears to be the single most important obstacle to human well-being. An overwhelming amount of evidence suggests that emotional conflicts, both within the individual and with other persons, contribute heavily to crime, drug abuse, alcoholism, accidents, and the majority of the symptoms of physical illness, as well as such obvious examples as divorce, school adjustment problems, and difficulties in employer–employee relationships.

As one would suspect of something of such singular importance, this worthy goal is receiving priority attention in those American schools where enlightened leadership prevails. Many such schools are putting heavy emphasis on wholesome personality growth within the general guidelines proposed by proponents of humanistic education, and virtually all schools make some effort to meet their responsibilities in this area. Although much progress has been made, the American educational system has come under increasing criticism for not doing more to encourage personality growth, which in lay terminology becomes "character" or "moral development." Regardless of how well the school performs in this area, it is always going to be asked to accomplish more. Much of the explanation for this situation lies in the fact that human personality growth tends to appear simple in principle, yet be anything but simple in practice.

It is all well and good to build up the self-concept of children with praise and to admonish them to be kind to one another, but this simplistic strategy soon becomes hampered by a whole host of competing priorities and goals. Society dictates not only that its members develop pleasant personal qualities but also that they "produce," and, to the child, production translates into school achievement with its inevitable personal and competitive pressure. Additional stress results from the need to "conform" to reasonable standards of behavior as exemplified by the old saying "your right to swing your fist ends where my nose begins." Most examples of personal interaction are not so clear-cut; it thus becomes easy for well-meaning children, and adults, to violate the rights of others without realizing the fact. The development of fair and equitable ways of dealing with parents, peers, teachers, and others involves ordinary cognitive learning as well as an appeal to the value-laden qualities of fair play and ethical standards.

THE MENTAL HEALTH PROGRAM

The responsibilities of the elementary school in the realm of mental health include providing (1) a healthful emotional environment in the classroom, in the cafeteria, on the playground, and in all other school settings; (2) appropriate mental health services, including the identification and referral of students who appear to need clinical treatment; and (3) direct instruction leading to the development of knowledge and skills related to mental health. Of these three areas of concern, the first clearly merits top priority. Good mental health is based on wholesome personality growth—a process that is influenced by a host of environmental factors. The school is second only to the home as the setting in which this process takes place. Relatively few children require such direct mental health services as treatment or counseling related to emotional conflicts in the form these services presently take; however, those children with overt emotional problems typically present the most urgent and pressing challenge within these three areas of responsibility, if not the most important. A more detailed discussion of the classroom teacher's role related to these two areas will be presented in subsequent sections of this chapter; this portion will be concerned with the educational aspects of mental health.

TEACHING MENTAL HEALTH?

The growth and development of a child's personality appear to be a continuous process that begins at birth and continues into adulthood at the very least and until death if one accepts the more recent philosophical swing toward the views of Erik Erikson and others of the lifetime development school.[1] Every experience—every emotional event—exerts some degree of influence, however large or small it may be. How then can a teacher hope to "teach" something that is so obviously a part of the child's everyday existence? The answer lies in one of the fundamental truisms of the educational process. Children cannot be "taught" anything—but they can be helped to learn. Carefully planned learning situations can facilitate their sharing with one another many important concerns regarding themselves and their relationship with the significant persons in their lives. They can become familiar with the basic pattern of personality development and thus gain valuable reassurance that they are indeed normal. Even the simple matter of acquiring useful terminology, of becoming familiar with the meaning of "self-esteem," "self-confidence," "trust," "anxiety," and "depression" is very helpful, as reasoning, insight, and good communcation are somewhat dependent upon vocabulary development. In these and other important ways, a relatively small amount of time spent in direct instruction in the area of mental health can yield disproportionately large benefits.

A POSITIVE APPROACH

Although some attention should be devoted to the study of mental illness in terms of its general characteristics, the single most important task of the mental health curriculum is to help children keep their personalities growing in a positive direction. The pursuit of this goal can yield direct benefits to more than 90 per cent of the children of any classroom who are normal or average in terms of mental health without doing any disservice to the occasional child with pressing emotional problems who must be accommodated within the group. Such a child needs treatment more than education. Moreover, if the survey findings of the mental health status of the general population are to be accepted, one must conclude that the average personality has plenty of room for improvement. The most widely quoted of these studies, The Mid-Town Manhattan Study,[2] identified 58 per cent of the population as "mildly to moderately disturbed." Similar investigations in such widely separated localities as Connecticut and Nova Scotia yielded basically the same results.[3] The conclusion that the average person suffers from low-grade mental illness may be challenged on the grounds that the

[1] See, for example, Erik H. Erikson, *Childhood and Society* (New York: W. W. Norton and Co.,) , 1963.
[2] Leo Srole et al., *Mental Health in the Metropolis: The Mid-Town Manhattan Study* (New York: McGraw-Hill, 1962) , p. 138.
[3] Bruce P. Dohrenwend, "II. Psychiatric Disorders in General Populations: Problem of the Untreated 'Case,'" *American Journal of Public Health*, Vol. 60, No. 6 (June 1970) , p. 1055.

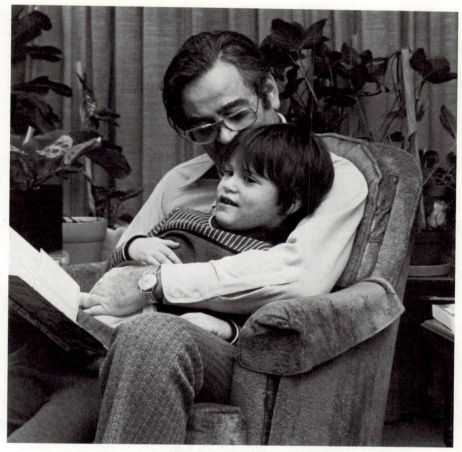

Figure 10.1. Developing Positive Feelings of Self-worth. (Sheila Bernstein)

standards were set too high, but regardless of what terms one chooses to apply, it seems clear that to be "average" or "normal" in our society by present-day criteria is no great accomplishment. Most children should aspire for something better.

CHILDREN'S INTERESTS as RELATED to MENTAL HEALTH

The investigation by Ruth Byler and her associates recorded many specific expressions of interests related to mental health on the part of elementary school children. A few representative comments and findings are included in this section to acquaint the reader with the way children of differing maturity levels approach this subject.[4]

Kindergarten Through Grade Two

• Interests of children of these ages as well as of all ages include seeking and finding congenial playmates. This involves interaction that gives rise to many aggravations and temporary concerns, some of which reach the teacher's ears. So strong is the drive to seek friends, and such a mark of basic well-being is the child's ability to play and work happily with other children, that teachers have learned to be concerned about the child who stands apart, or the child who seeks happiness in constantly running the show.

Grades Three and Four

• Third grade children reveal considerable confusion regarding the terminology and the substance of mental health. In answer to the question, "What is mental health?" third graders say: You are very weak and have to have a wheelchair. Sometimes people don't play with you. They think you are dull or stupid. . . . Why are some children mentals?
• Fourth graders ask numerous questions relative to understanding the self. These reveal self-examination, a desire to "see oneself as others see us": I would like to know what others think of me on the outside. They also begin to know the feeling of loneliness and its causes, and fear and its causes . . . .

Grades Five and Six

• Fifth graders ask: Why do my friends like me sometimes and sometimes not? Can we prevent from being liked or disliked [sic]? Why do some kids urge others into fights?
• Sixth graders ask: Why is there a scapegoat in every group of people? Why do some people have love and understanding in their hearts and some have hatred? Why are boys not supposed to fight with girls or say fresh things to them?

CONTENT OVERVIEW

The body of scientific information and theory that underlies the study of mental health and personality development is so vast that any attempt to deal with it within a single chapter must necessarily be restricted to the bare essentials. Furthermore, the general lack of consensus as to the nature of these essentials requires the authors of any such attempt to interject their

[4] Ruth Byler, Gertrude Lewis, and Ruth Totman, *Teach Us What We Want to Know* (New York: Mental Health Materials Center, Inc., 1969).

own personal values and idiosyncrasies to a significant degree. As always, readers are advised to interpret content suggestions in light of their own professional orientation and the realities of their own teaching situation.

ME and MY SELF-CONCEPT

The natural activities of children bring them in contact with a wide variety of people, objects, and situations. As these contacts accumulate, children amass a large body of information concerning themselves and the world in general. Also, as their neural systems mature and as they develop physically, the depth of their insights and the scope of their living experiences increase. Most psychologists, particularly those of the humanistic school such as Sidney Jourard,[5] maintain that children soon begin to organize the information they acquire into meaningful generalizations or concepts of those things of interest to them. For instance, a young child may become aware that a favorite toy is soft and brown, that it has black buttons for eyes, and that its name is "Teddy." The child may also understand that it is "my" teddy bear and that no one can (or should) take it away. All of this information is organized into the child's concept of the toy, and, in addition to this cognitive aspect, the concept includes all of the feelings that are attached to this object. The child may feel that "Teddy" is pleasant to squeeze, that he is good, that "he loves me" and "I love him."

In a similar fashion the child forms the far more important concept of himself or herself. This concept must be accurate and realistic in terms of skills, abilities, and responsibilities if the child is to make good decisions as to what tasks or situations are to be attacked or avoided. These cognitive or informational aspects are intimately related to the affective or valuing aspect of the child's self-concept, which consists of his or her beliefs regarding personal worthiness, virtueness, and lovability. All manner of good things happen when self-concepts are positive rather than negative. Life immediately becomes more pleasant—more worth living; self-concern and self-doubt fade into the background and the child's full attention and energies become available to meet the challenges provided by school, play, and social interaction. There is a tendency to reach out toward others in positive ways—to give praise and compliments, to help those in need, and to solicit and accept help from others. These behaviors contrast with the withdrawn child who thinks of himself as inept and unworthy and tends to keep to himself. He may feel, "Who cares what I might say anyhow?" "Who would want to help me?" "Who would want my help?" Another more outgoing child with a negative self-concept might reach out to others but in a very hostile fashion, acting on the rationale that "Because I am not worthy of anyone's love or care, I must use strength, fear, or trickery to get the things

[5] Sidney M. Jourard, *Healthy Personality* (New York: Macmillan Publishing Co., Inc., 1972).

I need." It is not difficult to see how either positive or negative patterns can feed on themselves as the reactions of others tend to confirm each child's basic impression of himself or herself.

SELF-LOVE. Perhaps the most important of the benefits of feeling good about oneself is the increased ability to form strong bonds of love and affection with others. Erich Fromm discusses positive feelings about one's self in terms of "self-love," which he places in opposition to "selfishness." He endorses the biblical injunction to "Love thy neighbor as thyself," and goes on to explain

> . . . love of others and love of self are not alternatives. On the contrary, an attitude of love toward themselves will be found in all those who are capable of loving others. *Love*, in principle, *is indivisible as far as the connection between "objects" and one's own self is concerned.*[6]

Children who feel themselves unworthy of love cannot fully receive love

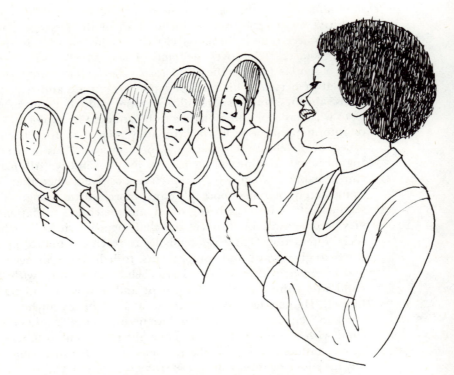

If they really knew what sort of person I am . . . . .

[6] Erich Fromm, *The Art of Loving* (New York: Harper & Brothers Publishers, 1956), pp. 58, 59.

from others. When others express love toward them, these children either question its sincerity or feel that it is based on misconceptions; they feel, "If they really knew what sort of person I am they wouldn't love me—someday they'll find out." The anxiety related to such a point of view tends to keep such individuals so preoccupied with their own problems that they have little of the time or energy that genuine concern for others requires.

FOSTERING POSITIVE FEELINGS. There are a number of important things teachers can do to help children develop valid, positive self-concepts. For reasons probably related to each human's long period of almost total dependency during infancy and early childhood, children tend to rely on the clues, reactions, and direct remarks of other people as they seek to judge what sort of persons they themselves are. Later, they will become more autonomous and self-reliant, but during their elementary school years they are quite vulnerable to the judgment of others. Teachers can structure discussions and other learning experiences where children are encouraged to say good things about one another and, because all persons have good points, such support can be sincere. Unfortunately, children in our society tend to be fair game for direct criticisms and negative innuendoes that would seldom be directed toward adults in similar circumstances. Consequently, they tend to hear far more of what is bad about themselves than what is good. Appropriate classroom activities can bring some balance to this situation.

SELF-DISCIPLINE. Compliments are most gratifying when they are preceded by honest revelations about oneself: "They know how I really am, yet they still think I'm OK!" Kindergarten–primary children tend to be quite open about themselves, although they are often honestly confused concerning their strengths and weaknesses. However, older children soon begin to "put on fronts" or "façades" in their attempt to appear more favorable to others and to themselves. It is inappropriate and sometimes dangerous for teachers to encourage young people to venture too far into the area of self-disclosure, but it is helpful for children to drop their defenses somewhat and admit that they were afraid or embarrassed by certain situations. This process actually helps them find out more about themselves, and, within a classroom situation where an atmosphere of honesty and trust has been established, they are often delighted to find out that neither the teacher nor their classmates think less of them for revealing a few of their weaknesses—the others understand because many of them realize they have similar characteristics.

GETTING ALONG with OTHERS

CRUCIAL IMPORTANCE. The ability to interact smoothly and constructively with other people is one of the most important factors in the determination

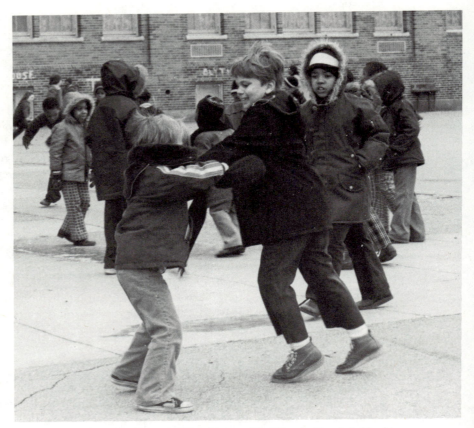

Figure 10.2. Getting Along with Others. (Carol Ashton)

of individual levels of well-being. At the personal level the deep human needs for affection and companionship require interpersonal skills for their fulfillment; in the business, professional, and vocational worlds the ability to deal effectively with superiors, peers, and subordinates is usually crucial to success; even in the somewhat chaotic world of theater and entertainment the most successful performers are often those who can quickly sense the audience's reaction—who can empathize with their fans and meet their expectations. At the opposite extreme we find bright children who fail at school because of "adjustment" problems, workers fired or passed over for promotion because they just don't "fit in," and bitter third-time divorced types who have concluded that the main thing in life is to "look out for number one because no one else really gives a damn." Although many of these examples are admittedly oversimplified, the importance of interpersonal skills in present-day society cannot be over emphasized.

SKILL DEVELOPMENT.   Much of how children get along with others depends as much on *who* they are as *what* they do. Children who are secure with themselves and who have had their own basic needs fulfilled tend to develop comfortable ways of interacting with others. Children who are drifting into a neurotic pathway for lack of companionship need some healthier person who can offer them companionship—meet their needs—despite their unfriendly behavior; the odds of such a relationship occurring are raised if these children can learn to make overtures and to reciprocate. Even if these efforts are clumsy and insincere at first, they may provide the opportunity for continued involvement and the development of honest companionship as time passes.

One of the most effective ways a teacher can assist the development of interpersonal skills is to utilize every reasonable opportunity to organize children into cooperative working groups for the completion of learning tasks. A social science unit on "Native Americans" might involve the construction of a model Indian village, with one group working on teepees or lodges, another on canoes, another on trees and scenery, and so forth. Here the friendless child—the social isolate—can be gently forced into a group in a highly structured and protected situation where each person knows what is expected of him or her and where classroom rules or norms prohibit excessive ridicule and encourage fair conduct. Here, the satisfaction and skills gained from interpersonal interaction may be of equal or greater significance than what is learned about the Indian village.

As important as these correlated learning experiences may be, some time should be spent in the direct instruction of interpersonal skills in a unit on personality and/or mental health. The unit content can be simply and effectively organized on the basis of the significant categories of persons with whom the children interact. Parents and siblings form important categories that may be dealt with either in the larger areas of family living or in the mental health area, depending on the local curriculum. This study is of obvious benefit to those children from intact families who have brothers or sisters; however, the only child also needs to know about sibling relationships and the role of the absent parent as part of his or her general knowledge of American society. Peer relationships comprise another highly important area of obvious value, as do teacher–pupil interactions. This latter category provides a model for many other leader–follower patterns in which children may become involved such as participation in clubs and youth groups, athletic teams, and music and drama groups. Relationships with strangers is another important category with many important ramifications including the need for caution in unprotected circumstances and the need for both courteousness and occasional assertiveness in other situations.

Although the appropriate applications may vary, certain general principles provide guidance in all human relationships. This task is clearly more of an art than a science, therefore, the various authorities may differ. However, a few of the more well supported factors are:

1. *Empathy.* As people become more emotionally mature, they develop the capacity to "put themselves in the other person's shoes" or "to get inside their heads" and become aware, not only of what they know but also of how they feel. This tends to encourage less resentment of those in authority ("now that I know what they are up against"), more skillful leadership of subordinates, and more sympathetic and helpful behavior in a variety of situations. Ideally, it should also help the child recognize when he or she is being "bullied" and thus encourage the assertion of personal rights.

2. *Honest Communication.* The development of the courage and skill to express one's true feeling is helpful in the formation of a valid self-concept. This quality also facilitates good interpersonal relationships. It is possible to be too expressive—to unnecessarily burden others with your feelings; however, the more common tendency is to "cover up"—to not broach a topic when discussion is needed. For example, one of a young girl's good friends might fall into a pattern of teasing her on a sensitive topic, with a consequent buildup of resentment. Often the relationship may be saved if the injured party will speak up and let the friend know that things have gone too far. A boy might truly feel that a teacher was treating him unfairly. If allowed to persist, such a situation could easily lead to poor schoolwork and a widening breach with the teacher. Such negative consequences can often be averted if the child will seek an opportunity to discuss the matter. Positive feelings should also be more frequently expressed. When children like what someone is doing or wearing, for example, it is good that they develop the habit of telling them about it. The child thus not only makes the other person feel better but also builds up a surplus of good will that may be needed later, on perhaps less pleasant occasions.

3. *Genuine Concern for Others.* It is probably impossible to *teach* children to be genuinely concerned for others. This quality appears to arise spontaneously among children who have developed a positive self-concept and the ability to empathize with other persons. However, the guidance and supervision of a mature person can lead to increased opportunities to exercise this skill and thus hasten its development. Both classroom activities that are planned purely for social interaction and activities that involve social interaction as part of some larger purpose, as in the Indian village project, can help children learn to depend on one another and appreciate the friendship and help they receive.

CARING for and FEEDING a PERSONALITY

Most children are quick to grasp the fact that they possess bodies that require proper care and nourishment if they are to grow tall and strong. But it is considerably more difficult for them to understand that their respective personalities are of equal or greater importance than their bodies and that personalities also have important needs that must be met if their potential for emotional and social growth is to be realized. Children often learn to take an active role in their physical development as they attempt to eat the proper foods, obtain healthful exercise, and observe certain safety precautions to avoid accidents or excessive stress, yet they tend to drift passively along the line of least resistance where social and emotional experiences are concerned.

It would, of course, be unwise to encourage school children to embark on a program of rigorous self-examination and character development. Personalities are not built—they grow. However, a basic understanding of this process can help children understand what the responsible adults in their lives are seeking to do for them. Also, they can begin to develop insights that will be helpful as they move toward adolescence and more independent decision making. Personality structure and development can be explained by use of any one of several acceptable theories, most of which give attention to the following general categories:

NEEDS AND GOALS. Virtually all psychologists accept the concept that humans possess certain innate needs such as those for food or sexual gratification that are either present at birth or that develop as a natural part of the maturing process. There is considerable disagreement as to the specific nature and extent of innate needs because of the difficulty in distinguishing between a need that is innate—inborn—and one that is acquired by living experience. The need for wealth and material possessions seems to be clearly learned or acquired, whereas the need for food is clearly innate. However, the needs for affection, power, and self-esteem are thought to be basically innate by the humanistic psychologists, whereas the behavioristic school feels these needs are learned. Although the issue of innate versus acquired needs is of great scientific interest, it has limited practical significance. Regardless of whether it arises from our genes or our early social experience, the human desire for affection, social recognition, and other common factors represents a near-universal characteristic that must be taken into account.

Basic needs are universal, but goals are more clearly human creations that can be reviewed and modified. However, once a child establishes proficiency in music or athletics as an internalized goal, it can become nearly as powerful as the need for food as a motivator of behavior and as a potential source of satisfaction or emotional stress. The formation of realistic goals is dependent on the validity of the self-concept, that is, on the ability to carry out a hard appraisal of personal strengths and weaknesses. It is obviously inappropriate to force school-age children into lifelong commitments; however, it is very useful for them to become familiar with the goal-setting process and to realize that they can take an active role in this process as opposed to the too-common process of drifting into unexamined channels.

VALUES. Although values are similar and may be identical to goals, they often carry moral or ethical overtones that tend to restrain or redirect behavior rather than to provide clear direction. The goal of academic achievement may encourage systematic study and close attention in class, but the value of honesty prevents the zeal for good grades from leading to cheating on exams. A 4-year-old girl might dearly wish to play with the children across the street but restrict herself to her own side in accordance with the wishes of her safety-conscious parents. Here we see the effects of the value of obedience to authority or obedience to parents. Values can clearly provide useful guidance to behavior; however, values, if they are to make their optimum contribution to the child's well-being, must be (1) constructive and worth holding and (2) clearly identified by the child involved. As shown in a following section, various classroom techniques exist that can help children identify and examine their own values without exerting any untoward pressure on them to change their basic beliefs.

SKILLS AND ABILITIES. The layperson seldom thinks of skills and abilties as a personality component, yet what children can do and how they go about it are factors that help determine who they are. The many skills and abilities that each child possesses can be organized into various broad categories according to the particular theoretical approach one chooses to follow. A serviceable model for introducing children to the topic is as follows:

1. *Basic Cognitive and Motor Skills.* This group includes such direct, forthright qualities as intelligence, reading ability, motor coordination, muscular strength, artistic ability, and so forth. The eventual level of performance that a child achieves in most of these attributes generally represents some interaction of genetic potential, formal and informal learning experiences, and personal effort. Each of these three factors provides important implications for the mental health curriculum. Children should learn to recognize and accept the fact that genetic factors provide some individuals with natural advantages over others; they should learn to understand the nature and value of environmental factors as they affect the development of human potential and develop an early allegiance to the American "core value" of equal opportunity for all; finally, they should come to realize the extent

236

to which concentrated personal effort can offset genetic or environmental handicaps. Although these concepts may seem somewhat abstract
and esoteric, kindergarten children already know these things in hazy
and often confused terms; with a little outside help they can begin
to sharpen and clarify these important points.

2. *General Strategies.* As people react to various situations, their behavior
tends to fall into typical patterns that can be identified and labeled as
aggressive, deliberate, dependent, and so forth. When presented with
new tasks, one child will typically attack them immediately with
independence, confidence, and enthusiasm, and will realize succes or
disaster depending upon the nature of each task and his or her
abilities. Another child, when confronted with the same task, will
typically ask many questions and request assistance and thus succeed
when a more deliberate approach was needed but fail in those situations requiring a quick response. These patterns carry over into interpersonal relationships. Here, one child who is treated unfairly by a
classmate may respond vigorously and aggressively, another may endure
the insult and "even the score" later in some "sneaky" way, another
may immediately run to a parent or teacher for justice, and still another may seek to negotiate a fair compromise. Ideally, children must
be guided toward a flexible pattern in which the response is appropriate
to the situation. However, children also must learn that there are
limits to this flexibility, that some people are more assertive and others
are more timid, some are more impulsive and others are more deliberate, and that there are advantages and disadvantages to each pattern.

3. *Coping Devices.* Because of deficiencies in ability or the limitations of
practical factors in the environment, children are frequently unable
to satisfy their needs by direct, overt behavior. Even in the most carefully organized school, for example, children are occasionally going
to be pressured to complete school tasks that are beyond their ability;
also, the rather fickle, unstable social world of the elementary schoolchild places severe emotional stress on virtually every child once in
a while. In many instances children face these disappointments directly
—they suffer the pain and either trim their expectations or intensify
their efforts to improve their academic or social skills. Their personalities grow as they are "toughened" by the "school of hard knocks." In
grows as they are "toughened" by the "school of hard knocks." In
other cases, however, the burden is too great and the child is forced
to use an emotional "crutch" in the form of a coping device or defense
mechanism. Although some of the minor devices such as gum chewing,
finger tapping, or the use of profanity are subject to a reasonable
amount of conscious control, other more important ones such as rationalization, projection, and fantasy appear to operate at the unconscious level.

Most elementary teachers are familiar with these common mental mechanisms but often overlook this automatic unconscious quality. True rationalization, for example, is not merely the offering of a plausible excuse for dubious behavior; an "excuse" may be effective in fending off the attacks of the child's teachers, parents, or peers but does little for personal feelings of guilt and incompetence. If anything, it intensifies anxiety; however, true rationalization has a near-magical quality because it alters the child's perception of the realities of the situation; it could cause a girl to believe that the severe beating she administered to her little brother was motivated by her desire to discipline him for some misdeed rather than by her jealousy of him as a rival for parental affection. There would be no feelings of guilt because she believed in her heart that she had acted properly.

Probably the teacher's most important responsibility with regard to coping devices is to handle school assignments and guide social behavior within the classroom in such a manner that the children are challenged but not overwhelmed and consequently forced to retreat into the use of these devices. From an educational standpoint there is considerable value in helping children gain a basic understanding of every person's capacity for self-deception. Although one is not able to consciously avoid the use of a major defense mechanism, it is possible to see evidence of its use "after the fact" in one's own behavior and in the responses of others. This ability tends to discourage excessively harsh judgments and leads to increased levels of empathy and insight.

SUGGESTED LEARNING ACTIVITIES

The following suggestions are presented in an effort to demonstrate how the content described in the preceeding section might be translated into effective classroom learning activities. They were designed to accommodate a wide variety of classroom groups provided that proper selection and adaptations are made according to the needs, interests, abilities, and maturity level of the particular children involved.

- Have the children cut out the word "PEOPLE" as they would if they were cutting out paper dolls. Shelf paper would be good material to use for this activity. As a class project, have the children fill in each letter with pictures they have drawn or cut out from magazines that represent those qualities that each person needs to get along with people such as a good sense of humor, kindness, honesty, and helpfulness. An initial planning session may be needed to discuss and list these characteristics. Using string, have the children hang their banner up in the school cafeteria.

- With the use of the opaque projector and construction paper, have each child make a silhouette of his or her head. When the children are finished, have them write on the silhouette all the positive things they feel about themselves.

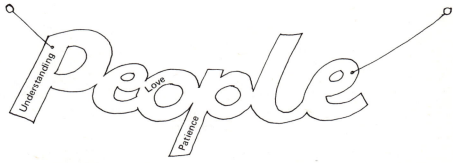

- Many people find different ways to handle their emotional conflicts. Have the children develop a list of all the ways they can think of to deal with emotions and conflict. When they have exhausted their list, have them write each method on a 3 × 5 card; color code and alphabetise these cards and put them in an "emotions" box. When the children feel they need a method to deal with their emotions, they can refer to the box. New ways to deal with emotions may be added to the box as they are discovered.

- Have the children select one day when they will give only positive feedback to anyone they talk to. At the end of the day, have them record how they felt when they said something nice to someone and what the other person's reactions were to their positive communication.

- To help the children learn how to get along with all types of people, have the upper elementary children volunteer their time to help out in the community in anyway that they can (e.g., read a story to a shut-in, clean someone's yard with no money involved).

- Many times we are able to tell how people feel by the look on their faces. Have the children look through magazines and cut out pictures of people expressing different emotions. If an appropriate picture cannot be found, write the emotion on a card. Put all the pictures and cards in a box labeled "Box of Emotions." Form the class into a circle; have one child select a picture or card from the box and role-play it for the entire class. Have the class members in the circle guess the emotion. Because we can usually tell a person's emotion by his or her facial expression, try putting a pillow case over the role-player's head and see if the students can guess the emotion without seeing the face.

239

- Have the children construct two "wheels of good and poor personalities." On one wheel hub they are to write "Good Personality" and then construct and label as many spokes as they feel there are traits for a good personality. They are to repeat the activity for the second wheel using the traits of a poor personality.

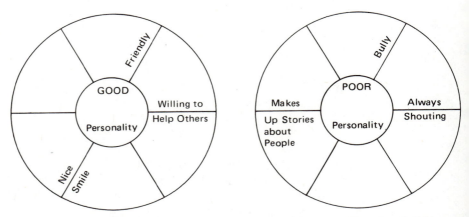

- Take an old white bed sheet and place it on the floor. Give the children crayons or magic markers and have them write on it all the words they can think of that say "PRAISE".

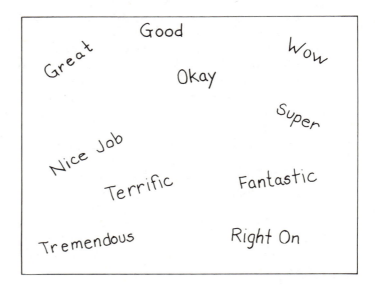

- Have the children print their first names vertically, one letter after the other. After each letter, have them write a feeling word describing themselves or draw a picture. The feeling word should start with the same letter as the letters in their names.

B - busy   A - ability
i - intelligent   n - nice
L - likeable   g - great
L - loveable   e - energetic
                  L - likeable
                  a - adventurer

- Have each child construct out of cardboard a large letter "I" approximately 1 foot wide and 2 feet high. Have them make a collage of how they feel about themselves on the "I." They may use any materials they would like (e.g., dried foods, pictures, yarn, buttons).

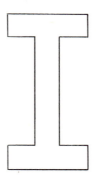

- One's feelings are never constant, they are ever-changing. Some of the situations that make our feelings change are passing a test you thought you failed, someone saying you have a warm smile, going to recess, etc. Because of this constant change throughout the day, the class and teacher often do not know how each other is feeling. The following activity will help correct this situation:

Construct a large "thermometer of emotions" and place it near the door. Have the children decide what feelings they would like on the thermometer. Then have each child print their names on arrows that will adhere to the thermometer. Have the children start the day by indicating how they feel in the morning. Whenever their feelings change, they are free to change their arrow on the thermometer.

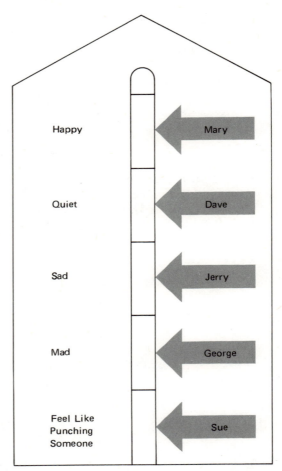

- Ask each child to make an outline of his/her hand on a piece of newsprint and fill it in with a "handfull of strong points." The most important personal quality should be written on the thumb, the next most important on the index finger, and so forth.
- Before the close of school each week, leave time for the children to share with the rest of the class their thoughts regarding the following statement: "This week I felt good when_____."
- Have the children design a plaque for themselves of the five most important things they would like to accomplish in life. You might want

242

to provide some common categories of life activities such as vocational, social, religious, educational, recreational, travel, and so forth. You may want to leave them on their own. Have the children discuss their plaques with the other children and then take them home to display in their bedrooms as a reminder of the things they would like to do or, as they grow and change, the things they would like to change from the original plaque.

- Have the children construct a mobile of what they think a friend is.
- Have the children design a mirror and cover the portion that would reflect an image with aluminum foil. On the aluminum foil have them stick the following letters: "My weakness I need to work on . . ." Once or twice a week have the children get into groups and share with the other members of the group the weakness that they have been working on. This will provide the children an opportunity to see that other people have weaknesses too and that all can do something to correct them.

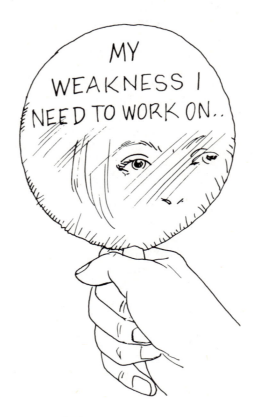

SUGGESTED RESOURCES

The learning resources listed in this section are a selected sample of materials with which the authors are personally familiar. Appropiate grade levels have been included when these were indicated by the source.

BOOKS

About Values
The Human Values Series
 (Grades 1–6)
Arnspiger, Brill, Rucker
Stech-Vaughn, Co.
Austin, Texas

Child Mental Health Core Library
National Institute of Mental Health
5600 Fishers Lane
Rockville, Maryland 20052

I Am Loveable and Capable
Sidney Simon
Argus Communications
Niles, Illinois 60648

Mental Health at School
National Institute of Mental Health
5600 Fishers Lane
Rockville, Maryland 20052

Promoting Mental Health in the Classroom
Handbook for Teachers
Karne Tood
National Institute of Mental Health
5600 Fishers Lane
Rockville, Maryland 20052

What Makes Me Feel This Way
Eda Le Shan
Macmillan Publishing Co., Inc.
866 Third Ave.
New York, New York 10022

CURRICULA

Dimensions of Personality Series
Cebco Plaum Publishing Co.
104 Fifth Ave.
New York, New York 10011

Human Development Program
Harold Bessell, U. Palomares
(Grades K–3, 4–6)
El Cajon, California

Life Skills for Health
Focus on Mental Health
(Grades K–3, 4–6)
Robert Frye
Drug Education Program
Division of Health Safety
State Education Department
Raleigh, North Carolina

FILM

The Kingdom of Could Be You
Encyclopedia Britannica
Educational Corp.
425 N. Michigan Ave.
Chicago, Illinois 60611

FILMSTRIPS

Nancy and Sluggo—Report Card Day
Colgate Palmolive Company

Sesame Street for Growing
Personal Growth and Development
(Grades K–2)
Guidance Associates
757 Third Ave
New York, New York 10017

GAMES/ACTIVITIES

Elementary Squirms
CDCC
P.O. Box 262
Campbell, California 95008

Helping Hands Value Game
(Grades K–4)
CDCC
P.O. Box 262
Campbell, California 95008

How Do You Feel Hats
(Grades K–1)
Six Role Playing Hats That Make Things Happen
Trend Enterprises
St. Paul, Minnesota 55165

I'm Glad That I Am Me
A Book of Activities
Dr. Frank Brouillet
State Superintendent of Public Instruction
Olympia, Washington 98504

100 Ways to Enhance Self-concept in the Classroom
Handbook for Teachers
Jack Canfield, Harold Wells
Prentice-Hall, Inc.
Englewood Cliffs, New Jersey

KITS

Developing Understanding of Self and Others
Kit of Activities and Materials
Designed to help children grow emotionally and socially
Don Dinkmeyer
Kit #1—K–3
Kit #2—4–6
Developing an Understanding of Self and Others
American Guidance Service Inc.
Publisher's Building
Circle Pines, Minnesota 55014

246

POSTERS

Moods and Emotions
Teaching Pictures
Grades K–3
Sylvia Fester
David C. Cook Publishing Co.
Elgen, Illinois 60120

RECORDS

Free to Be You and Me
Marlo Thomas
Bell Records
New York, New York 11972

TELEVISION SERIES

Inside Out Series
Grades 3–5
Agency for Instructional Television
Bloomington, Indiana
(Check your local public service TV station)

HEALTH SERVICE ASPECTS

Mental health services within the school are generally provided by a psychological services unit separate from other school health services, but often included with the health service unit and the attendance services under a department or division of pupil personnel services. The extensiveness of mental health services in a school, like the scope of any other school program, is determined by the amount of funds provided. Some building staffs will include a full-time guidance counselor and/or crisis teacher, others will not. Social workers, psychologists, and even psychiatrists may be available but are not generally assigned to elementary schools on a full-time basis. In addition, community mental health centers also provide psychological services to schools. The amount of professional staff time available from any or all of these sources is generally inadequate to meet the needs for service. Whereas school physicians and nurses are generally legally prohibited from providing diagnostic and treatment services to children, psychological services staff members are not thus restrained. What they can do is what the state of their art and the hours in a day permit them to do.

Case finding is almost always dependent on teacher observation of pupil behavior in terms of whether or not it conforms to that expected for the sex, age, and social group to which a given child belongs. The difficulty teachers face is in determining whether a given behavior is the result of naughtiness, which merits appropriate noncorporal disciplinary action, or of a socioemotional problem, in which case the pupil may need assistance. There are no set guidelines; the ability to distinguish between the two is acquired by the study of child psychology and by experience.

Teachers are expected to handle disciplinary problems by themselves or with the help of a designated person, usually an assistant principal, if they need it. A teacher who has the time to do so may also be able to help a pupil cope in a direct and healthful way with disturbing problems of a socioemotional nature. If not, or if the problem is complex or chronic in nature, then a referral to psychological services is usually in order. The problem is that acutely disturbed children as well as misbehaving ones need immediate appropriate adult responses. This is usually available only in schools with crisis rooms to which such pupils may be referred at any time. In such rooms, the crisis teacher may provide either help with a socioemotional problem or open disapproval of naughty behavior, depending on the needs of the child.

ENVIRONMENTAL ASPECTS

Disturbed and disturbing behavior is likely to occur less frequently in small schools, where the teachers and pupils know each other, than in large schools where pupils are relatively anonymous and adult behavior is depersonalized. A good school climate or socioemotional environment is enhanced by a balance between freedom and structure appropriate to the age of the pupils; this balance can be provided through opportunities for youngsters to practice self-discipline and assume responsibilities, by the provision of a variety of ways for pupils to learn, and by practices dictated generally by a humanitarian philosophy.[7]

REFERENCES

BERNE, ERIC. *Games People Play*. New York: Grove Press, Inc., 1966.
_____. *What Do You Say After You Say Hello?* New York: Bantam Books, Inc., 1972.

[7] Robert S. Fox et al., *School Climate Improvement: A Challenge to the School Administrator* (Bloomington, Ind.: Phi Delta Kappa, undated).

DOHRENWEND, BRUCE P. "II. Psychiatric Disorders in General Populations: Problems of the Untreated 'Case,' " *American Journal of Public Health,* Vol. 60, No. 6 (June 1970), p. 1052.

ERIKSON, ERIK H. *Childhood and Society.* New York: W. W. Norton and Co., Inc., 1963.

FROMM, ERICH. *The Art of Loving.* New York: Harper & Brothers Publishers, 1956.

HARRIS, THOMAS A. *I'm OK—You're OK.* New York: Harper & Row, Publishers, 1967.

JOURARD, SIDNEY M. *Healthy Personality.* New York: Macmillan Publishing Co., Inc., 1972.

MASLOW, ABRAHAM H. *Motivation and Personality.* New York: Harper & Row, 1970.

MENNINGER, KARL. *The Vital Balance.* New York: The Viking Press, 1964.

SKINNER, B. F. *About Behaviorism.* New York: Alfred A. Knopf, 1974.

————. *Beyond Freedom and Dignity.* New York: Alfred A. Knopf, 1971.

SROLE, LEO, et al. *Mental Health in the Metropolis: The Mid-Town Manhattan Study.* New York: McGraw-Hill Book Company, 1962.

The Birds and Bees and Me—Human Sexuality

As a vital part of the process of maturation, each young person must come to terms with his or her own sexuality in regard to both erotic impulses and the broader aspects of developing a suitable role as a man or woman. Within our own society there is considerable controversy concerning issues related to both these aspects; however, there is virtually unanimous agreement on their fundamental importance. It is clear that adult society in the form of parents, teachers, and religious leaders has a responsibility to provide children and youth with effective guidance with respect to their developing sexuality; it is equally clear that this responsibility is not being met in any effective manner. Surveys typically reveal that young people obtain the bulk of their information concerning sexual matters from one another. In contrast to areas of human conduct such as politics, economics, and science where the knowledge and wisdom of one generation is passed on to the next, sexual information, knowledge, and insights must be rediscovered by most young people with little help from their elders.

SOCIETAL TRENDS

Any analysis of the reasons for this gross educational void can become extremely complex; however, a brief consideration of the shifting attitudes toward sexual matters within society at large can provide elementary teachers with a suitable orientation to their proper role in school programs of sex education.

PARENTAL ATTITUDES

Few sexual problems that occur within American society result from parental apathy. Most parents are so concerned and emotional regarding sexual

250

matters that effective judgment and communications are hampered. Parents generally worry too much and do too little concerning the sex instruction of their children. They usually succeed in providing general moral and ethical guidance in the form of vague prohibitions of premarital sex, but this may be accomplished by attaching negative connotations to all erotic behavior regardless of the circumstances. Fortunately, many parents have become comfortable with their own sexuality and are thus able to provide their children with effective models that enable wholesome attitudes and behavior patterns to be "caught" even if not "taught" through open discussion. However, even in the homes where this healthy atmosphere prevails there is often a void in regard to specific knowledge and concepts.

PEER EDUCATION

In 1964 Kirkendall and Calderwood reviewed studies of the source of sex information and concluded that young people were still getting the "majority of their insights about sex from one another."[1] Since this disturbing observation parents have probably become more effective as purveyors of sex information, and the number of school programs has increased. But though the trend for these "official" sources may be upward, progress in general appears to be slow.

The more recent study of adolescent sexuality by Robert Sorensen revealed that

> 72% of the boys and 70% of the girls say that they and their parents do not freely talk about sex. In fact, most adolescents are at a loss to know what their parents want them to know about sex. They feel a great need to learn specific facts about techniques and problem situations rather than hear abstract discussions and morality lectures.[2]

In regard to school programs Sorensen found general support for the concept of sex education, with only 17 per cent of his sample agreeing with the statement that "Sex education courses in school are not valuable for young people." However, he found little evidence that the sex educational needs of this group were being met by such programs.

Both the lack of information and the quantity of overt sex-related behavioral problems among adolescents provide clear implications for elementary schools. The problems of this age group have their roots in misconceptions and unfavorable attitudes that developed during their earlier years as preschool and elementary school pupils. Much can be done during these

[1] L. A. Kirkendall and D. Calderwood, "The Family, the School, and Peer Groups: Sources of Information About Sex," *Journal of School Health*, Vol. 35, No. 7 (September 1965), p. 290.
[2] Robert C. Sorensen, *Adolescent Sexuality in Contemporary America* (New York: World Publishing, 1973), p. 84.

quieter times to prepare the young person for the more pressing challenges of adolescence. Moreover, the persistence and potency of the peer informational system are coming to be regarded as an advantage rather than an obstacle to the total school–community process of education. Most educators would be delighted with evidence that children frequently discuss literature and science among themselves; the educational task with respect to sex is to pump sufficient accurate information and constructive attitudes into the system.

MASS MEDIA

Although sex education as obtained from parents is apparently short on specific information, it nonetheless exerts significant influence in terms of a general moral orientation that tends to come into competition with the values and practices of the young person's peer society. More recently, the traditional rivalry between parents and peers has been complicated by the growing importance of the mass media as a third source of information and guidance. Sexual innuendoes are appearing to an increasing degree in the G-rated movies and ever more explicit sexual content is presented in the PG- and R-rated films that some children attend. The same pattern holds true to a somewhat lesser degree for television shows where the concept of "adult" versus "family" entertainment is opening the way for more forthright presentations of sexual situations. A visit to virtually any newsstand will demonstrate that the concept of sexual openness has accelerated since the pioneering efforts of *Playboy* magazine's Hugh Heffner in the early 1950s.

Children's literature, specifically children's fiction, reaches young people via both public and school libraries and commercial book stores and book clubs and thus tends to bridge the gap between the school and the mass media. In this case also there has been a less explosive but relentless trend toward the inclusion of more sexual content. As one authority notes, "The Hardy Boys Didn't Have Wet Dreams"; however, their more modern counterparts encounter all manner of sexual experiences within the pages of highly respected and often award-winning novels written for the upper elementary and junior high school levels.[8]

THE SCHOOL PROGRAM

The obvious changes in public behavior and attitudes in such an important area of conduct as human sexuality provide important implications for the

[3] Lorna B. Flynn, "The Hardy Boys Didn't Have Wet Dreams," *SIECUS Report*, Vol. 1, No. 2 (November 1972), p. 1.

school's role in sex education. However, as might be expected, the emotional and philosophical connotations commonly attached to this subject produce more than the usual degree of differences in interpretation of these societal trends. Some view the new freedoms in practices and expression as evidence of moral decay, whereas others view them as a welcome relief from the excessive repressiveness and hypocrisy of the past. Despite these differences, there is reasonably clear agreement on two important points: First, sexual matters may be discussed in public forums such as the classroom more easily than in the past; parents, administrators, teachers, and pupils are relatively more at ease with the subject even though it remains somewhat sensitive. Secondly, sex education must come early in the child's school career if it is to exert an appropriate impact in the formation of sexual concepts and attitudes. Health educators are nearly unanimous in their agreement that sex education should be presented at every school level.

PROGRAM DEVELOPMENT

Many public schools fail to include sex education in their curricula out of fear or reluctance to become involved with such a sensitive issue. However, a sizable minority of forward-looking school districts have instituted good programs that demonstrate both the willingness of parents to accept sex education in the elementary school and the type of procedures that are generally successful in gaining this acceptance. A brief review of this process can help prepare the new elementary teacher for possible involvement in such a curriculum development effort. The very real need for sex education together with the more favorable trends in public acceptance makes this involvement a very real possibility.

PLANNING. In the realm of curriculum development, as in the commercial world, good salesmanship depends on a good product. Consequently, the planning of a new sex education program often requires a year or more of concentrated effort. The philosophical approach and major goals are generally established by a broad-based committee, with parents, students, teachers, administrators, and health service personnel represented. Working groups are formed next; these usually require the recruitment of additional members. Their jobs are to formulate objectives, plan learning activities, and search for instructional material for specific grade or school levels. Outside consultants are frequently hired to assist with the organizational tasks and/or the technical aspects of subject matter.

ADOPTION. Although it must operate within the broad framework of state law, the board of education in effect establishes the curriculum within most school districts. Consequently, any newly proposed program of sex education should either be submitted to the board for its approval or be developed within the scope of the currently approved curriculum. This step protects teachers from any possible charges that they are teaching inappropriate subject matter. Dissident parents may still complain to the school administration; however, considerable pressure and legal jeopardy will have been removed from individual teachers.

PUBLIC APPROVAL. The school board has legal authority with respect to the curriculum, but from a practical standpoint the large majority of parents and interested members of the public must support any new program if it is to endure. The inclusion of parental representatives in the original planning group can go a long way toward assuring that this support as information is disseminated and rumors are squelched throughout the planning period. Once the work is complete, it is a good idea to schedule public meetings to explain the program and show examples of the instructional materials that will be used. Although it is occasionally necessary to modify the proposed curriculum at this point to accommodate public objections or suggestions, strong public approval is the more common result.

IMPLEMENTATION. In those instances in which only a single school or a limited number of schools are involved, all the teachers may be included in the planning process and thus gain the needed preparation for putting the new program into action in their classrooms. In larger systems, however, appropriate in-service training and orientation sessions are needed for those teachers who were not directly involved in the planning process. The amount of preparation needed is largely dependent on the professional background of the staff. Fortunately, an increasing number of teacher-training institutions train prospective elementary teachers in the handling of sensitive topics such as human sexuality as part of their normal program. Another development that can shorten the process of development and implementation is the growing availablity of "pre-packaged" model programs that planning groups may choose to use in whole or in part, thus avoiding the entire curriculum development task.

TEACHING APPROACH

Ideally, only those teachers who have had specific professional training in human sexuality should be assigned teaching responsibilities for this topic. Considering the crucial importance of good sexual adjustment to the welfare of both the individual and society, this standard surely merits serious consideration. The reality of the situation, however, is that most school districts are fortunate if a trained person can be found to provide program leadership and supervision. Specific training for the typical classroom teacher is usually lacking, but, before one seeks to use this lack of specific training as grounds for ruling out the elementary teacher as a sex educator, the full consequences of this action should be examined. In most instances sex education would then be left to the parents whose efforts are often very sparse and very late in coming, to the peers whose information is often inaccurate and based on immature reasoning, and to the mass media whose goals are more often geared to entertainment than to education.

Actually, the general training and background of classroom elementary teachers enable them to bring many useful assets to this sensitive teaching task. Most authorities in the field of sex education feel that the psychosocial rather than the biological topics of human sexuality are of uppermost importance. Here, the preparation in general psychology, educational psychology, and growth and development found in most teacher preparation programs provides an adequate foundation. Many of the common teaching skills such as discussion leadership and the use of role-playing and audio-visual materials are highly applicable to the teaching of sex education. A final and perhaps most important asset is the ability to establish rapport and gain the trust of children—a skill the prospective teacher begins to develop during student teaching and related laboratory experiences and seeks to refine during the early years on the job. The typical teacher who adds a reasonable amount of self-study in human sexuality to these general qualities will be able to do a creditable and worthwhile teaching job; with experience and/or specialized training this creditable performance can be raised to an outstanding one.

Once the emotional barrier is crossed and the new teacher becomes conditioned to the novelty of handling sexual content in the classroom, he or she will often find the task quite satisfying. Most elementary schoolchildren are very interested in sexual topics, yet not overwhelmed by them; they tend to adjust more quickly than most adults to the initial embarrassment and sensitivity associated with this topic. The subject matter is not highly technical and not difficult for the teacher to master. Also, effective and attractive teaching materials are available that ease the burden of the teaching task. In general, human sexuality should be treated as just another subject. Although some of the topics are quite sensitive or controversial, the same may be said for many topics of a political, economic, or cultural nature that any comprehensive school program cannot ignore.

CHILDREN'S HEALTH INTERESTS as RELATED to HUMAN SEXUALITY

Ruth Byler and her associates brought a strong measure of scientific support and precision to the common observation of most parents and teachers that school-age children generally are quite interested in a variety of sex-related topics. The relatively limited sample of verbatim comments and general findings reprinted in this section lack comprehensiveness but should provide the reader with a general impression of the attitudes of children of various maturity levels regarding this sensitive topic.[4]

Kindergarten Through Grade Two

- A kindergartner relates the story: Muddie had a baby in her stomach . . . and the doctor took Larry out. The doctor cut my mudder's stomach, but she didn't die because she still had her heart. . . . I wonder how he creep into her stomach?
- Incidents arouse curiosities which are related to the differences in sex roles. Conversations among second graders as they look at farm scenes showing cattle inevitably produce some comments such as: How can you tell which is a cow or a bull? Bulls have horns. . . . At a dairy farm, do they have just cows?. . . Is the bull the father of all those calves?

Grades Three and Four

- Third graders ask many questions about babies that revolve about these points: Where does a baby come from? How does it get out of the mother's stomach? Why can't newborn babies talk and walk?
- Fourth graders show interest in this subject but less so than third graders. Questions probe the cause of having babies, prenatal conditions and activity, birth, the characteristics of the newborn child, and infant abnormalities. . . . and for the first time, abortion is named.

Grades Five and Six

- The interest in babies, so strong in grade four, and which waned slightly in grade five, picks up again in grade six. . . .
- In regard to social–emotional development, fifth graders ask: Why do girls call and send notes? If you tell them to cut it out, they call more. (This from a group of boys. . . .)
- In regard to babies, sixth graders ask: How does a girl get a baby? Is it good to have a baby? Why can't you have a baby when you are not married?

CONTENT OVERVIEW

Although the underlying cultural and scientific knowledge related to human sexuality is vast and complex, an effective program for the elementary school can be based on a limited number of priority concepts. Perhaps the main

[4] Ruth Byler, Gertrude Lewis, and Ruth Totman, *Teach Us What We Want to Know* (New York: Mental Health Materials Center, Inc., 1969).

consideration is balance. It is more important that an awareness of the essential topics be developed than that a detailed study be made of any one of them. This point will be illustrated further as the major content areas are discussed.

THE SEX DRIVE

The development of some understanding of the erotic strivings and feelings that constitute the sex drive is perhaps the most challenging aspect of the sex education task. It is also perhaps the most important; as most boys and girls approach and enter preadolescence as fifth and sixth grade pupils, they are not so much concerned with their possible role as future parents as they are with their own current sexual feelings and behavior. In writing of the upper elementary years, L. Joseph Stone and Joseph Church observe that

> . . . there is a steady traffic among children in off-color stories, which may be poorly comprehended but are sure to elicit titters and giggles. Children likewise giggle together over the dictionary in which they look up words referring to sexual or excretory functions, or over the Bible in which they look up references to fornication.[5]

Children of this age need assurance that their growing personal interest in sexual matters, together with the interesting and often pleasurable sensations that occasionally accompany "touching experiences" that occur during "horseplay" or autostimulation, represent not evil or pathological tendencies but the early development of a normal drive toward involvement with the opposite sex. Also, the basic relationship of affection and love to physical attraction and gratification should be discussed in simple terms. The basic observation that both sexual and affectional needs are commonly satisfied in the same personal relationship, as in a happy marriage, can be made without becoming excessively involved in any complex analysis of the subject.

This effort to develop an awareness of the significance of the sex drive in its adult form in the upper elementary grades has a greater chance for success in those programs where the concept of affection as it occurs between parent and child is discussed in primary grades and preschool classes. Here, among other things, it can be pointed out that people who love one another often want to hug, squeeze, and kiss. Although love involves much more such as genuine care and concern for another's happiness, it is often expressed in physical ways that "feel good." This concept may be more appropriately presented in a unit on family living or mental health at these lower grade levels; however, it nonetheless provides the foundations for the

---

[5] L. Joseph Stone and Joseph Church, *Childhood and Adolescence* (New York: Random House, 1968), pp. 396–397.

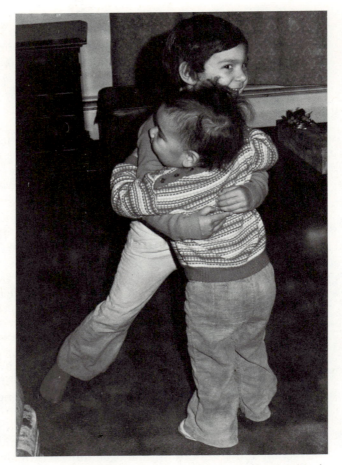

Figure 11.1. Hugging Makes Me Feel Good. (Carol Ashton)

preadolescent to understand how these same basic feelings begin a shift in direction from the parent toward friends of one's own age group.

SEX ROLES

The study of sex roles may be divided into two distinct but interrelated categories. The first includes factors related to sexual orientation or gender that may affect the development of the typical heterosexual pattern, with sexual interest focused on the opposite sex, as opposed to some form of homosexuality. The process by which one's specific orientation is established has only recently received significant scientific study and is as yet poorly understood. Currently, the more widely supported hypotheses focus on parent–child relationships during the preschool and early school years as the crucial determinant, but thus far few reliable guidelines are available as to how parents and teachers can help the child with this task.[6]

SEXUAL ORIENTATION.   Present-day attitudes in American society are becoming more constructive in regard to those with atypical sexual orientations, and any comprehensive program of sex education should deal with this issue; however, its serious consideration is not usually advocated for the elementary school years. Perhaps the best way the elementary teacher can prepare children for dealing with this topic at a later maturity level is to do a good job with the standard topics so that the children will become comfortable with the general subject. Also, as will be noted in the section on health services, the feminine boys or the girls with "tomboy" tendencies may need some attention to protect them from excessive teasing or ridicule.

SEXUAL EQUALITY.   The second category of subject matter relative to sex roles includes the more generalized aspects of human behavior as it is affected by individual concepts of maleness or femaleness. Although the activities of feminist organizations have, over the past decades, brought a high degree of public attention to various forms of sex discrimination, sex roles have been undergoing significant changes throughout most of the current century. The work of Susan B. Anthony, which contributed to the establishment of women's suffrage as a constitutional right in 1920, and that of Margaret Sanger, which helped break down the barriers to birth control, are notable examples of these many earlier achievements. The feminist movement during the 1970s has centered on economic issues, particularly with regard to gaining equal opportunities to enter male-dominated professions and vocations and to earn promotions and receive equal pay for equal work.

Although women have been the apparent benefactors of the recent trends, the road to change has not been a one-way street. Just as we are seeing more female truck drivers and police officers, we are also seeing more male nurses, elementary teachers, and airline flight attendants. Just as we are seeing a necessary reduction in the time devoted to housekeeping and child-rearing responsibilities by working wives, we are also seeing pressure on working husbands to increase their share of these responsibilities. Just as we are seeing women encouraged to give vent to their assertiveness in both the vocational and social spheres, we are also seeing men encouraged to express their tender feelings more freely.

These changes within the larger society provide certain important implications for the elementary school program. Depending on the particular locale, for example, children may come predominantly from homes where the mothers work full-time at outside jobs, where the mothers adopt the

[6] For an interesting and authoritative treatment of this topic, see Richard Green, "Children's Quest for Sexual Identity," *Pychology Today*, Vol. 7, No. 9 (February 1974), pp. 45–51.

traditional housewife role, or where both patterns exist to significant degrees. Each of these, together with the gradations in between, creates its own set of educational needs that must be met if children are to adjust to the situation in their homes and develop tolerance and understanding for the different practices found in the homes of their classmates. These objectives require some understanding of the basic factors that affect each mother's decision to work, such as her concept of a job as a means of fulfillment, the size of the father's income or the amount of support he provides if divorced or separated, the number and ages of her children, and the quality and availability of baby-sitters or day-care services.

A woman's decision as to whether to assume or share the breadwinner's task is, of course, only one of many aspects of the study of sex roles. On further exploration of this topic, children will find that parents vary considerably as to what they feel is appropriate for boys as compared with girls concerning the type of recreational activities they should pursue, household chores they should be assigned, clothes they should wear, and social behavior and mannerisms they should display. It seems clear that both the variations in attitudes among different families and decade-to-decade changes in social consensus regarding sex roles are likely to continue. In such a situation the school's responsibility is to help children become aware of sex roles and the dimension along which they may vary as opposed to lobbying for any particular point of view.

In addition to the immediate goals of adjusting to current practices, some attention should also be devoted to helping children think realistically about their future roles as men and women. This requires some emphasis on the direction of current trends and logical projections as to what the situation may be when the children reach young adulthood. Also, a shift in focus is needed from a mere adjusting to the views that exist within each child's home and neighborhood, over which he or she has little control, to an examination of personal feelings and preferences as to the way things should be. This study overlaps to some degree the concept of "career education," which is currently popular in many school districts, but extends beyond the narrower concern with occupational choice to encompass a consideration of future life-styles. Obviously, the choices individual children make will normally change many times before they become old enough to act upon them; however, the experience they gain in the process of monitering trends and opportunities and relating such to their personal situation is extremely valuable regardless of the tentative nature of their conclusions.

HUMAN REPRODUCTION

As one critic so aptly observes, the old sex education could have been more appropriately termed "reproduction education."[7] In reaction to this tradi-

[7] Kirkendall and Calderwood, op. cit.

tional imbalance, the authors have thus far sought to emphasize content of more immediate value to children; however, in the move toward modern relevance one should not discount the importance of the plain, old-fashioned "birds and bees" aspect of this subject. The basic concept of sexual reproduction can be effectively presented at the kindergarten–primary level by use of teaching materials focusing on animal reproduction or, better yet, by maintaining mating pairs of gerbils, guinea pigs, or other pets in the classroom.

PREGNANCY AND BIRTH.   At these grade levels simplicity is the key to effective teaching. Children need to learn that babies grow in a special place inside the mother after the male has placed sperm inside her body to join with her egg. Any additional content presented normally consists of more refinement of this basic theme. The eggs produced by animals are small and soft; they do not have shells. The male's sperm comes out through his penis, which he places inside the female during a process termed mating. The babies receive food and oxygen, the important part of air, from the mother's body. When the babies have grown large enough to live in the outside world, they are forced out of the mother's body and nourished by milk she produces in her breasts. Once these basic facts have been established, the balance of the time devoted to the biological aspect may be spent in clearing up the naive misconceptions and satisfying the innocent curiosity typical of this age. Once teachers of the kindergarten–primary grades "take the plunge" and present these simple concepts, they are often surprised and relieved by the relatively unemotional way they are received by the children.

At the upper elementary level, children are ready for (1) a more detailed study of human reproduction, including menstruation; (2) a basic study of the development of secondary sex characteristics that accompany the onset of sexual maturity; and (3) a more complete description of sexual intercourse, including the basic concept of sexual arousal.

SEXUAL MATURATION.   To first grade pupils, sperm are produced by the male's body when he grows up, but to fourth graders, sperm are produced by the testes after their development has been stimulated by hormones from the pituitary gland. A similar release of hormones by this gland in the maturing female causes her ovaries to develop and release one or more eggs each month, which are carried to the uterus through fallopian tubes; the ovaries themselves also now begin to release chemicals that stimulate the uterus to develop a thick lining designed to nourish the egg if it is fertilized by a sperm. Although these examples illustrate an appropriate increase in complexity, the technical aspects have still not progressed beyond the pamphlet stage and are still well within the grasp of anyone whose college training included a basic biology or general science course. The informational voids and gross misconceptions common to this area enable simple,

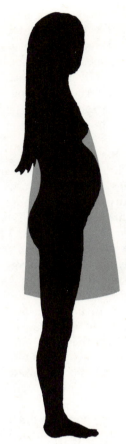

Figure 11.2. Children Need to Learn That Babies Grow in a Special Place Inside the Mother.

accurate descriptions to appear as something approaching the "wisdom of the ages."

Menstrual education per se within a comprehensive program of sex education normally occupies a relatively minor role. The most important goal within this topic is to help prepubescent girls develop a basic understanding of the process and to view it as a normal, natural phenomenon. Boys, too, need this information in order to demystify the process and offset the many folk tales they hear. Somewhat secondary to this general need is the narrower topic of menstrual hygiene, which includes the practical mechanics of handling the menstrual flow and the occasional dysmenorrhea (menstrual pain) and other problems that the newly menstruating girl may encounter. These will be discussed in the following section on health services. The training of most school nurses enables them to serve as highly useful resource persons for this phase of the topic. Also, of course, those nurses who have received specialized training in classroom teaching techniques can be called upon to play a larger role in the teaching of human sexuality and other health topics.

SECONDARY SEX CHARACTERISTICS. Closely related to the study of reproduction with its focus on the primary characteristics of maleness and femaleness is the need to help children understand the more generalized physical changes that accompany the onset of sexual maturity. Termed secondary sex characteristics, these include the broader shoulders and deeper voice of the male, the wider pelvis and breast development of the female, and the growth of axillary and pubic hair in both sexes. These should be explained as resulting from the release of male and female hormones into the bloodstream by the now functional testes or ovaries of the early adolescent. One of the more urgent objectives is to acquaint the children with the wide variations in the normal age at which these changes take place so that markedly early or late maturers do not become unduly concerned.

COITUS. Even if one chooses to adopt one of the more extreme interpretations of current trends in adolescent sex activity, most elementary school pupils are still some years away from their first sexual intercourse, yet they are definitely curious about this process. It is precisely this combination of interest yet remoteness from any undue pressure to participate that creates a good teaching situation for this topic in the upper elementary grades. Here again, simplicity is the watchword. The thoughts of sexual participation, together with the touch and view of the partner, trigger reflex action within the male that increases the blood supply to the penis to effect an erection. Similar stimuli lead to vaginal lubrication and enlargement in the female that facilitate the insertion of the penis. The desire for increased pleasure and excitement leads to pelvic movements that generally cause a climax or ejaculation in the male, with a consequent release of a fluid termed semen. The female sometimes experiences a parallel reaction at the peak of her excitement that is termed an orgasm. Either of these reactions is sometimes produced in other ways such as manual stimulation, which is termed petting if by a partner or masturbation if by oneself.

The presentation of information on this simple and basic level within the context of suitable classroom learning activities will do much to "defuse" this subject in the minds of typical fifth grade pupils, for example. They can then respond more constructively to the inevitable sexual innuendoes of the mass media and misconceptions of the peer culture. They will presumably be able to put sexual issues in proper perspective as they apply to their age group and to redirect their energy and interests to the many other unanswered questions concerning their environment.

263

SUGGESTED LEARNING ACTIVITIES

The following suggestions are presented in an effort to demonstrate how the content described in the preceding section might be translated into effective classroom learning activities. They were designed to accommodate a wide variety of classroom groups provided that proper selection and adaptations are made according to the needs, interests, abilities, and maturity level of the particular children involved.

- Many upper elementary schoolchildren as they approach puberty think that their personal feelings and experiences about their sexual development are unique. However, through a process of sharing their sexual experiences and feelings with others, they are often relieved to discover their feelings and experiences are rather common and ordinary. To help your students discover how personal attitudes about their sexuality develop, have them rank those people they would feel most comfortable talking with about their sexual development (1, most important; 7, least important).

  _____ teacher
  _____ friend (s)
  _____ member of their church
  _____ doctor
  _____ parent (s)
  _____ brothers and sisters

- To show the children how much they have grown from birth to their present age, have them bring in clothes that they wore as a baby at birth, 1 year old, 3 years old, etc.

- Divide the class in half. Ask one group to watch the various commercials on TV and select those that they feel are using some form of sex to sell their product. Allow time for them to compile their findings. Ask the other group to select advertisements from magazines that they feel are selling their product through the use of sex-related appeals. After both groups have reported their findings, have them discuss why this particular technique is used and whether they feel this method is effective.

- To show the primary children the differences in the sizes of people and various animals at birth, take pieces of yarn and mark every foot of length with a plastic curtain ring. This will show the children as they unwind and expand the yarn across the room the various sizes of animals at birth. Have the children compare a human baby to a giraffe, monkey, elephant, dog, etc. Have the children look up their own height (length) at birth and make a life line for comparison with the other children in the class.

- Have the children draw pictures of themselves. When they have finished their pictures, have them describe how they feel about themselves in words around the picture.

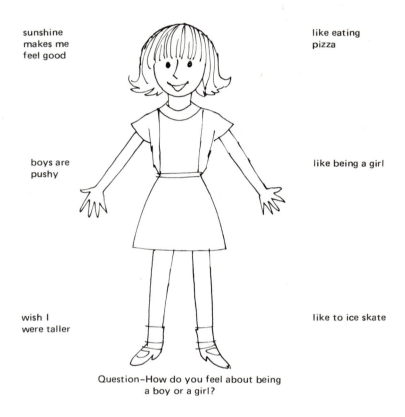

sunshine makes me feel good

like eating pizza

boys are pushy

like being a girl

wish I were taller

like to ice skate

Question—How do you feel about being a boy or a girl?

- In order for your students to gain a better understanding of their physical characteristics, have them stand in front of a full-length mirror at home and carefully study their bodies (e.g., shape of their head, size of their fingers, posture, color of eyes). This activity should be experienced in the primary grades. As puberty begins, many physical changes (especially of a sexual nature) are taking place. To help your students discover and practice self-disclosure about these sexual changes, have them think about and examine their bodies without their clothes. With their hands and eyes, have them explore the curvatures, texture of skin of each part of their body, and the general outline of their genitals. Have them think about their feelings while engaged in this activity, especially as it relates to themselves as boys or girls. Note: This activity should be used only with parental permission within the context of a comprehensive, administratively approved program.

• Put the children into groups and give each group a sheet of newsprint with the words "Love" printed in the middle of it. Have the children write on the newsprint around the word all the meanings that they feel there are for the word. Have the groups discuss their definitions and see if the class can agree on one definition.

• In Chapter 4, the children studied the various parts and organs of the body. If the genitals were not included, discuss them now. When you have finished, have the children share with the other members of the class other names that they have heard or learned for the genitals. Discuss why they feel these names are given instead of their regular names. Note: Be sure this activity has official approval.

• As our bodies grow and change at puberty, we experience many new feelings. Have the students draw a sail boat with a rudder. Around the sailboat, the students draw gusty wind clouds. In the clouds have the students write the pressures and feelings that they are experiencing at this time in their life. If they can think of something that would help their boat to keep on a good course in life, have them write it on the rudder.

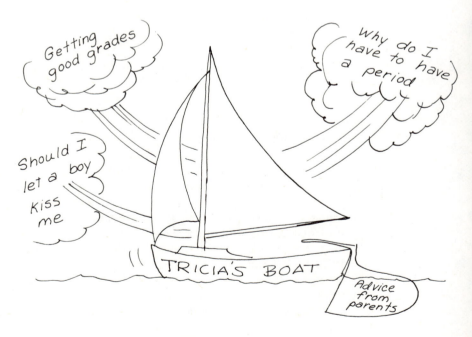

- Have the children complete the following statements:
  When people hug me I feel_____.
  When I touch my genitals_____.
  Being a girl is_____.
  Being a boy is_____.
  Men crying makes me_____.
  My height_____.
  Acne is_____.
  When I see two people of the same sex kissing_____.
  Sex is_____.
  Dancing makes me_____.
  When I grow up I would like to be_____.
  My brother makes me_____.
  My sister makes me_____.

- Have the students make a 1-foot "ruler of life" from construction paper. Ask them to mark their ruler into thirds, with each section representing a period of their life. In each section of the ruler, have the students write in events in their lives that they can remember (good or bad). If they are unsure of a certain period of their lives, have them ask their parents. When their rulers are complete, have them share them with the rest of the class and see if there are any similarities or differences in their life patterns. Ask them to discuss the possible reasons for these findings.

SUGGESTED RESOURCES

The learning resources listed in this section are a selected sample of materials with which the authors are personally familiar. Appropriate grade levels have been included when these were indicated by the source.

BOOKS

Girls Are Girls
Boys Are Boys
So What's the Difference?

Sol Gordon
John Day
666 Fifth Avenue
New York, NY 10019

Human Growth
Lester Beck
Harcourt Brace Jovanovich, Inc.
757 Third Avenue
New York, New York 10017

The Human Story
Facts on Birth, Growth and Reproduction
S. Hofstein
Scott, Foresman and Co.
Glenview, Illinois 60025

Valuing in the Family
Herbert Brayer and Zella Cleary
Pennant Press
San Diego, California

Yertle the Turtle
Dr. Seuss
Random House, Inc.
New York, New York

FILMSTRIPS

Growing into Womanhood
Growing into Manhood
Grades 5–8
Guidance Associates
757 Third Ave.
New York, New York 10017

Human Growth—There's a New You Coming
    —for Boys
    —for Girls
Marsh Films
Shawnee Mission, Kansas 66028

ENVIRONMENTAL ASPECTS

Perhaps the most important contribution of the school environment to education about human sexuality is the presence of adult models who exemplify desirable qualities of maleness and femaleness, and the appropriate ways in which men and women behave toward one another. The difficulty is that the traditional norms for such modeling behavior are no longer entirely appropriate in light of the emerging egalitarianism, and new norms have not been developed. It is clear that women teachers are no longer expected to act or be treated by men as though they were helpless, but rather as competent and worthy peers. The egalitarian model also requires that both women and men be placed in positions at all levels of the administrative hierarchy in the school. Love affairs between teachers also contribute to sex education; however, the appropriateness of various ways such pairs may have of expressing their affection in public, and especially in the school, is not well established. On the other hand, the culmination of a faculty romance in a wedding is also educational, as is the pregnancy of a teacher and her absence for the delivery and a period of providing infant care. Pupils take great delight in such events, especially if they are invited to the wedding or have an opportunity to see the baby.

If animals are used as subjects for sex education experiments, appropriate provision must be made for their caging and care. Appropriate caging varies with the gnawing ability of the animal—some will escape from even a sturdy wooden cage. For these a cage constructed of metal and heavy wire mesh is required. Children need protection against bites, which may be provided by a covering of mesh fine enough to prevent insertion of a child's finger. For the protection of any animal, handling by children must be limited. Food, water, and clean litter appropriate to the needs of the animal must be provided. Classroom pets are usually boarded out to a pupil's family over weekends and vacations and disposed of by adoption. Making all such arrangements in advance of the acquisition of the animal makes life easier for the teacher in the long run.

Although live models, whether human or of some other species, are most effective sex education devices, learning is also facilitated by books and other materials. Materials that present sex-role stereotypes or inaccurate information about sex should be replaced as soon as possible. Both children and adults tend to believe anything they see in print.

Toilet rooms in schools should be equipped with fixtures appropriate to the sex and age of the pupils who use them. Boy's rooms are equipped with urinals, for example, and those for older girls are equipped with dispensers of menstrual hygiene materials. These differences can be shown to the children, and the reasons for them discussed.

HEALTH SERVICE ASPECTS

Health service professionals in elementary schools are rarely faced with cases of pregnancy or venereal disease. Although some young children are sexually abused, usually by a parent, relative, or family friend, the rarity of these occurrences dictates that they be handled on an individual basis. Fortunately, school nurses and physicians are not only better prepared to deal with such cases than they formerly were but also have access to more and better community services for referrals. In most states, there is now no age limit for abortions or other birth control services or for VD treatment services, nor is parental consent required. Both legal and medical services for rape victims are being improved as the result of efforts by women's groups.

The main role of health service professionals in the area of sex has traditionally been that of providing such sex education as children receive in some schools. The sex education thus provided is probably better than no education at all, but the content is usually limited to teaching girls about menstruation and the use of tampons or sanitary napkins and to teaching boys about wet dreams, masturbation, and the dangers of impregnating a girl. Typically, all fifth grade girls were herded into the auditorium and shown a film and given a lecture by the school nurse. A male school physician or physical education teacher did the same thing for the boys. Occasionally, these sessions were held in the evening, with the same-sex parents invited to attend. This traditional pattern still prevails in some schools, the chief improvement being that menstruation is no longer presented as a richly rewarding emotional experience, and masturbation is no longer condemned as sinful or as a cause of mental or physical disease. But large, segregated presentations still lead pupils to wonder what those of the opposite sex are being taught, and encourage attitudes that set sex apart from the rest of life as something sinful, dangerous, or dirty.

In schools enlightened enough to have moved sex education into coeducational classrooms where it belongs, school nurses and physicians have become invaluable resource persons to the regular teacher who has now assumed the responsibility. At the least, the nurse and often the physician are available to provide information to the teacher and to review resource materials for their factual accuracy. Once a unit has been initiated by the regular teacher, the nurse and sometimes the physician may accept an invitation to a class session in the role of a visiting expert, either to present some special aspect of the subject or to answer questions prepared beforehand by the class.

In addition to their roles in sex education, school health service professionals are often called upon to provide individual counseling and guidance to students, and sometimes to teachers, when individual problems arise or when sex education has been deficient. For example, a few girls are likely to experience their first menstruation well before the others do and before they have received instruction at home and school. The nurse is usually called upon to provide reassurance, information, and hygiene supplies when this occurs.

The most common sex-related problem seen in the health service is dysmenorrhea, or painful menstruation. There are two types of dysmenorrhea, primary and secondary. Primary dysmenorrhea has no identifiable cause, but it can often be prevented or alleviated by exercises designed to strengthen the abdominal and pelvic muscles, as can some of the cases of secondary dysmenorrhea, also. Such exercises can be taught either by the nurse or by the physical educational teacher. Another helpful technique is to reduce salt intake for a week before menstruation to reduce water retention. It is also helpful to avoid emotional tensions. The occasional use of small doses of aspirin to relieve discomfort helps victims function at home and school, but does nothing to relieve the basic cause of dysmenorrhea. Large and frequent doses increase the menstrual flow. Most over-the-counter medications sold for the relief of menstrual pain are only glorified concoctions of aspirin. Heat applications and avoidance of overexertion are nondrug ways of relieving dysmenorrhea. Secondary dysmenorrhea has one of a number of basic physiological causes that require medical identification and attention. These include pelvic inflammatory disease, which often results from untreated gonorrhea, and displacement of the uterus. Therefore, a medical referral, preferably to a gynecologist, should follow failure of exercises or other simple methods to relieve the problem.

Observable masturbation may be of some concern to teachers, but in most cases it does not signify a medical problem. Children do need to know that masturbating in public is not acceptable social behavior. Some retarded or emotionally disturbed children masturbate frequently and openly, but these will manifest their basic problem in many other ways as well. Misinformed children often worry about their masturbatory behavior, but teaching that it is a common and harmless way of relieving sexual tension also relieves concerns that may be associated with it.

271

REFERENCES

DEMAREST, ROBERT J., and JOHN J. SCIARRA. *Conception, Birth and Contraception*. New York: McGraw-Hill Book Company, 1969.

FLYNN, LORNA B. "The Hardy Boys Didn't Have Wet Dreams," *SIECUS Report*, Vol. 1, No. 2 (November 1972), p. 1.

GREEN, RICHARD. "Children's Quest for Sexual Identity." *Psychology Today*, Vol. 7, No. 9 (February 1974).

KIRKENDALL, L. A., and D. CALDERWOOD. "The Family, the School, and Peer Groups Sources of Information About Sex," *Journal of School Health*, Vol. 35, No. 7 (September 1965).

LERRIGO, MARION, and HELEN SOUTHARD. *Parents' Responsibility*. Chicago: American Medical Association, 1970.

————. *A Story About You*. Chicago: American Medical Association, 1971.

McCARY, JAMES LESLIE. *Human Sexuality*. New York: D. Van Nostrand Company, 1973.

STONE, L. JOSEPH, and JOSEPH CHURCH. *Childhood and Adolescence*. New York: Random House, 1972.

12

Pills and Booze— Psychoactive Substances

The subject matter related to the general area of psychoactive substances provides another example of the many interesting, zesty, and challenging topics that characterize any serious study of health. However, like the substances themselves, the classroom study of drugs can be either used or abused. At its worst, drug education becomes highly simplistic: drugs are uniformly bad substances that young people abuse for frivolous reasons— for kicks—because the others do it, or as a reaction to too many TV ads for cold remedies; education thus becomes a preachy sing-song in praise of abstinence as the ultimate solution. Although this approach appeals to many parents and a small percentage of students who would probably never abuse drugs under any circumstances, the available evidence suggests that it actually encourages drug use, if not abuse, among the more susceptible students.[1] However, in its best form, drug education becomes yet another effective vehicle for developing an awareness of basic human needs and constructive modes of need satisfaction, as well as effective ways to cope with the many drug use situations that one inevitably encounters in modern-day American society.

DEFINING DRUG EDUCATION

The views (1) that drug use is inextricably bound up with basic human needs and (2) that drug use situations are inevitably encountered in our society lie at the heart of the new, promising approach to drug education. In contrast to the typical efforts of the past, this new approach requires that

[1] Richard H. DeLone, "The Ups and Downs of Drug-Abuse Education," *Saturday Review of Education* (September 11, 1972), p. 28.

273

psychoactive substances be studied in a far broader context as applied to all their basic aspects.

PSYCHOACTIVE SUBSTANCES

According to the older view, the name *drugs* was restricted to such substances as marijuana, heroin, LSD, the amphetamines, and the barbiturates —drugs that are commonly used illegally. Such "legal" items as coffee, tobacco, and alcohol were regarded as being somehow quite distinct from the "street drugs" and thus required quite different treatment as a classroom topic. The concept of legal versus illegal drug use is undeniably important and merits serious attention; however, the tendency to structure the entire study of drugs on this basis tends to fragment and obscure some of this topic's most important concepts. For example, an effective understanding of drug dependency requires that the student view it as a phenomenon that can occur with legally purchased alcohol, legally prescribed sleeping pills, and legally purchased laxatives as well as with illegal street drugs. This larger view not only equips the student to recognize drug dependency in its more subtle forms but also provides the foundation for a more comprehensive view of dependency as applied to food, work, or TV viewing as the addicting agent.

HUMANISTIC ORIENTATION

The "old" drug education centered on a pharmacological analysis of all the common troublesome substances. Drug A is virtually harmless; drug B is habituating but not addicting; drug C is mildly addicting; and drug D is severely addicting. However, the "new" drug education recognizes that addiction, dependency, or intoxication occurs in people, not in drugs; thus the focus shifts from dependency-producing *drugs* to dependency-prone *people* and dependency-provoking *situations*. Drug dependency is seen not as the inevitable result of some chance encounter with an addicting substance but as a symptom of severe emotional stress that has its roots in some deep personal conflict or some unmanageable problem or situation. In another person or in another environment the same factors might have yielded vandalism, sexual indiscretions, or fanatical devotion to religious worship or schoolwork. Efforts to prevent drug abuse thus shift from a negative focus on the dire consequences of drug use to a comprehensive attempt to help the student develop a sound, stable personality and personal strategies for managing emotional stress.

THE DRUG USE CONTINUUM

The new drug education not only broadens its scope to the study of personality and environmental stress but also moves away from the old narrow concern with drug dependency, intoxication, and drug-related accidents to a more comprehensive study of drug use in all its common forms and varieties. This means that the coffee that gets one started in the morning, the aspirin that alleviates the headache, and the cocktails that "break the ice" come in for as much attention as mainlined heroin. This broader scope offers two distinct advantages, neither of which places coffee drinking in a more negative light or heroin use in a more positive light. First, the dynamics of drug use are presented in more familiar terms, a practice with obvious pedagogical advantages. Second, popular hysteria to the contrary, the large majority of children in the average classroom are not destined to become drug abusers regardless of the quality of the education they receive; however, virtually all will become drug users and all will encounter other

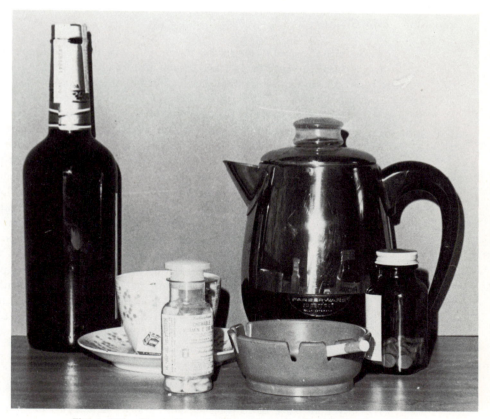

Figure 12.1. Drugs Come in Many Common Forms. (Carol Ashton)

275

drug users. The quality of their lives can be significantly affected by their skill in dealing with drugs within the realm of normal, legal use.

APPLICATION for the ELEMENTARY SCHOOL

As in the case with most health topics, the majority opinion among health educators is that students need drug education throughout their total school careers. Cornacchia and his associates in their text *Drugs in the Classroom* state that "it [drug education] should begin in kindergarten, although it should start earlier in districts that have preschool programs." [2] Drug use and abuse are obviously related to deep-seated attitudes and values related to personal goals, health in general, and specific drugs and use patterns. Such attitudes are formed over a long period of time, with the early experiences being the most crucial; thus the elementary school years become perhaps the most important of all.

BASIC GOALS

Many formalized statements of long-range objectives or goals for school drug education programs have been developed; however, these can be reduced to three major, universally desired outcomes:

1. *Prevention of Drug Abuse.* Once viewed as the only purpose of drug education, this traditional goal retains an important place despite the addition of other more positive objectives. As noted above, however, the strategy for achieving this goal has shifted from a fear-provoking emphasis on the dire consequences of drug abuse to more generalized efforts to foster wholesome personality growth. The overlap of this aspect of drug education with the area of mental health and with the teacher's efforts to maintain a healthy emotional climate in the classroom become quite obvious, as does the relationship to good support services in the area of counseling and guidance. Thus most of what a truly good school provides in the realm of drug abuse prevention does not appear as drug education per se but as good teacher–pupil relationships; good curricula and good instruction leading to feelings of accomplishment and success; classroom experiences directed toward the humanistic goals of a positive self-concept; good interpersonal skills based on love, trust, and honest communications; and good counseling as needed to prevent the development of unmanageable personality conflicts.

[2] Harold J. Cornacchia, David J. Bentel, and David E. Smith, *Drugs in the Classroom: A Conceptual Model for School Programs* (St. Louis: The C. V. Mosby Co., 1973), p. 133.

2. *Fostering Intelligent Drug Use.* The intent here is not to encourage drug use but to equip students to handle more intelligently the drug use situations they will surely encounter. These situations include their exposure to coffee, aspirin and other over-the-counter drugs, prescription drugs, and alcohol, as well as their encounters with friends and relatives who use alcohol and/or other psychoactive substances. This goal is based on the fact that drug use is an integral part of modern American society and even totally abstinent persons must understand certain concepts pertaining to these substances if they are to function at optimal efficiency.

3. *Encouraging Civic Responsibility.* Virtually every person acquires certain responsibilities for other persons and for civic action in regard to drug use or abuse. Examples of such responsibilities range from the 6-year-old child who should know that a 3-year-old brother should not be snooping in the family medicine cabinet to the adult who has to vote on whether the drinking age should be lowered to 18 years. The prevention and control of drug abuse requires the active participation of the total population; those who are not personally prone to drug problems can be particularly helpful in their individual or collective action in behalf of others. At the elementary or secondary level it is often the nonabusing friend who guides an abuser toward help or who discretely informs parents or school authorities of the problem; at the college level peer counseling organizations often function to good advantage; and within the larger society voters at the local, state, and national level are often called on to form public policies and support prevention and treatment programs.

DEVELOPMENT of the DRUG EDUCATION PROGRAM

As with all significant health topics, drug education is best planned as part of a comprehensive health curriculum that is presented in concert with a program of school health services and with consideration for a healthful school environment. As noted, the overall emotional climate of the classroom and of the school in general is commonly regarded as more important than education in the prevention of drug abuse. Within the realm of health services, teachers, school nurses, counselors, and other school personnel have responsibility for the early detection and referral of drug and other socio-emotional problems. And in regard to education per se, those activities directed toward the fostering of mental health in general are of paramount importance. Within this broad context the presentation of learning experience related specifically to drugs serves a vital if somewhat secondary role.

PRINCIPLES

Cornacchia and associates support this approach through their set of guiding principles for the school drug program. The following seem particularly applicable at the elementary level:

1. The school atmosphere should focus on the improvement of the quality of human interaction and human relatedness, especially between teachers and students. This approach is usually referred to as the humanistic emphasis. Schools, and especially teachers, need to be more concerned with pupils than with the content they teach. The drug problem is a human problem.
2. The educational program should be graded and sequential in order to reach all students. It should begin in kindergarten, although it could begin earlier in districts that have preschool programs.
3. The school program must include more than just education. Some students will need special counseling, guidance, and assistance.
4. School activities must be related to and coordinated with those efforts taking place outside the school and should involve the participation of the community, including parents.
5. The nature and extent of the drug problem in each school and school district must be identified, and attention must be given to the variety of physical, psychological, social, and spiritual needs of the users and nonusers of drugs.[3]

APPROACH

The teaching of drug education at the elementary level does not require a unique philosophical approach or a special effort to create a particular type of emotional climate in the classroom. All the general imperatives for good teaching apply. The selection of specific topics should be determined by the interests and genuine educational needs of the pupils. Balanced attention should be given to the attitudinal, value-laden aspects and the factual, cognitive aspects. Active pupil involvement in the selection and implementation of learning activities should be fostered within the limits of their level of maturity. An even-handed treatment of controversial issues should prevail. And the values, feelings, and beliefs, that make each child unique should be respected at all times.

This thumbnail sketch of program principles gives the initial impression that drug education is something special, but all these requirements apply equally well to the study of American history, ecology, or reading. What is needed is simply a good teaching effort. Drug education is "just another

[3] Ibid., pp. 132–133.

subject," but the good teacher seeks to make every subject interesting, useful, and meaningful.

ORGANIZATION

Within a comprehensive program of health education, the specific makeup of the drug education component could vary considerably according to the content of other related units, particularly those for mental health. The development of a positive self-concept and a repertoire of constructive strategies for coping with stress represent the most promising long-term approach to the prevention of drug abuse. If a strong effort is made toward these goals in a unit on mental health, the drug education unit can be restricted to a more conventional study of specific drug issues; however, if these vital learning experiences are not provided elsewhere, then the drug unit must bcome the vehicle for their presentation.

The consumer health area of the curriculum typically includes material on the hazards and pitfalls related to the unwise use of over-the-counter drugs as well as some attention to the activities of the Food and Drug Administration and the Federal Trade Commission in the protection of the consumer. Here again, the need to avoid overlapping content is quite obvious. The opportunities to present drug-related content as part of the study of social science, general science, and other areas outside the health curriculum should also be considered. The entire drug education curriculum could be integrated into other subject matter areas if any one of a variety of effective organizational patterns, or the presentation of drug education experiences in other fields could be used to supplement and enrich a specific drug education unit. The quality of the specific learning experiences is more important than the particular type of curricular organization.

CHILDREN'S HEALTH INTERESTS as RELATED to PSYCHOACTIVE SUBSTANCES

In their analysis of the findings of their study of health interests, Ruth Byler and her associates list smoking, alcohol, and drugs among the subjects to receive at least some attention at every grade level. However, as might be expected, their findings reveal more interest in this subject among children of the higher grade levels. A few representative comments and findings are included in this section.[4]

[4] Ruth Byler, Gertrude Lewis, and Ruth Totman, *Teach Us Want We Want to Know* (New York: Mental Health Materials Center, Inc., 1969) .

Grades Three and Four

- Third graders express slight concern about drugs and smoking, and none about alcohol.
- Fourth graders show familiarity with the names of today's harmful drugs, particularly LSD, accompanied by abysmal ignorance of how they are used, and wild probing as to the effects on the individual. . . .
- Fourth graders ask: Is marijuana a dangerous drug? How does it affect you? Why do so many people smoke? Is it hard to give up smoking?. . . Why do people drink so much?. . . What would happen if I should drink some whiskey?

Grades Five and Six

- Regarding alcohol: This topic received little attention in either grade. The sixth graders say: Teach about the effects of alcohol early; then they'll be more intelligent teenagers when they are 15 or 16 and not lose their heads and drink.
- Questions show rising curiosity in both grades about what drugs are, how people use them, and what the effects are. Fifth graders wonder whether, as they grow older, they might come to like and use them. Sixth graders reveal a deepening perception of why people use them and what the effects are. . . .
- Toward smoking, fifth graders seem to become quite emotional. Many questions show repugnance and puzzlement that anyone would smoke, knowing the hazards. Concern is shown about parents who smoke. . . .
- Sixth graders say: Smoking is our greatest health problem. When you start smoking, why can't you stop? Why do they sell cigarettes? . . .

A CONTENT OVERVIEW

As with most health topics, the content available on psychoactive substances for selection and incorporation into a particular school curriculum tends to be overwhelming. Moreover, there has been so much drug information in the mass media in recent years as to give the impression that everyone knows all they need to know about drugs. Although public hysteria has abated, because of fatigue if nothing else, the problems are as severe as ever. The public may know more about drugs, but this information does not seem to be leading to better decision making in terms of either personal practices or public policy. Random, diffuse information is not enough; facts must be (1) focused around useful generalizations or concepts that provide guides to the decision-making process and (2) made real or vital through learning experiences designed to reach the pupils at the feeling, valuing level in regard to these major concepts. In this section an attempt will be made to identify the content of highest priority.

MOTIVATIONS for USE

Although the various psychoactive substances commonly used in our society vary greatly in their relative potency, in their basic effects, and in their potential for destructive effects, users commonly report similar reasons for their involvement with these substances. When asked why they began the use of cigarettes, alcohol, or illegal drugs, they commonly cite "curiosity" or a desire to "follow the crowd" and join in an activity with their friends or that seemed to be popular within society in general. Closely related to both these reasons is the prevalence of drug-related information and advertising as presented in television, magazines, and other mass media.

Every normal person seeks to acquire and enhance his or her ability to cope with the world—to learn about things and to develop useful skills. The twin motivations of curiosity about one's environment and the tendency to model one's behavior after that of others, particularly those that seem to be "ahead of the pack" in the coping game, generally serve the individual very well. Much of what is done in good programs of education and child rearing has the effect of intensifying environmental curiosity and the tendency to follow worthy examples of behavior. There is obviously no way to extinguish these basic motivations without doing great harm to the individual; however, they can be made more useful and constructive in their application.

Fortunately, the same natural tendency to grow into a more efficient, capable person that motivates many people toward drug experimentation also leads them away from drug abuse in the large majority of cases. As the average new user begins to see evidence of the hazards of intoxication, dependency, accident risk, and conflicts with authority, drug use tends to moderate or cease entirely. It is very easy to overlook this simple fact, yet studies of our most widely used psychoactive substance, beverage alcohol, shows that 90 per cent of the users do not develop abusive patterns. The figures for marijuana, although not as reliable, show a similar pattern. In our hysteria over the "drug problem" we tend to overlook the average, healthy person's tendency to avoid self-destructive behavior. Cigarette smoking represents a possible exception to this general rule. Here, the untoward effects are so slow and insidious in their onset that the individual has a well-established habit before experiencing any harmful effects.

PATTERNS of DRUG USE

Of the vast numbers of persons who are prompted to sample a popular substance such as alcohol, which may be used legally, or marijuana, whose use is socially condoned in many groups, a sizable percentage will eventually become regular users. The more widely accepted surveys generally reveal 30 to 40 per cent of the adult population as users of alcohol at least once a week. The data for marijuana, although less reliable, frequently reveal 20 per cent or more of regular users within adolescent and young adult population groups. The large majority of these persons avoid serious drug problems and thus constitute a "user" category as distinguished from abstainers or abusers. This group includes literally millions of people who are regularly involved with potent drugs; however, little reliable information is available as to their motives or the positive or negative effects this use may have on their lives. Thus far, most scientific study has centered on the abuser.

The obvious facts concerning users are (1) there is something in the substances or the conditions surrounding their use that is attractive to them—that keeps them coming back—and (2) there are enough positive or protective factors in the situation that enable them to avoid drug dependency and other serious abuse. The motivation in some cases may be purely a matter of taste; the individual may prefer wine at meals or beer to slake the thirst of a hard day's work rather than other inert beverages. Here, we have drugs used as a dietary substance. More often, the user is probably consciously or unconsciously seeking the degree of relief from everyday tensions and pressures that a mild dose of some drug such as alcohol can provide. Closely related to this pattern is the regular use of a drug as a "social lubricant" to ease the initial stiffness of a social gathering. Drugs in these cases appear to be used as coping devices.

A third category of users is formed by those who appear to enjoy "getting high" on a regular basis. When asked why they have adopted this pattern, the answers may range from a rather frivolous "just for kicks" to a sincere but presumably misguided belief that their instances of intoxication can lead to profound insights concerning themselves and/or the universe. This is often called "mind expansion." A more widely accepted explanation for this general pattern of use is that there is something lacking in the lives of persons who are otherwise quite well-adjusted persons. Those members of these categories wih more serious emotional difficulties escalate into the abuser categories; however, many continue in a stable pattern of regular use for years.

DRUG DEPENDENCY

The issue of personal susceptibility seems to lie at the heart of the drug dependency problem. Of the vast numbers of people who are prompted to sample various drugs because of curiosity and a desire to follow the behavior patterns of friends, parents, and public figures, only a small percentage will be susceptible to drug dependency and abuse problems. Why the same initial exposure will produce disenchantment in one individual and strong desire for further use in another remains the object of much research and controversy. Although several logical theories and suppositions exist, there are few well-established facts.

Individual personality factors and their interaction with the unique set of social–cultural pressures and forces that affect each person appear to be the main causes of drug abuse; however, the possibility of simple biological susceptibility cannot be discounted. Some persons tolerate their first cigarette very well, and after a few more trials they begin to reap the pleasures and satisfactions that make this habit so popular, whereas other more fortunate individuals react so adversely to their first encounter with tobacco that they are never tempted to try it again. Similarly, at the opposite end of the drug continuum, most first-time heroin users report a pleasant, euphoric reaction; however, a significant minority report either a "zero" reaction or an unpleasant nausea.[5]

But even these apparently "tissue-related" reactions appear to be affected by personality or situational variables. It has long been noted that an individual's reaction to a drug experience varies with the mood or feelings at the time. In reporting his experience with cocaine in 1885, Freud observed:

> If one takes a minimally active dose while in excellent health and does not exert any special exertion thereafter, one can hardly perceive any surprising effect. It is different, however, if this dose of cocaine hydrochloride is taken by one whose general health is impaired by fatigue or hunger. After a short time, he feels as though he had been raised to the full height of intellectual and bodily vigor, in a state of euphoria. . . .[6]

It should be noted, however, that Freud later became thoroughly disenchanted with this drug following some adverse responses to it among his patients.

Similar differences have been noted in hospital situations with depressant drugs such as morphine. The rehabilitation of patients who were accidently addicted by medical personnel is relatively simple in most cases; however, when the patient has a preexisting emotional condition with tension and anxiety symptoms, it is typically more difficult to avoid a long-term drug problem.

The implications of these various observations are clear. The best defense against drug dependency is the fostering of positive mental health. Although not infallible, this approach to control is analogous to immunizing children against polio. It is virtually impossible to prevent exposure to the dangerous agent; therefore, the most practical course of action is to build up each child's resistance to infection or, in this case, addiction.

---

[5] Oakley S. Ray, *Drugs, Society, and Human Behavior* (St. Louis: C. V. Mosby Company, 1972), p. 202.
[6] From Sigmund Freud, "On the General Effects of Cocaine," lecture before the Psychiatric Union on March 5, 1885. Reprinted in *Drug Dependence*, Vol. 5, No. 17 (1970).

Good mental health can be reasonably well defined and there is much that can be done within families, school, and society at large to promote this desirable status. However, it is equally clear that anything close to perfect mental health will remain an ideal rather than a realistic objective for the large majority of our population (see pp. 226–227). Within the foreseeable future, the average child will always carry some degree of susceptibility to drug dependency and other forms of self-destructive behavior.

The consequences of becoming dependent on a potent drug such as alcohol, heroin, or the barbiturates are well known. These include the increased exposure to accident risk, the overdose, the tissue damage that can result from a deterioration of health habits, and the long and intense use of a toxic substance in the case of alcohol or the hazards of unsterile needles and consequent infections in the case of heroin.

Although these tissue-related threats are very real and should not be discounted, they should not overshadow the more common and equally devasting consequences on the behavior and personality of the abuser. The drug-dependent person typically spends a significant portion of his or her waking hours either intoxicated to some degree or preoccupied with thoughts and plans for the next occasion of drug use. Anything close to full attention to one's work or social interaction with others becomes impossible and performance in these areas soon begins to deteriorate. Academic, vocational, and/or social skills fail to develop, and relationships become damaged, both with schools, employers, friends and loved ones, and, perhaps most important, with oneself as self-confidence is lost. All this can occur long before any physical damage becomes evident.

THE CHARACTERISTICS of DRUGS

A drug is commonly defined as any substance other than food that can alter the structure or functioning of the body. Within this necessarily broad category those drugs that are psychoactive—that effect changes in mood, feeling, and/or behavior—merit particular attention because of their high potential for abuse. The various schemes for classfying drugs can become extremely complicated; in terms of clinical use there are analgesics, antidepressants, sedatives, narcotics, hypnotics, soporifics, just to mention a few of the more common categories. From a legal standpoint psychoactive drugs are placed in five somewhat illogical categories mainly on the basis of their supposed potential for abuse; another more logical, yet complex system is based on the chemical structure of these substances.

Although somewhat oversimplified, it is more useful to divide drugs into three categories according to their basic effects on the individual.

DEPRESSANTS.   A wide variety of drugs function to slow down such bodily processes as heart rate, respiratory rate, reaction time, and muscle tone, and thus may be termed depressants. Subjective reactions are typically experienced as relaxation, a reduction in inhibitions, and often a drowsy euphoria. The better-known members of this category include the opiates such as heroin, morphine, and codeine; the synthetic opiates such as methadone and demerol; the barbiturates such as phenobarbital and seconal, often termed "downers"; and beverage alcohol in its many forms. Tranquilizers are similar to the depressants; however, they are more specific in their effects. When used in proper amounts they tend to reduce anxiety without causing any general depression of bodily functions. All the major depressants carry the threat of death by respiratory failure in case of an overdose (O.D.), and all can lead to severe forms of physical addiction. In addition to the desirable feeling of relaxation or euphoria, significant doses also produce varying degrees of temporary impairment of cognitive functions including judgment, reasoning, and memory.

STIMULANTS. As the name implies, stimulants speed up bodily processes and, from a subjective standpoint, tend to make the individual feel and act more energetic; when taken in intoxicating amounts a euphoric high often results, but with different qualities than with the depressants. The most important examples of drugs in this category are cocaine and the various amphetamines (uppers). Regular use commonly leads to a low-grade physical dependency characterized by lethargy and fatigue in the absence of the drugs; lethal doses produce death by either cerebral hemorrhage or heat stroke. Amphetamines are frequently used on the campus to maintain alertness while studying for exams. Although the majority of students no doubt gain some immediate benefits without incurring any serious harm, involvement with stimulant drugs carries the risk of (1) becoming dependent on them to avoid chronic feelings of fatigue and (2) a consequent habit of barbiturate use to "come down" for relaxation and sleep.

HALLUCINOGENS. Such drugs as LSD, the lesser-known mescaline and peyote (derived from cactus plants), and psilocybin (a variety of mushroom) tend to produce changes in perception and cognition with few major effects on bodily processes and are thus classed as hallucinogens. Marijuana, although generally milder in its effects, is also commonly placed in this category. The effects of any of these drugs vary widely according to (1) the amount and potency of the particular drug involved, (2) the nature of the situation or the circumstances surrounding its use, and (3) individual differences in the neural system and/or personality structure of the individual involved. However, alterations in the judgment of time and the perceived size, shape, and color of objects are frequently reported with the ingestion of large doses, as are overt auditory or visual hallucinations.

The occasional use of marijuana in social situations probably involves no more real risks than the normal social use of alcohol, other than the threat of legal consequences. At the other extreme, use of the more potent LSD has, on occasion, led to serious accidents, suicide, and severe psychotic reactions to "bad trips." But as with the other drug categories the overall impact on the users' quality of life depends not so much on the particular drug used but on the way it is used. Some persons no doubt can use any one of the common hallucinogens for years without any untoward effects. However, these drugs pose the same common threat as do all other drugs that produce significant psychoactive effects. Highly susceptible individuals may develop use patterns that involve frequent, perhaps daily, intoxication; when this pattern persists over months and years, a steady erosion of the individual's social, recreational, and/or vocational life frequently ensues.

OVER-THE-COUNTER DRUGS. A wide variety of mild psychoactive substances are available without prescription in any drugstore and most supermarkets. Aspirin in appropriate doses commonly provides significant relief from occasional headaches and the fever and achiness of colds and similar infections; however, excessive use can lead to significant stomach irritation. Also, it is still the leading cause of accidental deaths due to poisoning among children. A variety of antihistamine compounds are marketed as relievers of cold symptoms. Although many people gain a measure of relief from symptoms, the side effects involved can produce problems in certain instances. Drowsiness is the most common side effect; this is capitalized on when the same basic compounds are prepared in higher doses as aids to relaxation and sleep.

SUGGESTED LEARNING ACTIVITIES

The following suggestions are presented in an effort to demonstrate how the content described in the preceding section might be translated into effective classroom learning activities. They were designd to accommodate a wide variety of classroom groups provided that proper selection and adaptations are made according to the needs, interests, abilities, and maturity level of the particular children involved.

- Ask the children to be "people peepers" for one week. Have them use an invisible magnifying glass to detect ways either their friends or adults get their "kicks" out of life. Before you send them on their investigation, have them discuss what the word *kick* means to them.
- Have the students decorate a wastepaper basket or cardboard box with the letters "Basket of Dependencies." Have them write on slips of paper all those things that either they, their parents, brother or sister, or other people seem dependent on (e.g., vitamins, watching TV, food, aspirin). List only one dependency on each slip of paper. During the

week have the children select slips of paper and discuss them with the class. Ask them if these dependencies could be given up.

• Have the children draw a tree and write on its branches some of the problems they are currently facing (e.g., use of marijuana, alcohol, or cigarettes, obesity, lack of friends). Many times these are not the real problems but symptoms of other less obvious ones. The roots of their tree are to represent those problems of which the children may not be aware but which may actually be the main cause for the problem on the branches (e.g., parents, separation, failure to make the school's hockey team, failing grades). If they cannot fill in the roots at first, don't press them but work with them on seeing the real causes/reasons for the branches.

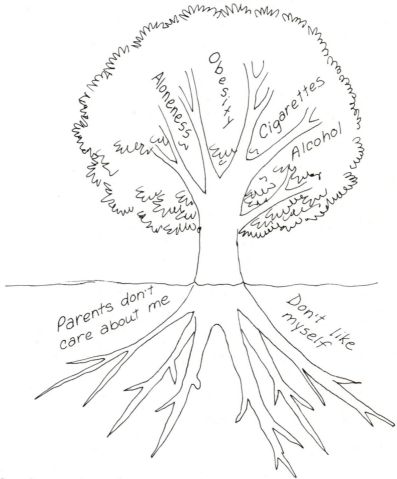

• Select four or five students from the class and have them wear the same clothes, fix their hair the same way, and so forth. If you have

287

a set of identical twins either in your class or at the school, they may be used for your discussion. After these students have been presented to the class, have a group discussion on how they are really different even though they look alike. How is it that, even though we may be brought up in the same family, our values and ideas may be different? Another way to present the concept of how things are really different when they look alike is to use the activity "Lemon Game" from the *Handbook of Structured Experiences for Human Relations Training*, by Pfeifer and Jones, University Associates, La Jolla, California.

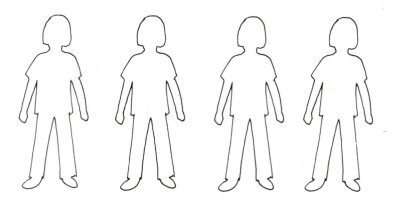

- Have the students take a dinner-size paper plate or a paper bag and draw their faces to represent how they feel about themselves. On the reverse side have them complete the following statement: "There is no one in the world like me because_____."
- Have the children bring in different-colored pieces of felt large enough to make a banner. Have the students design a banner for their room that describes them.
- Each year "National Smoking Education Week" is held during the month of January. Have the children design a paperweight with each side representing reasons why people should not smoke. Have the children present the paperweight to someone they know who smokes as a reminder of what can happen to their life if they continue. If they do not know of anyone who smokes, see if either one of the other students or you can help them locate an individual that they could present their paperweight to.
- Boredom is one of the major reasons that individuals give for turning to alcohol, drugs, etc. Have the children create a "Community Resource Box" of all the activities that their school, youth groups, churches, etc., have to offer. Have them make a record for each activity as to when it is

offered, fees or other costs involved, the telephone number, address, and times they are open. Place the box in a central location so that all the students can benefit from it. Along with the box, they could also create a monthly calendar of events.

• On construction paper have the children draw a large pair of eyeglasses. On the lenses, have them write about how they feel when people smoke. When they have completed their projects, have the students share their glasses with the class. As each one of us looks through our glasses, we can see that our own personal values cause us to see different reasons why people feel differently about people smoking.

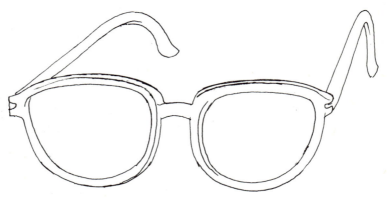

How I feel when people smoke.

• Place written descriptions of various situations inside a grocery bag. These should be the open-ended descriptions that need endings. Ask volunteers to role-play each situation. Stop each one before closure and ask the class to provide an appropriate ending.

Situation 1:

Your sister has been to the school dance and she calls home for a ride. Your older brother arrives on his motorcycle to pick her up. She discovers that he has been drinking and has a can of beer with him. What should she do?

Situation 2:

You are in the school's lavoratory when you are surrounded by a group of students. They hand you a glass jar with various-colored pills in it. They encourage you to take one. You refuse and try to leave when they corner you and start chanting, "Take one, take one." What should you do?

Situation 3:

Your parents just finished entertaining some guests before going to

289

a play. While helping to clean up you noticed that someone left a pack of cigarettes behind. You have always wondered what it would be like to smoke a cigarette, so you take one and you are just about to light it when_____.

- Have the students create a scale like the one represented in the picture. On one side of the scale have the students place paper disks representing events they feel cause *pressure* in peoples' lives. On the other side, have them place disks representing things that can help alleviate pressure in peoples' lives (ways to cope with problems).

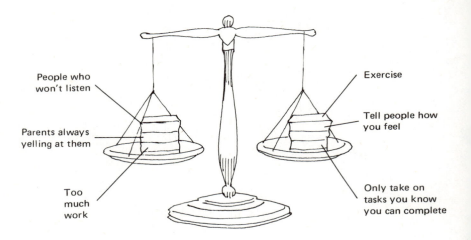

People who won't listen

Parents always yelling at them

Too much work

Exercise

Tell people how you feel

Only take on tasks you know you can complete

- Ask the children to think of the last time they felt restless, sad, or bored and the way they were able to change these unpleasant feelings. Invite them to share these experiences.
- Have the children create pictures or word descriptions to represent all the reasons they feel good about life. Take a piece of yarn with clip-on clothespins, hang their creations for everyone to see. Have them take their project home to hang in their room as a reminder of how important life is and the importance of keeping it happy and healthy.
- Have the children design a wishing well. Have them make anonymous wishes either for themselves or for their parents, brother, sister, friend, etc., write them on a piece of paper and place them in the well. Just before lunch each day, select one of the wishes and share it with the rest of the class. Through hearing the wishes of other students, they may begin thinking about things they had never thought of before.

On their sheet of paper
complete: "I wish. . . . . ."

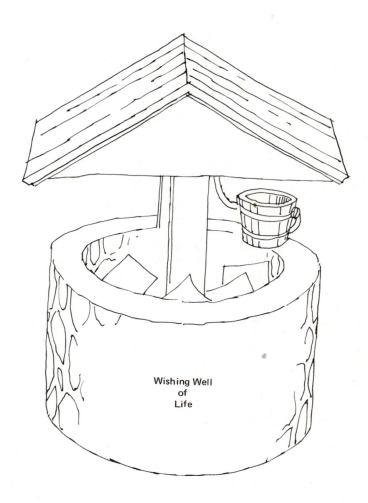

Wishing Well
of
Life

SUGGESTED RESOURCES

The learning resources listed in this section are a selected sample of materials with which the authors are personally familiar. Appropriate grade levels have been included when these were indicated by the source.

ALCOHOL

BOOKS

Alcohol
Scott, Foresman and Co.
S. Hofstein
Glenview, Illinois 60025

Alcohol and Alcoholism
Marvin Block
Wadsworth Co.
Belmont, California

Basic Concepts of Alcohol
Laidlaw Brothers
A Division of Doubleday and Company
Thatcher and Madison
River Forest, Illinois 60305

Facts About Alcohol and Alcoholism
National Institute on Alcohol Abuse and Alcoholism
5600 Fishers Lane
Rockville, Maryland 20852

National Clearinghouse for Alcohol Education
P.O. Box 2345
Rockville, Maryland 20852

You and Alcohol
Choose for Yourself
Dr. Maurice Ames
Ramapo House
235 East 45th Street
New York, New York 10017

You and Your Alcoholic Parent
Edith Hornek
Public Affairs Pamphlets
381 Park Ave. South
New York, New York 10016

CURRICULUM

A Programed Unit on Facts About Alcohol
Julius Shevlin and Isidor Goldberg

Allyn and Bacon Inc.
Boston, Massachusetts

FILMSTRIPS

Alcohol and Children
Educational Activities, Inc.
Box 392
Freeport, New York 11520

What Are You Going to Do About Alcohol
Grades 5–8
Guidance Associates
757 Third Ave.
New York, New York 10017

PAMPHLETS

Alcohol and You
Channing L. Bete Co.
Greenfield, Massachusetts 01301

Teaching About Drinking
NIAAA
Superintendent of Documents
U.S. Government Printing Office
Washington, D.C. 20402

What Teacher Should Know About Children from Alcoholic Parents
Alcoholics Anonymous
Local Chapter

DRUGS

BOOKS

Bensley, Marvin
Values Education—A Promising Approach to the Drug Problem
Curriculum Trends
Croft Educational Services, Inc.
New London, Connecticut

Dennis the Menace Takes a Poke at Poison
Grades 3–6
U.S. Department of Health, Education, and Welfare
Washington, D.C.

Drugs and Your Safety
Scott, Foresman and Co.
Glenview, Illinois

Katy's Coloring Book About Drugs and Health
U.S. Department of Justice
Washington, D.C.

Super Me
Bi-Lingual Drug Abuse Prevention Activitity Book
NCCDE Publications
726 Jackson Place, N.W.
Washington, D.C. 20506

Tuffy Talks About Medicine
Grades K–3
Coloring Book
Aetna Life Insurance Company
151 Farmington Ave.
Hartford, Connecticut 06115

CURRICULA

Coronado Plan
Grade K–6
Pennant Press
Progressive Playthings
San Diego, California 92120

Teaching About Drugs
A Curriculum Guide K–12
American School Health Association and
the Pharmaceutical Association
Kent, Ohio

FILMSTRIPS

Drugs—Friend or Foe
Marsh Films
P.O. Box 8082
Shawnee Mission, Kansas 66208

Me, Myself, and Drugs
Grades 4–6
Guidance Associates
757 Third Ave.
New York, New York 10017

Squeeze Learns About Drugs
Marsh Films
P.O. Box 8082
Shawnee Mission, Kansas 66208

POSTERS

National Tar Headquarters
359 National Press Building
Washington, D.C. 20045

GAMES/ACTIVITIES

Drug Attack Game
Lockheed Education Department
Technicon Medical Informational Services
Mt. View, California 94040

SMOKING

BOOKS

About You and Smoking
Houser, Richmond, Harrelson
Scott, Foresman and Co.
Glenview, Illinois 60025

Morris the Mule
Comic Book
York Toronto
Tuberculosis and Respiratory Disease
157 Willowdale Ave.
Willowdale, Ontario M2N4Y7

The Story of a Cigarette
Coloring Book
Grades K–3

American Cancer Society
Lindsey R. Curtis, M.D.
Contact your local society

You and Smoking
Dr. Robert Spellani
Ramapo House
235 East 45th Street
New York, New York 10017

FILMSTRIPS

Decision for Mike
Grades 5–8
American Cancer Society
Contact your local society

What Are You Going to Do About Smoking?
Grades 5–8
Guidance Associates
757 Third Ave.
New York, New York 10017

GAMES/ACTIVITIES

Think and Do Sheets
Signal Press
1730 Chicago Avenue
Evanston, Illinois 60201

PUZZLE

Smoking Puzzle
American Lung Association
Contact your local chapter

ENVIRONMENTAL and HEALTH SERVICE ASPECTS

As indicated in the preceding discussion, the emotional climate of the school probably has much to do with the extent to which drugs are used or abused by pupils. There are two aspects that may be important, one positive, the other negative. The positive aspect has to do with the opportunities present in the school for self-fulfillment. These include such things as the use of student art rather than commercial art in the decoration of the building. It also includes the involvement of all students in preparations for major activities such as field days, PTA fairs, science fairs, and the like. These things enhance the feeling pupils may have that "This is my school, and I am an important part of it." The negative but still useful aspect is an attitude shared by a solid majority of both pupils and teachers alike that says that "The use of certain drugs is not tolerated within the school or on its grounds. We understand and tolerate drug users, but we don't allow them to use their drugs here."

Putting both these attitudes into practice is strongly abetted by replacing large schools, which are inherently impersonal and dehumanizing, with very small ones, where everyone knows and watches the behavior of everyone else, and in which all teachers and pupils come to know and be interested in one another.

Occasionally, a child will appear in school who is high on a drug of some kind. Unless signs of respiratory or circulatory difficulty, including deep anesthesia, appear, knowledgeable health service professionals will generally provide the time, rest, and reassurance that finally bring recovery. Such instances not only are rare in most schools but also most often signify only that these youngsters have been experimenting with a drug. Only a very few of them have a drug abuse problem and many of them experiment with relatively harmless drugs that rarely cause dependency, such as marijuana.

The discovery of the rare youngster who has become dependent on a drug presents two very real problems. The first is that our present harsh drug laws generally cause more harm than they prevent, and if the police are called in they may deal with the youngster in ways that are legally appropriate but socially inappropriate. Elementary-age youngsters are provided a degree of protection by their legal status as juveniles, but the juvenile justice system in the United States leaves much to be desired.[7] In cases where intervention by legal authorities occurs, it is important that the school have a well-defined policy governing such interventions designed to protect the rights of both children and parents. Such a policy must, of course, be worked out jointly by school and police officials, but it usually requires that students may be interrogated by police on school property only in the presence of their parents.

The second problem is that, with the exception of well-designed methadone maintenance programs, the treatment of drug-dependent behavior has not proven to be highly effective. However, neither the school health nor the school psychological service is the appropriate agency to determine whether a drug problem exists and to treat it. It is their business to know the

---

[7] See Lisa Aversa Richette, *The Throwaway Children* (New York: Dell Publishing Co., Inc., 1969) .

sources of help available in the community and to make the best referral possible.

Given the general ineffectiveness of both the legal and treatment apparatus, it does not seem appropriate for schools to engage in drug abuse case finding through screening tests or searches of pupil possessions. These approaches tend to destroy any confidence pupils may have in school staff members as helping and trustworthy adults. A more desirable approach is to seek to find students who show any signs of generally disturbed behavior, which may include drug use, and try to help, while avoiding labeling them as drug problems.

REFERENCES

BLOOMQUIST, EDWARD R. *Marijuana*. Beverly Hills, Calif.: Glencoe Press, 1968.

CORNACCHIA, HAROLD J., DAVID J. BENTEL, and DAVID E. SMITH. *Drugs in the Classroom: A Conceptual Model for School Programs*. St. Louis: C. V. Mosby Company, 1973.

DELONE, RICHARD H. "The Ups and Downs of Drug-Abuse Education," *Saturday Review of Education* (September 11, 1972), p. 28.

FREUD, SIGMUND. "On the General Effects of Cocaine." Lecture before the Psychiatric Union on March 5, 1885. Reprinted in *Drug Dependence*, Vol. 5, No. 17 (1970).

LINGEMAN, RICHARD R. *Drugs from A to Z*. New York: McGraw-Hill Book Company, 1974.

McGRATH, JOHN H., and FRANK R. SCARPITTI. *Youth and Drugs*. Glenview, Ill.: Scott, Foresman and Co., 1970.

MILES, SAMUEL V. (ed.). *Learning About Alcohol*. Washington, D.C.: American Association for Health, Physical Education, and Recreation, 1974.

PLAUT, THOMAS F. A. *Alcohol Problems*. London: Oxford University Press, 1968.

RAY, OAKLEY S. *Drugs, Society, and Human Behavior*. St. Louis: C. V. Mosby Company, 1972.

part 4

The Plan

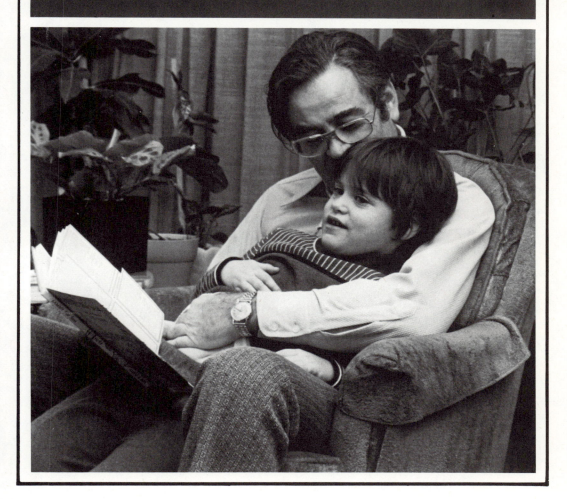

Health Curriculum— The Structure

As beginning teachers face their first teaching job, they normally exhibit far more interest in *how* to teach than *what* to teach. They assume with considerable justification that the curriculum has been established prior to their arrival and that the content to be covered in the fourth grade, for example, will be reasonably well specified in some sort of curriculum guide. Consequently, in the authors' experience, teachers show great interest in obtaining new teaching materials such as films, filmstrips and pamphlets, slightly less interest in learning new (to them) teaching techniques such as values clarification and role playing, and very little interest in initiating or participating in efforts to revise the curriculum.

PASSIVE ACCEPTANCE

In most school situations it is appropriate for teachers to accept the curriculum as it is for the first year or two while they are adapting to their profession if this is their first job, or to a new school if they have had previous teaching experience. Behind this pattern of acceptance should lie the willingness and ability to play a part in future decisions as to what should be taught at particular grade levels and what the general direction of the school's program should be. This imperative applies both to the total school curriculum and to specific areas within the curriculum such as health education. Unfortunately, the way things should be is seldom the way they are in the majority of schools with respect to curriculum revision.

Both veteran and beginning teachers typically accept the assigned content as given and apply their energies to the teaching tasks without seriously questioning why the decision was made that it should be taught at their grade level. And, worse yet, supervisors and other administrative personnel

301

with specific responsibilities for the orderly revision of the curriculum assign this task a relatively low priority in comparison with personnel matters, budget concerns, and other aspects of school management. Therefore, it is possible that a new sixth grade teacher in the 1970s may find that some harassed committee working after school in the 1960s decided that health education at his or her grade level should consist of the study of cleanliness and grooming, communicable disease, and nutrition. And without much stretch of the imagination one might find that the committee of the 1960s, feeling somewhat overwhelmed by the task of establishing a health curriculum from scratch, had used the well-known "cut and paste" method of curriculum development and borrowed largely from a neighboring school district's program that had been established in the 1950s.

Most school districts, of course, will not allow a major portion of the curriculum to go 20 years without revision; but too often revisions are merely superficial in nature rather than a basic review of the content itself. In some cases a committee will merely alter the format and update the terminology. "Principles" of nutrition become "concepts" of nutrition; "attitudes" toward nutrition become "values" regarding nutrition; old-fashioned educational outcomes such as "to help pupils develop the ability to select a balanced meal" are reworded "the pupil selects a balanced meal when given a choice of several foods" and relabeled as behavioral objectives. Another committee might leave the format and jargon essentially unchanged and direct its effort at updating the content within the topic, consequently, references to cod-liver oil and the advantages of brown over white bread might be dropped in favor of information concerning government-mandated enrichment programs. But neither committee would dare challenge the basic idea that nutrition, communicable disease, and cleanliness and grooming are the priority topics for the sixth grade.

SPECIAL HANDICAPS

The problems described here tend to be found throughout all areas or subjects of the curriculum; however, they tend to be particularly acute where health education is concerned. Although the reasons for this are not entirely clear, certain factors appear as particular obstacles to good curriculum development in health. Two of these that are quite specific to the task of curriculum development will be considered here.

PROBLEMS OF SEQUENCE. Unlike mathematics and reading, whose content tends to suggest an orderly sequence, health education sometimes develops as a somewhat formless collection of topics that seem to contain few logical starting points. In the realm of mathematics it is logical that children learn about the place value of numbers before they attempt to study decimal fractions. Teachers who violate the inherent discipline imposed by the sequential aspects of mathematics will soon find that they have a class of thoroughly frustrated children. But although health content should be arranged in a logical sequence, one can get by with little thought to this important aspect of curriculum structure. Fifth grade pupils may study the anatomy and physiology of the body, for instance. In the sixth grade these same pupils may study human reproduction, where the whole concept of hormones and endocrine control of body functions either will be taught over again, or will be ignored completely, with such comments as the "uterus engorges with blood because it must get ready for the egg." Somehow, in most health lessons no one asks how the uterus was smart enough to "know" that the egg was coming.

PROBLEMS OF PERSONNEL.   Some teachers and administrators tend to regard health education as something outside the regular curriculum, something that exists purely as some adjunct to health services. As a subject, they view it as mysterious and complex, one that contains aspects over which parents sometimes become emotional; therefore, the safest thing to do is to leave all decisions in the hands of nurses and physicians. The programs may not then become very dynamic, so the reasoning goes, but at least we cannot be sued for teaching medically unsound content. The problem, of course, is that physicians and nurses, although highly trained and knowledgeable in the treatment of specific illnesses and injuries, often have difficulty in determining what aspects of their knowledge would be of most value to the average laymen, and have even greater difficulty in relating these aspects to the educational needs of elementary schoolchildren. A common exception to this generalization is the school nurse who is also trained as an educator; such a person combines the best of both worlds. Unfortunately, there are few such persons available. Therefore, in most school situations it is particularly important that teachers and health professionals work together in planning the health curriculum.

CURRICULUM STRUCTURE

Other than the need to recognize these specific obstacles, the curriculum development task within the field of health education is virtually identical to that of any other field. Theoretically, there would be no need to discuss the structure of the health curriculum because it would be identical to that for social science, for example, although the content within the structure would obviously vary. However, there is some value in reviewing the general task of fitting health education content into the standard framework, if for no other reason than to provide some assurance that it does indeed fit. Furthermore, because the curriculum seems to be a pervasive influence within the school (to understate the case) that no one appears to fully understand or control, the authors cannot resist the temptation to try to reduce this complex topic to understandable terms.

THE SCHOOL'S PHILOSOPHY

Most schools or school systems have a statement of philosophy; however, many of these documents were written years ago by persons who have long since retired, moved on, or passed away. This in itself is no great fault, as the nation is still being served quite effectively by the authors of our constitution, long deceased as they are. However, in contrast to the living constitution of the nation, most school philosophies were not all that meaningful in the first place and subsequently served no practical purpose in the years the school was supposed to be functioning in harmony with their provisions.

Most school personnel are vaguely aware of this somewhat silly situation and, unfortunately, react in ways that further confuse the matter. Administrators often try to preserve the original illusion. They may dig the statement out of the files, dust it off, and maintain that it does indeed guide the major decisions relating to the school. A more common reaction is to shrug one's shoulders and say, "I really was never much of one for philosophy—I'm more of a practical, commonsense type of a person." The problem with both of these reactions is that they ignore the fact that schools have real philosophies as constituted by the composite beliefs and values of those that carry out their programs. These beliefs may be very diverse and consequently operate at cross-purposes on frequent occasions, but they are just as likely to be reasonably homogeneous as those who do the hirings consistently search for "our kind of people."

It is important to recognize that regardless of what "your kind of people" may be, a program of health education may be devised that will conform with the general point of view of the school or the school system. Health educators have philosophies; it is to be hoped that the perceptive reader has noticed a humanistic theme throughout this text, for example. However, health education as a curricular area is not bound to any single point of view. If an individual curriculum committee or a school or school system favors the "good, hard subject matter" approach with emphasis on basic knowledge from the scholarly disciplines, it can develop a health curriculum based on the basic principles of physiology, psychology, and anthropology, for example. If the people involved are more interested in process than in conventional subject matter, a discovery approach may be adopted with the assurance that the broad and inherently relevant field of health will provide many promising topics for individual exploration. If a school is located in a poverty area and "does not have time for these curricular games," so to speak, the people involved will find that health education

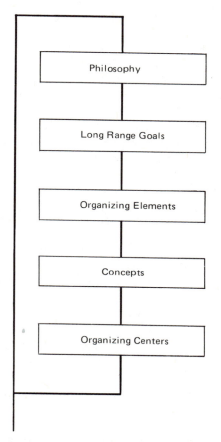

Figure 13.1. Curriculum Structure—General Components.

is eminently compatible with a program focused on economic and cultural survival.

Health education may always have a practical tone to its subject matter because it is inherently directed at the more basic human needs. This is as it should be, but it is also important that health education be viewed as a subject that fits into the mainstream of the school's curriculum. It has not been well served in situations where it is treated as something distinct from other school subjects.

LONG-RANGE GOALS

The first step in the long and arduous task of translating a general philosophy (which may or may not be in written form) into real classroom experiences is the formulation of long-range goals or, as they are sometimes called, "aims" or broad "objectives." Although the terminology may vary, the purpose of this component of the written curriculum is to express the values and beliefs, that is, the philosophy, in terms of the educational effects on the learner. These may be very general and somewhat vague, such as "the development of good citizenship," or they may be more specific, such as "the learner develops a valid self-concept that contributes to emotional stability."

Another somewhat related characteristic of long-range goals is that they may be developed for a total school or district program in a tight, highly integrated curriculum structure that features various subject matter areas (mathematics, science, etc.), all of which are planned with a view toward contributing to a single, broadly stated set of goals. The first example above concerning citizenship would be appropriate to such a structure. In other cases separate sets of goals are developed for each subject matter area, with all these individual sets of goals presumably designed to be compatible with some guiding philosophy. The second example above might be found among goals formulated specifically for a health education program.

It is true, unfortunately, that many statements of long-range goals are so full of meaningless clichés that they provide no direction to teachers or to those charged with the responsibility to develop teaching materials designed to implement these goals; however, it does not have to be this way. An example of a good long-range goal for the curriculum in health in the authors' opinion would be

> The learner exhibits tolerance toward persons whose health behavior differs from his/her own.

A teacher or curriculum development group seeking to construct a teaching unit on the topic of "alcoholic beverages," for example, would have to use some care in order to take proper cognizance of this particular aim. If the group was operating in a typical community where two thirds of the parents used alcohol on occasion, including one third who drank on a weekly or a daily basis, it could not restrict the unit content to a long list of alcohol-related problems without also giving proper attention to the 90 per cent of the drinking population who do not have these problems. Similarly, a unit on weight control, although appropriately highlighting the health values of slimness, would also point out that many overweight people lead happy, satisfying lives and do not spend all their waking hours agonizing over their excess pounds.

Another example of a goal in the same philosophical realm might be

> The learner feels comfortable and self-assured with his/her pattern of health behavior.

306

Most modern health educators as well as educators from other fields believe that children should learn to perceive discrepancies between what they believe in and how they behave; this is one of the fundamental purposes of values clarification. With this awareness they are better equipped to heal this "behavioral gap," cognitive dissonance, or whatever is labeled. The ultimate thrust of this general strategy is the development of children who do more and worry less about their health.

These are two examples of long-range goals for a health program that might negate the too-common tendency to ignore the individuality of each child when it comes time for health instruction. Very often, teachers throughout the course of a school year will convey the impression to children that in terms of politics you might wisely choose to be a Republican, a Democrat, or perhaps even a Socialist; in terms of religions you might wisely select Catholicism, Methodism, or Mormonism as your religion. But, in regard to health, only stupid people choose to be other than slim, muscular, nonsmoking, nondrinkers who always finish their milk.

MAJOR CONTENT AREAS

Once a guiding philosophy has been established and translated into long-range goals, the next step is to set up the major divisions of the curriculum as content areas, topical areas, or, in the language of pure curriculumese, *organizing elements*. When the elementary school curriculum is viewed as a whole, such subjects as social studies, language arts, and mathematics are examples of organizing elements. The definitive characteristic of these components is that they are broad enough and relevant enough to appear within the curriculum at each grade level or within the K–12 context at least at each school level. Social studies, for example, meets these criteria as it commonly is taught each year, although it may take the form of "My Neighborhood" with first graders and "Friends from Other Lands" with sixth graders. U.S. history normally would not qualify; this topic is so narrow it might appear at only one or two grade levels.

Health as an area of study becomes an organizing element of the curriculum of many elementary schools, and, like other such components, is commonly divided into organizing elements of its own within the health curriculum. Within this specific segment of the curriculum the same criteria apply; thus "Disease Control" becomes an example of an *organizing element* within the health curriculum, because learning experiences from this relatively broad area may appropriately be presented at each grade level or school level. "Heart Disease" and "The Body's Resistance to Disease" would not be organizing elements because they might receive visible emphasis only at one grade level. The organizing elements extend vertically through the curriculum from K to 6 if planning is restricted to one school level, or

K–12 in a systemwide format. The typical content areas presented in Chapter 1 (pp. 22–24) to describe the scope of health education as an area of study are also examples of a relatively comprehensive set of organizing elements.

These were

1. Structure and Functions of the Human Body
2. The Natural Environment
3. Nutrition
4. Disease
5. Safety
6. Consumer Health
7. Psychoactive Substances
8. Mental Health
9. Human Sexuality
10. Family Living

There is no one official list; each one tends to reflect the special beliefs or priorities of its creator or, if a committee product, its creators, and this example devised by the authors is no exception. Note that both "Human Sexuality" and "Family Living" appear, for instance; many health professionals would feel that this represents unnecessary duplication of content in these related areas. However, the authors believe that much of what is important about sexuality has little to do with families and much of what is important about families has little direct relationship to sexuality yet is vitally important to human well-being; thus both would appear as major organizing elements if these views prevailed. A common favorite, "Community Health," does not appear simply because it was felt that content related to this admittedly important area of study is best integrated into each of the designated areas. Thus study of the Food and Drug Administration area might occur with the study of consumer health, the U.S. Public Health Service with the study of disease, and so forth. The rationale presented in support of these choices is not so important in itself, as good curricula take many specific forms, but it does provide a good sample of the type of reasoning that must occur if a well-balanced and coherent curriculum structure is to be developed.

Perhaps a more relevant example is provided by the organizing elements of the officially adopted Maryland State Education Curriculum; it is organized into six major strands as follows:

1. Natural Conditions
2. Man-Made Products and Services
3. Social Forces
4. Sensory Stimulation

5. Assimilated Substances
6. Genetic Perpetuation [1]

Once again, one can find evidence of the specific views and priorities as expressed by a particular curriculum development group. An interesting innovation in this curriculum is the combining of the study of nutrition and psychoactive substances into a single strand termed "Assimilated Substances." The group no doubt felt that some of the same social and emotional factors that affect food choices and weight control, for instance, also determine personal behavior with respect to alcohol and tobacco products. Also illustrated is the tendency of curriculum development groups to alter the titles of relatively standard categories in efforts to more clearly designate the various elements. Thus what others might call the "Natural Environment" here becomes "Natural Conditions" and an area commonly termed "Consumer Health" here becomes "Man-Made Products and Services," perhaps to provide an early indication to those using the guide that they will be called on to deal with a broader range of subtopics than they might otherwise expect.

Although the organizing elements of various curricula are usually expressed in the form of labels or titles of broad areas of content as in the examples above, in one of the more highly regarded curriculum models within health education, that of The School Health Education Study, the organizing elements of their curriculum were expressed in such statements as

- There Are Reciprocal Relationships Involving Man, Disease, and Environment
- The Family Serves to Perpetuate Man and to Fulfill Certain Health Needs [2]

The first statement provides a mandate for the study of society concerns within the closely related topics of disease and environment and, in addition, places special emphasis on the reciprocal aspects. A simple example might be that human beings affect the environment by activities that pollute the air, and the environment, thus altered, affects them by contributing to the development of respiratory diseases such as emphysema. The second statement calls for the study of human reproduction, i.e., the perpetuation of man, within a family context that should obviously cover other family functions, e.g., the fulfillment of certain health needs. These interpretations may seem rather obvious and simple minded; however, whoever seeks to implement the work of any curriculum committee or group must read its document carefully and apply honest effort to the interpretation of its meaning. Many

---

[1] *Health Education: A Curricular Approach to Optimal Health* (Baltimore, Md.: Maryland State Department of Education, 1973).
[2] School Health Education Study, *Health Education: A Conceptual Approach to Curriculum Design* (St. Paul, Minn.: 3M Education Press, 1967), p. 22.

good curriculum development efforts have gone for naught because action-oriented teachers and supervisors have "gone off half-cocked" so to speak after a cursory review of a new curriculum guide.

CONCEPTS

The organization of the health curriculum into a group of broad content areas provides an immediate indication of its general scope as well as significant clues to the subject matter priorities of the developing committee. However, the information to be gleaned from a review of the content areas alone is very limited. One may see, for example, that nutrition will be taught, but one must look to the more specific components of the curriculum to see what content will be emphasized within this broad area of subject matter. Many curriculum groups have found the formulation or selection of concepts to be very worthwhile because of their value as organizers of the planning process and as a means of communicating to teachers the specific intentions of the curriculum development group.

Concepts, by Asahel Woodruff's widely accepted definition, are complete and meaningful ideas that exist within persons' minds. As such, they are unique, individualized constructs that are influenced by each student's previous learning experiences and the specific characteristics of his or her perceptual and cognitive equipment. A unit on drug education might include the study of alcoholism as a specific component or concept to be developed, for example, and although teachers might encourage all their pupils to develop a uniformly valid concept of this health problem, a pupil with parents who drink in moderation will form a quite different concept than a classmate with an alcoholic parent. Even if the alcoholism concepts of these two pupils contain similar cognitive content, they would very likely differ along their affective dimension. The child with nonalcoholic parents is not going to feel the same about this disease as the child who lives with the problem each day.

It is this quality of combining the cognitive and the affective into a single meaningful idea that makes the "concept" a highly useful planning component. As the attention of the class is directed to each new concept, each pupil is led into learning activities that challenge him or her with the questions (1) what do I know about this thing and (2) how do I feel about it. Both knowledge and feelings related to a particular concept must conform in a harmonious way with reality and with the other important aspects of the pupil's conceptual structure if it is to serve him or her in a constructive manner. This brief discussion of the underlying dynamics of concept formation should also identify the concepts that appear in curriculum guides as not true concepts but mere verbal descriptions of concepts that pupils

310

and students will be encouraged to develop. Although these "paper concepts" are but dim reflections of the rich and vital idea that may have been in some curriculum worker's mind, they still can prove useful as a means of communication among professionals who understand the full significance of this useful curriculum component.

MEANINGFUL FOCAL POINTS

Thus far, considerations involved in the decisions made in the typical curriculum structure under discussion have been related to what might be called long-range strategy—to the organization of the curriculum structure as it extends over the full 6 or 7 years of the conventional elementary school, or the 13 years encompassed by a K–12 curriculum plan. Horizontally, the concern has been with the full breadth of health as described by all its subareas or organizing elements. These decisions are important if children are not to study the same "dumb" things each year, sometimes even including the same "dumb" movies, and if there is to be genuine progression in the form of sequential experiences designed to capitalize on prior learning. But, as important as these strategic decisions are, the classroom teacher is likely to show far more interest in the week-to-week and day-to-day "tactics" of curriculum implementation.

The planning task comes down to earth, so to speak, when an *organizing center* is selected around which to focus the designated learning experiences for a particular organizing element at a particular grade level. This curriculum component often takes the form of a teaching–learning unit or series of units as described in Chapter 14. As such, it represents the level at which the theoretical considerations that formed the curriculum structure are translated into practical terms for presentation in the classroom. On the basis of interest studies and the overall requirements of the curriculum with respect, for example, to nutrition, it might be logical to select the fourth grade as the most appropriate level for the study of food selection and the makeup of a balanced diet. Digestion might be emphasized in the fifth grade and weight control in the sixth grade, but food selection per se is slated for the fourth grade. It might be approached through a theme of "Meals Around the World" to provide an interesting format for the study of widely varying menus, all of which meet the criteria for good, balanced nutrition.

The main characteristic of a good *organizing center* is that it provides an interesting focal point around which a variety of essential learning experiences can be studied. Menus of various ethnic restaurants could be brought to class for analysis in terms of the basic four food groups, and a "tasting party" could be organized in which various exotic items are sampled. Toward the end of this series of experiences, study could be focused on food selection in contemporary America. Within a well-organized curriculum food selection per se might be dealt with through the seventh grade even though other aspects of nutrition would receive attention at the interest levels.

In this particular example the time allotment for nutrition at grade four might provide for only one unit of study; if more time is available, two or more teaching units might be presented within the framework of a single center. If "Disease Prevention" were the organizing center for disease in grade five as opposed to the "Nature of Disease" in grade four and "New Ways to Treat Disease" in grade six, for example, then two teaching units might be presented, one for communicable disease and a second for chronic disease. Although the planning of these curriculum components must be carried out with respect for the discipline of the organizing elements, "the organizing centers determine the essential character of curriculum." [3]

THE MIDPOINT

The examination of the curriculum in this chapter began with general philosophy, then proceeded to long-range goals, content areas, and concepts and organizing centers. This encompasses the first half of its organization. The focus has been on the "heavy" elements that are the traditional concern of formal curriculum committees and that are often ignored by the many action-oriented teachers who may find themselves so busy trying to teach the curriculum that they never examine its general structure and content with a critical eye. Although it is natural that they should be more concerned with the "trees" of day-to-day teaching than with the "forest" of the overall program, teachers should always remember that the material they find in their various curriculum guides was planned by fallible human beings. Each teacher has a responsibility to follow the established guide and a parallel responsibility to contribute to its continual development with constructive criticism.

In addition to becoming equipped for an active role in curriculum matters, the teacher who takes the trouble to become familiar with the broader components of the curriculum will also be able to deal more intelligently with his or her primary task of translating its abstract goals into concrete classroom learning experiences. This action at the operational level commonly involves behavioral objectives, specific content, and learning activities, as will be discussed in the following chapter.

[3] John I. Goodlad, *Planning and Organizing for Teaching* (Washington, D.C.: National Association of the United States, 1962), p. 28.

REFERENCES

BLOOM, BENJAMIN S. et al. *Taxonomy of Educational Objectives—Handbook I: Cognitive Domain.* New York: David McKay Company, Inc., 1956.

FINE, MORTON. "Health Instruction Practices and Problems of Selected New York City Elementary School Teachers," *Journal of School Health,* Vol. 45, No. 3 (March 1975), pp. 165–171.

FODOR, JOHN T., and GUS T. DALIS. *Health Instruction: Theory and Application.* Philadelphia: Lea Febiger, 1974.

FRANKEL, JACK R. *Helping Students Think and Value: Strategies for Teaching the Social Studies.* Englewood Cliffs, N.J.: Prentice-Hall, Inc., 1973.

GRONLUND, NORMAN. *Stating Behavioral Objectives for Classroom Instruction.* New York: Macmillan Publishing Co., Inc., 1970.

HONE, ELIZABETH, and EDNA M. CHAPMAN. "Walk Through Your Heart," *Instructor,* Vol. 75, No. 1 (August-September 1975), pp. 164–168.

KRATHWOHL, DAVID R. *Taxonomy of Educational Objectives—Handbook II: Affective Domain.* New York: David McKay Company, Inc. 1964.

LEIGH, TERRENCE M. "Will the Real Health Education Please Stand Up," *School Health Review,* Vol. 5, No. 2 (March-April 1974), pp. 10–14.

MAGER, ROBERT F. *Preparing Instructional Objectives.* Palo Alto, Calif.: Fearon Publishers, 1962.

14

Curriculum Planning at the Classroom Level

It is difficult to describe the classroom teacher's task in the planning of health education learning experiences because the factors that influence it vary greatly from situation to situation. The more important of these factors are those related to the quality and thoroughness of the more generalized planning that has taken place above the classroom level. In the ideal situation the incoming teacher will find that health education has been planned for the entire school system on a kindergarten-through-grade-twelve basis, with topics selected for emphasis at each grade level based on the characteristics of the pupils and the demands of subject matter progression. If the quality of this planning has been good, the topics selected will be interesting and relevant; if it has been thorough, the facts, concepts, skills and other expected outcomes for each grade level will be clearly expressed, generally in the form of behavioral objectives, and a number of alternative learning experiences will be made available as well as other suggestions for teaching materials and specific means of evaluation.

THE CURRICULUM GUIDE

When effective planning help is provided for classroom teachers, it most often takes the form of a curriculum guide. The format and general characteristics of these documents vary considerably; many of the terms used to designate the various categories of these guides are confusing because many different words or phrases are applied to essentially the same components by different curriculum development committees. For example, one of the important sections of almost all guides is one that contains suggested learning activities in the forms of appropriate written assignments, discussion topics, field trips, art projects, role playing, and so forth. Depending on

314

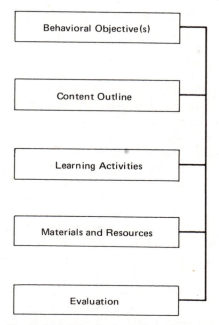

Figure 14.1. Curriculum Structure—Operational Components.

the preferences of particular curriculum committees, these may appear under the headings of "Learning Activities," "Learning Opportunities," "Teaching Activities," "Teaching Suggestions," "Suggested Activities," or simply "Methods." The key to handling such a proliferation of terminology as well as the basic task of fully utilizing the proferred guide lies in recognizing the common components by what they contain rather than by how they are labeled.

GENERAL FORMAT

The major components of a well-organized curriculum guide for any subject may be organized into two broad categories on the basis of their role as (1) definers of the general structure and philosophical thrust of the program and (2) guides to the day-to-day activities of the classroom.

"STRATEGIC" COMPONENTS. Most health curriculum documents begin with a statement of philosophy and/or a statement of long-range goals. The next step down in the hierarchy is a set of content areas or organizing elements that divide the study of health into six to twelve topics of study. On the

315

border between the "strategic" and operational categories are the organizing centers that establish subtopics to be emphasized at specific grade or school levels. These components were discussed in some detail in the preceding chapter.

OPERATIONAL COMPONENTS. Because all components probably exert some effect on the instructional activities of any given classroom on any given day, the decision to designate any particular group of components as operational is somewhat arbitrary. However, the behavioral objectives often provide the primary guides to the day-to-day activities of health instruction. These components are designed to provide the teacher with a clear understanding of what the pupils are to achieve. The more helpful guides, in the minds of most teachers, are those in which these objectives are stated in reasonably precise terms such as "Given a brief narrative of the activities of a specific family, the pupils can identify incidents that illustrate at least three basic family functions." A second major component commonly found is a series of *content outlines* or concepts that parallel the behavioral objectives and that provide both a clearer interpretation of the objective and added help in planning the presentation. To continue the example, the outline might contain basic information on "Meeting Affectional Needs," "Providing Companionship," "Child Rearing," "Meeting Recreational Needs" and so forth as typical family functions. Succeeding sections on *learning activities* and *materials and resources* are normally provided; these contain, in most cases, more suggestions than any single teacher could use and thus allow for a personal selection. Learning activities and materials are closely interrelated; a sound film, for example, can be both an activity and a resource; consequently, these sections are sometimes combined into a single section. A final section on *evaluation* normally includes specific suggestions for determining if the pupils are able to demonstrate the behavior described in the related objective.

Depending on the degree of emphasis or specificity the developing group sought to provide, a typical section such as family living might contain from five to fifteen behavioral objectives, each with its supporting components. Each of the other divisions of the health curriculum would be similarly represented. Usually only three or four major topics are covered at a grade level, particularly in the upper elementary grades where greater depth is desired for a topic such as "Mental Health." Therefore, the total curriculum could be covered in grades four, five, and six, for example, in a cyclical pattern, with sections of the guide simply designated as "Upper Elementary" or "Level II" rather than divided into sections for each grade level. If a similar guide was provided for the K–3 level, a school or system might cover a small portion of each major topic at each grade level in a continuous-emphasis type of organization. However, this would require considerable improvision because the suggested learning activities would have to be applied over the broad range of maturity levels encompassed within the primary grades.

THE SPECIFIC COMPONENTS

The various sections of the typical guide as just described are obviously not unique to the field of health education; they either are identical or have similar counterparts in other teaching fields such as science and social studies. However, because each field has its unique aspects, each component will be discussed in terms of its particular application to health education.

BEHAVIORAL OBJECTIVES. Every educational program is based on the simple concept that a learning experience changes one's behavioral capacity; that after pupils have learned something, they can do something they could not do before, even if it is as simple as reciting a definition of a "communicable disease" or citing examples of such diseases. Most educators feel that it is not logical to encourage naive pupils to simply study whatever might happen to strike their fancy at a given moment; every program has certain objectives for the pupils involved even though these may be highly non-directive, such as "The pupil selects a health topic of his/her own levels of ability and interests." If the teachers are to do their job, they must assist the pupils in their efforts to learn in accordance with these objectives. A good educational program in the minds of the majority of teachers, parents, educational authorities, and probably the pupils themselves if one would pose the question to them in understandable terms, represents a balance between mature guidance and direction on the one hand and the encouragement of pupil initiative and decision making on the other. Behavioral objectives can serve as a useful tool for communicating to teachers essentially what they are to help the pupils accomplish.

The single definitive characteristic of a behavioral objective is that it states the expected outcomes of instruction in terms of learner behavior; everything else is secondary, at least in the minds of the authors. And it is this "everything else" that appears to lie at the heart of much unnecessary controversy. If this essential feature is kept in mind, the use of behavioral objectives offers many advantages. Some of the major examples are as follows:

1. *The focus of the planning process is shifted from the teacher to the pupil.* In the past it was quite popular to state objectives as in these examples:
   - To present the basic facts of weight control.
   - To encourage the maintenance of proper body weight.
   Presumably, once the facts had been presented or the weight main-

317

tenance had been encouraged, then the objective was realized, regardless of whether any change had been affected within the pupils. In behavioral forms these same objectives might appear as follows:

- The pupil can relate the basic facts of weight control.
- The pupil accepts the value of the maintenance of proper body weight.

These objectives clearly indicate that the main concern is with what the pupils accomplish rather than with what the teacher does. And, although these examples are rather loosely stated, they still provide clearer indications for evaluation than do the first pair. These advantages are not momentous, but they do represent a significant improvement.

2. *Accurate evaluation is facilitated.* The task of evaluation is a difficult one that commonly produces considerable differences of opinion and some emotionalism. Regardless of one's particular feelings concerning this issue, the first step in the evaluative process is an accurate statement of what the educational program is designed to accomplish. Although they are no panacea, behavioral objectives appear to provide the best available device for the accurate expression of these intentions. The key to their usefulness both as guides to the instructional processes and as facilitators of evaluation is the fact that the form of the objective may be varied to accommodate the basic philosophy of the program. For example, if a school is committed to a discovery-type approach where pupils have considerable freedom in selecting their specific topics for study, then the objectives cannot be expressed in terms of *content* to be mastered because there is no way to predict what content will be studied. Programs of this type are typically concerned with the *processes* of investigation and consequently must be expressed in these terms. Similarly, those of a humanistic bent who typically are concerned about moods, feelings, values, and so forth must express their objectives in affective rather than cognitive terms, as will be discussed below.

3. *Virtually all possible types of educational outcomes or expectations may be accommodated.* Because of the pioneering work of Benjamin Bloom,[1] David Krathwohl,[2] and their associates, categories and related terminology for educational objectives have been standardized to the point that both curriculum planning and general communication among educators have been greatly facilitated. One caveat for this optimistic assessment must be recognized, however. These taxonomies, as they are called, are somewhat complex and their usefulness is restricted to those who take the trouble to understand them; much con-

[1] Benjamin S. Bloom et al., *Taxonomy of Educational Objectives—Handbook I: Cognitive Domain* (New York: David McKay Company, Inc., 1956).
[2] David R. Krathwohl, *Taxonomy of Educational Objectives—Handbook II: Affective Domain* (New York: David McKay Company, Inc., 1964).

fusion and unnecessary criticism have been produced when this understanding is lacking. For a review of the cognitive and affective domain in terms of health education, see Figure 14.2.

As can be seen in Figure 14.2, the cognitive domain is designed to accommodate intellectual behavior of all degrees of complexity and independence of action, ranging from the simple memorization of frequently used terms to the independent study, interpretation, and assessment of a social problem with multifactored causes and consequences. The affective domain, in a similar fashion, can accommodate a wide range of feeling tones or degrees of personal commitment regarding a particular object or idea ranging from a simple willingness to recognize its existence to an all-embracing desire to accept it as the guiding force of one's everyday life. Because of this inclusion of a category for commitment strong enough to carry over into personal behavior the affective domain effectively deals with objectives that deal with actual health practices. For example, Krathwohl lists "Obeys the playground regulation," [3] to illustrate the type of objectives included in a subcategory under *Responding* (2.1 Acquiescence in Responding); the *Valuing* categories include prominent examples of overt behavior,[4] and the highest category, Characterization, is one in which by definition, "The individual acts in accordance with the values he has internalized . . . ." [5]

There is one type of expected outcome of health instruction that is not encompassed by these two domains of behavior, namely, the learning of specific physical skills. These would be included under a third major domain, the psychomotor, which at this time has not yet been well analyzed and divided into categories. This lack, however, is of little practical significance to health education as physical skills do not play a large part in the meeting of health needs, at least as they are commonly defined. The exceptions that readily suggest themselves are raised to certain aspects of first aid such as "can splint a simulated closed fracture of the lower arm" or "can use the fireman's carry to transport a simulated victim of equal body weight." These are interesting from a theoretical standpoint but are seldom taught in the elementary school program.

CONTENT OUTLINE

Before behavioral objectives became popular among curriculum makers, the content outline was often the major component of curriculum guides and served as the principal means to inform the teacher as to what should be covered. This encouraged an ineffective mode of instruction where the teacher simply plowed through the outline in a series of verbal discussions with the pupils or, in extreme examples of abuse, merely read the outline

[3] Ibid., p. 179.
[4] Ibid., p. 181.
[5] Ibid., p. 184.

Cognitive Domain

Knowledge	The student can define the term "blood alcohol concentration." (B.A.C.)	
Comprehension	The student can restate the definition for "blood alcohol concentration" (B.A.C.) in his/her own words.	
Application	Given the basic facts concerning a drinking incident, the student can estimate the B.A.C. of the person involved.	
Analysis	Given the case study of an alcoholic, the student can identify the most probable factors causing this condition.	
Synthesis	The student can suggest a logical program of public education and legal restraints designed to reduce alcohol problems.	
Evaluation	Given a description of a series of drinking patterns, the student can assess the probable effect of each one on long term living effectiveness.	

Affective Domain

Attending	The student demonstrates an awareness of the various problems caused by alcohol abuse.	
Responding	The student accepts responsibility for his/her own behavior in regard to alcohol.	
Valuing	The student values the qualities of reasonableness and moderation in one's behavior regarding alcohol.	
Organizing	The student reviews various patterns of drinking behavior in terms of their possible effects on his/her life.	
Characterization	The student regulates his/her behavior in regard to alcohol according to the demands of total living effectiveness.	

Figure 14.2. Representative Examples of Behavioral Objectives Dealing with Health Content from the Major Categories of Educational Taxonomies.

to the class. This was a very good way to "cover" material but a very poor way to make any lasting impact on pupils, other than perhaps developing a strong aversion to formal schooling. The advent of specific objectives well defined in terms of pupil behavior has since provided some firm stepping stones upon which teachers pick their way through otherwise overwhelming morasses of facts, figures, and definitions; furthermore, the use of concepts, as will be discussed in the following chapters, has provided beacons or landmarks to give proper guidance to this figurative journey. These developments have greatly facilitated the planning process even though many problems remain in the task of putting curriculum plans into action.

This progress has necessitated a change in the role of the content outline as applied to most modern curricula. The content outline is now more a resource to be used rather than a set of imperatives that must be covered. Also, the content outline can supplement the behavioral objective in the process of communicating to the teacher exactly what should be taught. For example, a behavioral objective within the area of consumer health might call for the ability to "distinguish between the various major procedures communities use to control the spread of communicable disease." The objective, when viewed alone, could leave the teacher somewhat perplelxed as to just what types of procedures were intended; however, the accompanying content outline might appear as follows:

I. Treatment of water supply
  A. Procedures
    1. Sand filtering—which removed large particles of impurities
    2. Chlorination—which killed most remaining germs of all types
  B. Diseases controlled entirely or in part—cholera, dysentery and typhoid
II. Control of insect and animal carriers
  A. Procedures
    1. Spraying of mosquitoes
    2. Rat-proofing and fumigation of ships; rat-proofing of warehouses and other dock and harbor facilities
  B. Diseases controlled
    —Malaria, yellow fever, plague, and various forms of mosquito-borne encephalitis (brain infection)
III. (Other sections on immunization, treatment, and quarantine would be included.)

This combination of behavioral objectives and content outline spells out what the curriculum development group had in mind while allowing "major" topics to be added or deleted as the needs of children and demands of social change, or as technological changes occur. These procedures give the curriculum materials built-in updating factors that greatly extend their useful life.

LEARNING ACTIVITIES

The learning activities that the teacher selects as the vehicle for the accomplishment of the behavioral objective are perhaps the most crucial components of the entire curriculum plan. It is the "moment of truth" when the products of the planning process first come into contact with the pupils for whom the program is intended. The most highly relevant and well-organized content can have zero or a negative impact on the pupils if poorly selected or poorly conducted classroom activities are used to present it to the class. In extreme cases, for instance, teachers may simply outline material on the blackboard and require pupils to copy it in their notebooks for lesson after interminable lesson; no content can survive such treatment. Poor learning activities can thus totally disable an otherwise well-devised program; however, good learning activities alone cannot guarantee success. A good teacher can be very effective in presenting outdated, inaccurate, or irrelevant content; through clever use of films, role playing, values clarification, and other techniques an enjoyable time can be had by both teacher and pupils even though the resulting experiences have no practical application to real life. As fruitless as such a situation is, it at least preserves the interest and morale of all concerned and thus keeps the door open to future improvements.

A well-developed curriculum guide will make several suggested activities available for each behavioral objective to accommodate the variety of teacher situations that may occur among the potential users of the guide. A number of factors can affect the conditions that surround various teachers. The teacher may or may not be well informed concerning the particular topic at hand; the resources available to the teachers in terms of materials, equipment, and facilities may vary considerably; the time allotment for health may vary considerably from school to school; the amount of preparation time the teacher can or will devote to the health lesson may vary; and the manner in which the children respond to various teaching approaches may be unique to their specific class.

In addition to a variety of suggestions an effective curriculum guide will also include a thorough enough description to provide teachers some indication of how the activities might work in an actual situation. The thoroughness of the description tends to vary considerably from one guide to another and even within the same guide. Consider these two examples from the state health education guide for Maryland, for example. Both were provided for the following behavioral objective for the primary level:

> Given a natural condition, the learner will be able to describe how man utilizes, conserves, adapts to, and controls it to support life.[6]

[6] *Health Education: A Curricular Approach to Optimal Health, Volume I* (Baltimore, Md.: Maryland State Department of Education, 1973), p. 6.

One rather sketchily described learning activity for the objective offers this suggestion:

> Take a neighborhood walk and look for interesting uses of the land in the immediate environment; e.g. uses of a vacant lot.[7]

This activity might work quite well assuming that there was a reasonable amount of variety in the use of land within the involved area; however, it would have been better to provide teachers with a few more examples beyond the single "uses of a vacant lot." Although every neighborhood is, of course, different, other examples such as use of land for a backyard vegetable garden, a parking lot, a small park, a shop, or an industrial establishment would serve to stimulate their thinking in regard to their own situation. Another suggested activity from the same page of this guide serves to illustrate how a more detailed description can make an activity more appealing to teachers and make it easier for them to use it effectively. This example is for the same objective and is as follows:

> Make a large map of the neighborhood, indicating various uses for the land; e.g. factories, housing, parks, playgrounds. Include the children's houses in the map. Discuss the proper use of streets, crosswalks, intersections, highways, alleys, driveways, and corners, and the meaning of traffic signs. Show how you would come to school and the safety precautions you must take in various weather conditions.[8]

Creative or innovative teachers might still wish to modify these activities to fit the requirements of their situation more closely; however, this quite thorough description would provide a better understanding of the curriculum committee's orginal intentions and thus facilitate useful modifications or even development of entirely different activities that would achieve the same effect.

Information concerning the actual selection and applications of various types of teaching methods will be presented in Chapter 16.

MATERIALS and RESOURCES

Few things are of more value to a busy teacher than a good, current list of films, filmstrips, pamphlets, and other such items that were carefully selected to. coordinate with the content of the curriculum. Unfortunately, such lists are difficult to compile and even more difficult to update as new aids to instruction become available. Even the more responsible curriculum development groups often do not or cannot take the time to preview all

[7] Ibid., p. 7.
[8] Ibid.

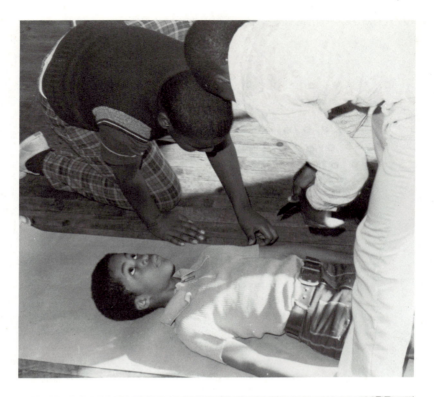

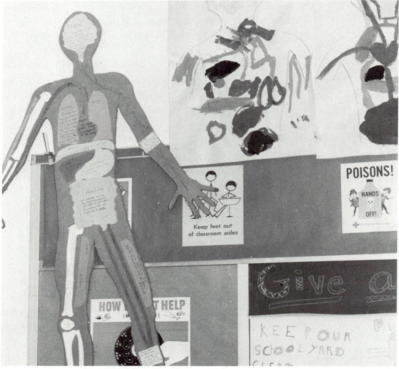

Figure 14.3.   Learning Activities Are the "Moment of Truth" for the Planning Process. (Carol Ashton)

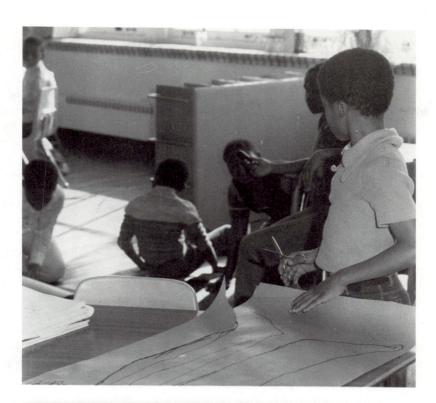

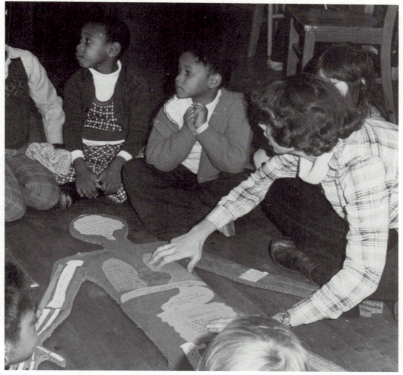

the items that they recommend. Also, because of time pressure or other obstacles, curriculum groups often are not able to make a thorough search of the vast numbers of instructional materials that are always available for health instruction. Consequently, many otherwise helpful curriculum guides may be deficient in the materials sections.

Because of the intrinsic problems with resource lists, teachers are advised to use them as starting points in their search for materials rather than relying on them as their only source of help. After reviewing these offerings, which in recently developed guides may be quite good, teachers should next check with the school librarian and/or learning center director as to what is available within the school or district. If health is well established as an important part of the curriculum, the local learning center may have in its collection may useful items. The more energetic teachers who have the time and inclination to search further will find that a whole host of voluntary health associations such as the American Cancer Society, governmental agencies such as the local public health department, and commercial organizations such as the American Dairy Association regularly produce a veritable river of instructional aids, many of which are free for the asking. More specific information on this task will be presented in Chapter 16.

Occasionally, teachers may find themselves serving on committees to prepare resource lists for health instruction. Such committees should keep in mind that with so many groups producing health instructional aids, the main task is to sort through the many offerings, previewing the more promising titles and recommendations and presenting these, together with addresses and local phone numbers, if available, of the major sources of materials. Too often such committees list everything remotely connected with the curriculum topic and thus overwhelm teachers with a multitude of ill-chosen recommendations.

One bright note in the often difficult area of teaching materials is the many good sources available to teachers to improve their personal background in the subject matter of health education. Most college and public libraries are well stocked with texts on such standard health topics as nutrition, disease, and the natural environment, and many of these are quite readable. The Time-Life Science series,[9] for example, is widely available, and with such titles as *Health and Disease, Growth, The Body, The Mind,* and *Food Nutrition* composes a veritable health science library for the teacher. The coverage of most health topics as provided in the major encyclopedias provides more information than can be covered in the typical elementary school classroom and thus constitutes a source that teachers should not ignore. Also, all segments of the mass media including maga-

[9] René Dubos, Henry Margenan, and C. P. Snow, consulting editors. *Life Science Library* (New York: Time, Incorporated) .

zines, newspapers, and television commonly devote considerable attention to most health matters of any significance.

EVALUATION

The achievement of a truly valid and administratively feasible evaluation of learning outcomes related to as broad and diverse a subject as health remains one of the major unsolved problems of this teaching field as it does in so many others. Moreover, health is also burdened in most programs with a heavy emphasis for immediate, practical results in the form of improved health behavior outside the classroom; this emphasis is commonly stronger than comparable expectations for other subjects such as language arts, where most educators are satisfied with good classroom performance as the main criterion for program evaluating. Health authorities become quite philosophical and emotional in their stress on practical results, often to the extent that they set impractical goals that cannot be achieved by the educational process alone. This issue will be discussed further in Chapter 17; therefore, this section will be restricted to comments regarding the use of the suggested techniques as commonly presented in curriculum guides for the evaluation of classroom performance.

One of the hallmarks of good planning in education is a close parallel between the behavioral objective or objectives for a given lesson or unit and the evaluating procedures used to assess the outcomes of instruction. Furthermore, this criterion can be applied without doing violence to any reasonable philosophical approach. For instance, some teachers may complain that when they are required to evaluate in terms of the specified objectives they tend to become too involved with fragmented ideas and isolated facts as pupils are asked to "list five examples," "define specific terms," or "sort selected items into categories." Where such a situation prevails, the fault obviously lies not with the evaluation process but with the irrelevance of the original objectives. Teachers who have the initiative and latitude of action to ignore highly structured cognitive objectives recommended for their grade level and to adopt a values clarification approach in a given situation, for example, obviously are setting up new objectives of their own even though they may not state them explicitly. In such cases it is these implicit objectives that should provide the basis for evaluation.

This example is related to another worthwhile generalization that can be applied to the process of evaluation, namely, that the degree of specificity or accountability should normally be varied to accommodate the nature of the subject matter. In a neighborhood where most children of the primary grades walk to school, for instance, a teaching unit on safety might include six or eight basic rules for pedestrians to use crossing streets, obeying crossing guards, and so forth. It would be reasonable to expect every child to memorize these rules, particularly if the local traffic situation was especially hazardous. This would set the stage for a tightly formulated behavioral objective that might be worded as follows:

> With no outside help or prompting, the pupil can list the six pedestrian rules devised for his/her neighborhood using words and phrases that in all cases conform to the original intent of the rules.

Objectives such as these are often informally termed "Magerized," after Robert Mager, who popularized highly specific behavioral objectives that commonly include the conditions of evaluation (with no outside help), the behavior (can list), the content (six rules), and a criterion for acceptable performance (conform to the original intent).[10] Like most objectives that lend themselves to strict accountability, this one deals with a relatively small portion of subject matter but, in this case, one highly relevant to the children involved.

Within this hypothetical unit on safety it would be logical to include an objective related to the attitude of the children toward traffic safety, that is, to their personal feelings about the importance of avoiding accidents and their acceptance of the usefulness of the proffered rules in accomplishing this. The behavioral outcome of instruction would be very difficult to "Magerize" within any reasonable restriction of practicality or feasibility. Under most conditions one would have to settle for something like the following wording:

> During normal classroom discussions and recitations on the topic of traffic safety, the pupil consistently exhibits an acceptance of the role of safety rules (as presented in the unit) as highly important and useful aids to accident prevention.

Those who favor strict accountability might think that such an objective has little value because it cannot be properly assessed. They would ask: "Specifically how will the pupil exhibit his/her acceptance?" "What are your standards for consistency?" and "Just how important is 'highly important' "? However, it seems far more reasonable, to the authors at least, to maintain that the attitudes of pupils toward the general topic of safety and safety rules are at least as important as their knowledge of safe procedures and thus must remain as an important objective regardless of the accountability problem. Teachers who are not sensitive to the feelings and developing values of their pupils are not going to accomplish much of

---

[10] Robert F. Mager, *Preparing Instructional Objectives* (Palo Alto, Calif.: Fearon Publishers, 1962).

lasting value in health education; when this sensitivity is present, classroom teachers will be able to make a reasonably accurate judgment as to how their pupils are accepting the usefulness and importance of the material they are studying. This is not to say that structured planning and structured evaluation should be abandoned so that teachers may simply "wallow around" in their subjectivity, but merely to recognize that evaluation is the "art of the possible." It should be as accurate as is feasible, but its limitations should not lead to the deletion of relevant subject matter.

THE RESOURCE UNIT

Some schools provide teachers with resource units to use as a basis for their classroom planning. In other cases where curriculum guides are provided, teachers are expected to develop resource units of their own based on the guide. Resource units are similar in many respects to curriculum guides in that they commonly include objectives, content outlines, suggested activities, lists of materials, suggestions or actual test questions, rating scales, and so forth for evaluation. Where such units are developed by officially sanctioned curriculum committees for a school system or individual school, they can guide teachers quite effectively by providing help in the actual planning process.

Resource units usually differ from curriculum guides in that they are organized around a smaller segment of the curriculum. Curriculum guides in health education commonly focus on the major topics of the health curriculum such as mental health or disease control. These were discussed in Chapter 13 as "organizing elements." Resource units commonly focus around much narrower topics such as "Getting Along with Others," Interpersonal Relationships," or "Smoking and Health," "The Role of Tobacco in Chronic Disease." These will be discussed later as "organizing centers." This narrower focus is often accompanied by greater detail in the suggestions offered, such as providing a series of test questions to use in evaluation rather than merely suggesting that "multiple choice questions be devised," as do many guides.

Perhaps the next most obvious difference between guides and resource units is that the latter are in some respects more closely geared to the dynamics of the learning process. Their narrower scope permits the use of some engaging themes as suggested by such unit titles as "Family Life in Other Lands," "Muscles for Strength—Muscles for Beauty," and "The Neighborhood Environment—Fighting Pollution at Home." In addition to the use of such focal points for the development of pupil interests, units commonly include activities designed for each of the classical phases of the teaching–learning cycle. For instance, several activities to be used to initiate a unit of study are usually offered that were selected because of their high interest value such as an attractive film on some phase of the topic or one that provides an overview of the topic to be studied. Next, activities may be suggested for the development of the unit. The selection of these activities is based on the assumption that the pupils have achieved a reasonable degree of motivation and involvement, and they are designed to provide comprehensive and sometimes ambitious learning experiences such as doing individual experiments. Finally, culminating activities are suggested such as the presentation of a demonstration or playlet by the pupils to other classes or the school as a whole, or a simple class luncheon prepared and eaten in the classroom as a fitting climax to a unit on nutrition.

Resource units for health topics come from a wide variety of sources and vary greatly in their sophistication and degree of completeness. As noted, they are sometimes the medium by which the official curriculum is described. They are sometimes developed informally by teachers over the years as they accumulate materials and ideas related to a commonly taught subject; in this form they may be tightly structured or may consist of a loosely organized resource file, which may nonetheless serve its creator quite well. Another common type are those prepared and distributed by various health agencies and organizations or health-related commercial groups. These, of course, have no official status but, like all resource units, contain a variety of suggestions designed to be helpful in the planning process.

TEACHING–LEARNING UNITS

Although it is virtually identical in format to the resource unit, the teaching–learning unit represents a refinement in the planning process. It is commonly designed for a specific class or a quite narrowly defined population of children. Teaching–learning units are often constructed by curriculum groups for total schools or total school systems where tight control of the curriculum is maintained by the school administration; ideally, they are constructed by individual teachers and are thus tailored to their particular style of teaching and to the characteristics of the pupils that they normally encounter. As such, they are relatively "lean" creations devoid of superfluous activities that might be impractical or inadvisable in the specific situation for which the unit was designed or of suggested resources that are unavailable or inappropriate. A teacher may develop a teaching–learning unit from suggestions in a curriculum guide, from a resource unit that provides suggestions appropriate to a variety of teaching units, or, in the absence of help from these sources, from "scratch." The end result should be a detailed plan for the teaching of a relevant topic that is entirely feasible and appropriate for a specific teaching situation.

LESSON PLANS

The task of planning individual sessions of health instruction differs little from that of planning for other subjects within the elementary school curriculum; however, there are a number of factors that tend to make planning for health instruction particularly important. Distressing as it may seem to those who feel that the health of children should receive the highest priority, health education is regarded as a "supplementary" or "minor" subject in many elementary schools. When relatively small amounts of time are alloted to it, perhaps 30- or 60-minute sessions once or twice a week, it is obviously important to make every minute count. Another reality of health education as applied to the elementary school is the typically shallow subject matter background of the teacher, who will seldom complete more than two college health courses. This handicap can be readily overcome with a reasonable amount of self-study; however, good planning and advanced preparation of lessons are especially important as this background is being accumulated. Finally, health content occasionally includes controversial issues such as alcoholic beverage use, birth control, water fluoridation, and human evolution. Much of what is worthwhile in such subjects as health, social studies, and even science is controversial and can be handled effectively with the use of the basic precepts of fairness, together with skills in discussion leadership that most good teachers possess. However, controversial aspects can be handled much more fruitfully and gracefully when they are anticipated by good advanced planning.

Many different formats for lesson plans exist; and teachers commonly develop unique variations of their own as they develop their individual style of teaching Almost all lesson plans, regardless of the subject or grade level for which they are designed, contain certain important components. Jack Fraenkel suggests five essentials that teachers need to consider in planning lessons:

1. A clear idea of what they wish to accomplish by the end of the lesson (i.e., a clear purpose or objective) . . . .
2. A clear idea of the procedures and activities they will use to help students attain the objectives they have in mind . . . .
3. Ensuring that the materials (books, newspapers, magazines, records, tapes, etc.) that students will need to obtain information are available . . . .
4. A clear idea of the *order* in which they will proceed to use the materials and activities . . . .
5. Provision for some means to evaluate whether or not the objective for the lesson was achieved . . . .[11]

[11] Jack R. Fraenkel, *Helping Students Think and Value: Strategies for Teaching the Social Studies* (Englewood Cliffs, N.J.: Prentice-Hall, Inc., 1973), pp. 380–381.

Using these five points as guides, a sample lesson plan for a first grade health lesson on the topic of family living might look like the one shown below. This lesson was based on the suggestions provided on p. 219.

SAMPLE LESSON PLAN

Mon., May 6,   Health—Family Living
                                                                          Grade I

Objectives
   The pupils:
   1. demonstrate an awareness of a wide variety of family patterns in terms of size and memberships.
   2. can list one advantage and one disadvantage of any family pattern.

Activities

5 min.
   1. Show series of *overhead transparencies* (3M # 00,00 and 00) depicting various family patterns—ask children to tell how each one differs from the others.

10 min.
   2. Distribute one large piece of *art paper* to each pupil. (Divide each paper in two sections by drawing a line across from side to side before lesson begins). Ask each pupil to draw as good a picture of his/her family as they can in five minutes on the top half of the paper using *crayons.*

10 min.
   3. Ask the class to stop and listen to new instruction—ask the pupils to think of another family they know and would like to visit or go on a picnic with for a full day— After making sure that every pupil understands and has thought of a specific family then ask them to draw this family in the bottom half of the paper.

15 min.
   4. Ask the class to put their crayons away and get ready to tell about their picture.
      a. ask two or three volunteers in turn to describe their family.
      b. ask three or four volunteers to tell (i) something good about the size of their family and (ii) something not so good (e.g., no sisters to play with, or my big brother picks on me, etc.).
      c. ask class to do the same for their friends and family.

Evaluation

10 min.
   Give each child one piece of *scratch paper.* Ask each child to draw quickly three different families they saw in the lesson including only the heads of the various members. Then ask them to mark an X for each good

thing they can think about the size of each family, then an O for each bad thing.

Although this plan might appear sketchy to anyone without significant teaching experience, it is far more detailed than those used by the large majority of veteran teachers. Experienced teachers usually do not need this much detail because they develop their own shorthand and after thinking the lesson through they need only brief notes to remind themselves of key points. However, this more complete plan would not be unreasonable in its detail in those schools where health is only taught once or twice a week.

Among the details, note that any reference to materials is underlined in this particular format so that the teacher can readily identify the items needed and assemble them after school or during preparation time on the day preceding the lesson. Note also the time allotments; most teachers find it best to make these generous as there are always unforeseen things that add to the time needed. There may be an interruption from outside the class, someone making an all-school announcement or a message reporting a phone call. Also, class discussion may run a bit long if a particularly relevant point happens to catch the interest of the class. It is a good idea to build in some flexibility in the lesson with an optional item. In this case the evaluation activity could probably be dropped because the final discussion provides a good indication of how well the pupils grasp the main ideas. This would not be pupil-by-pupil evaluation, but such coverage is not necessary on every lesson.

REFERENCES

BROWN, GEORGE ISAAC. *Human Teaching for Human Learning: An Introduction to Confluent Education.* New York: Viking Press, 1971.

FODOR, JOHN T. and GUS T. DALIS. *Health Instruction: Theory and Application.* Philadelphia: Lea & Febiger, 1974.

GOODLAD, JOHN I. *Planning and Organizing for Teaching.* Washington, D.C.: National Education Association of the United States, 1963.

Health Education: A Curricular Approach to Optimal Health. Baltimore, Md.: Maryland State Department of Education, 1973.

"Opening Things Up: Alternative Curricular Designs" (special series of seven articles), *Educational Leadership,* Vol. 28. No. 5 (February 1971), pp. 455–483.

School Health Education Study. *Health Education: A Conceptual Approach to Curriculum Design.* St. Paul, Minn.: 3M Education Press, 1967.

333

TABA, HILDA. *Curriculum Development: Theory and Practice.* New York: Harcourt Brace Jovanovich, 1962.

TANNER, DANIEL, and LAUREL TANNER. *Curriculum Development.* New York: Macmillan Publishing Co., Inc., 1975.

TYLER, RALPH W. *Basic Principles of Curriculum and Instruction.* Chicago: University of Chicago Press, 1950.

WOODRUFF, ASAHEL D. *Basic Concepts of Teaching.* San Francisco: Chandler Publishing Co., 1961.

Developing the Health Education Program

15

This is a chapter for teachers who are "not willing to mind their own business"—who tend to be "activists" in the constructive sense of the term. In Chapter 1 the point was made that the classroom teacher was the child's last line of defense against dangerous play equipment, chained fire doors, and other such items of neglect and faulty planning. This professional responsibility applies even more clearly to curricular matters. Although the threats are not so obvious, the long-term consequences of neglect and faulty planning as applied to the instructional program are equally as serious as those produced by fires or accidents. Teachers do not, of course, control the curriculum in a legal sense; this power resides in state legislatures and local school boards. However, most board members, superintendents, consultants, and others in the administrative hierarchy of the typical school system recognize the classroom teacher as one who combines professional training with a first-hand knowledge of the reactions of the pupils to the current program. This unique status provides both the power and the responsibility to participate in the continual task of program improvement.

THE TEACHER'S PLANNING ROLE

The classroom teachers' opportunity to have a voice in curriculum planning will vary greatly from school system to school system. At one extreme there may be so many curriculum meetings for teachers that they may long for less "democracy" and more time to plan tomorrow's lessons; at the other extreme the school administration may seek to deny teachers any voice at all in this important process. Although this broad range of situations still exists, there appears to be a general tendency these days for parents and other groups of laymen to be gaining greater influence in deciding what content should be emphasized, and, where this occurs, the teachers often become influential middlemen in resolving differences between the community and the school administration. Also, the advent of collective bargaining for teacher salaries and "work rules" has often provided the teachers with more power to influence the curriculum.

THE GOOD PROGRAM

The general thesis of this text is that the elementary school pupil needs and deserves a good program of health instruction. Teachers who accept this point of view and the responsibilities that it entails first need to assess the existing program in their school to determine if it meets acceptable criteria. Perhaps the only valid indicator of this is evidence of good health behavior in the pupils currently enrolled and in the "alumni" in higher grade levels; however, the task of evaluating out-of-school health is extremely difficult and usually beyond the ability of any single concerned teacher. Fortunately, the external characteristics of a good program are easier to observe. Among the more common of these are (1) the availability of a health supervisor, resource teacher, or other effective helping person; (2) a comprehensive updated curriculum plan, usually in the form of a written guide; (3) the availability of suitable teaching resources such as text books, films, and transparencies; and (4) an adequate time allotment for health instruction. These will each be discussed in greater detail.

THE HEALTH SUPERVISOR

Much has been written about the technical qualifications of health supervisors or coordinators, as they are often termed, but in the final analysis such a person must be committed and enthused about classroom health education, and knowledgeable about teaching elementary pupils and meeting their health education needs. The periodic visits of a health supervisor bring to the classroom teacher concrete evidence of community and school administration support of health education. It means that "Someone out there (or up there) cares about my efforts to teach my pupils something about health." The provision of this support, although intangible, is perhaps the most important function of the visiting specialist.

As important as is this emotional support, both the teachers and the taxpayers rightfully expect something more. Ideally, the health supervisor provides direct help in the form of information on new films and teaching aids, suggestions on teaching approaches to particular health topics, often with a demonstration lesson, and clarification of the more complex health principles or concepts that the classroom teacher may not thoroughly understand. The visit of such a person to each classroom, even two or three times a year, can provide an important "lift" to the teacher's health teaching and do much to strengthen the overall program.[1]

THE CURRICULUM GUIDE

Somewhat like the health supervisor, the health teaching guide provides both tangible and intangible support to the classroom teacher. In school districts where there is genuine concern for health instruction, the teacher is seldom told "teach whatever you wish" in health. Where there is concern, there is planning; and when planning occurs, written documents are the visible result. The professional training most elementary teachers receive in health is often superficial compared to such areas as language arts and mathematics; therefore, a curriculum guide with well-described content is very important. In the absence of such a document the health program becomes textbook centered at best, and at worst it disappears completely. The general structure of a curriculum guide was described in the previous chapter.

SUPPORTING RESOURCES

A few well-organized programs may dispense with the standard health text-book in favor of the intensive use of more current and flexible learning materials; however, in most cases the provision of a modern, carefully selected textbook for each pupil fills the need for his or her access to a comprehensive and readily available learning resource. There is also a need for a wide variety of films, filmstrips, slide-tapes, pamphlets and other instructional aids described in Chapter 16. Many of these materials may be constructed, borrowed, or otherwise obtained by the teachers on their own initiative; however, when suitable materials are commercially available it is a great convenience to teachers if these are purchased and made available through the school or district instructional materials center. The task of teaching four to six subjects each day makes heavy demands on the conscientious teacher's time; therefore, materials that are not readily available are often not used.

[1] For a specific account of the value of such a person, see Floss Fenton, "The Helping Teacher," *The School Health Review*, Vol. 4, No. 1 (January-February 1973), pp. 24–25.

TIME ALLOTMENTS

The most finite resource of any school district is time; even those few systems blessed with a rich tax base cannot buy more of this precious commodity. Consequently, the supporters of the various curriculum areas typically engage in fierce competition over the matter of time allotments, and there seems to be no way for those concerned with health education to remain above this unseemly battle. A single vivid dramatic health lesson may produce a remarkable change in health behavior for a few days, but long-term behavioral change toward favorable health habits requires thorough study and consistent reinforcement over extended periods of time.

Fortunately, the elementary teacher has alternatives that are not often available to secondary teachers to reduce the need for large time allotments. Within the self-contained classroom time can often be used more efficiently. If a particular health lesson involves a somewhat "messy" art project, with poster paints, dirty brushes, and paper scraps, for example, this class can often extend beyond the alloted time to finish the project with only one time-consuming distribution of art material and only one clean-up period; the next health period can be correspondingly reduced or canceled to keep the budgeted time in balance.

Another option open to the elementary teacher is that of teaching health concepts within the context of other content areas such as science and social studies. This practice, known as integrated or correlated health instruction, can be used to gain additional time for the health program, or, in some school situations it can be used as the basic pattern for all health instruction. This arrangement works well in the self-contained classroom where a single teacher handles all the content areas. However, careful planning is essential to do justice to all areas, and the practicality of this scheme is dependent on the objectives of the content areas with which health is to be merged. The success of a program of integrated or correlated health instruction virtually demands the presence of a health coordinator with good qualifications as a subject matter specialist.

Every elementary school schedule normally allows extra time for the discussion of special events and announcements. Some of this time can be used for health instruction concerning school and community health happenings such as a current flu epidemic or new cafeteria regulations. This incidental health instruction, as it is termed, can be a good supplement to the regular program; however, it is in no way a substitute for the systematic health education that every child needs.

Authoritative recommendations for time allotments for health in the elementary school program tend to be rather vague, with the most common one being that health education receive the same amount of time as other standard content areas. Actually, most health educators would be content with 20 to 30 minutes a day for direct health instruction throughout the elementary school grades. This, of course, is best regarded as an average

338

figure, with the option left open to consolidate instruction into two or three regular lessons per week.

THE TEACHER and PROGRAM DEVELOPMENT

The primary responsibility of the classroom teacher is to implement or put the instructional program into action in the classroom by use of well-selected materials and teaching activities. Although somewhat secondary to this obvious role as implementor, the teacher's responsibilities in the area of curriculum and program development, as alluded to at the beginning of this chapter, are almost equal in importance. And, as is the case with most professional tasks, the nature of these tasks varies considerably from school to school.

TEACHER as PARTICIPANT

Elementary teachers who take jobs with districts that have good health programs will find their planning and development responsibilities simplified. Presumably, a well-organized curriculum has already been planned and implemented and the heavy task of building a new program "from scratch" has been completed. The need to update content materials, and techniques by periodic curriculum revision and other modifications will still remain, but the presence of a competent and well-trained health education coordinator can do much to expedite these activities and see that they are carried out in an efficient manner. Where such leadership exists, teachers can restrict themselves to their natural roles in the planning process as grade level specialists who can provide information as to the immediate needs and capabilities of their pupils. Some of the details of this general curriculum development or revision process will be discussed later in this chapter.

TEACHER as INSTIGATOR

In those school districts with weak or nonexistent programs of health education, elementary teachers who are concerned about the needs of their pupils in this content area face a difficult task. Those of us committed to the field of health education would, of course, like to see all elementary teachers in such situations demand a good kindergarten-through-grade-twelve program, but, although individual teachers may react in such a manner, it is unrealistic to expect the majority of elementary teachers to take this major task upon themselves; therefore, some more conservative measures will first be considered.

339

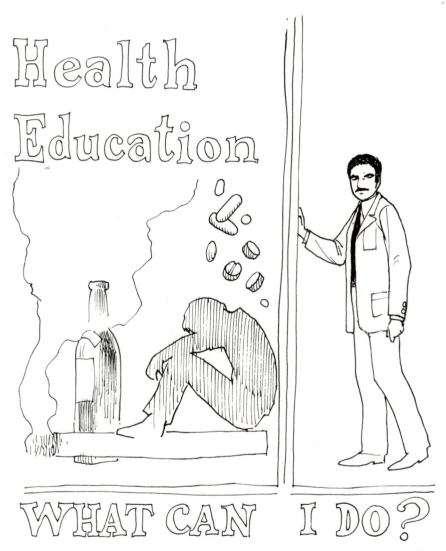

Health
Education

WHAT CAN I DO?

INCIDENTAL HEALTH INSTRUCTION. Even in the absence of a formalized program of health education, elementary teachers can develop considerable health knowledge in their pupils and promote good attitudes toward health through incidental instruction. Every school has health and safety rules and information concerning health services that must be conveyed to the children. In some schools these are deliberately correlated with the health curriculum; but in any event, the concerned teacher can utilize these and other health-related occasions to go beyond the mere transmitting of facts and discuss with the pupils the underlying reasons and concepts pertinent to these items. This constitutes a meager program at best, but considerable learning can go on during these "teachable moments"; it is certainly far better than nothing.

SOLO PROGRAMS.   A significant step beyond the minimal incidental program is taken by classroom teachers who find the energy and the opportunity to develop their own programs of health instruction. This can often be accomplished with little or no reduction in the time devoted to other content areas by working health content into the learning activities planned for these other areas. As mentioned previously, science and social studies provide the most frequent opportunities for the integration of health content; however, similar opportunities also exist in mathematics, language arts, art, and virtually any other area of study.

When there is time in the weekly schedule, it is simpler and more effective to teach health directly in its own designated time allotment. Regardless of the curriculum pattern selected, teachers who take the initiative to develop health education programs within their own classrooms should follow the same general planning steps needed for a district-wide planning effort, although these would be carried out on a smaller scale; this general process will be discussed later in this chapter. One very important note: any plans to add health education content to one's instructional program should be cleared with the building principal or other appropriate administrative representative to be sure that it comes within the general scope of the authorized curriculum. There is seldom any problem with the majority of health topics but the unauthorized teaching of material related to sex education or death and dying, for example, could produce serious repercussions. In any event, all new content should be cleared.

TEXTBOOK PROGRAMS.   Some school districts provide their elementary teachers with health textbooks for their pupils and with a time allotment, even though other essentials of a good program, such as a curriculum plan and assigned health supervisor, may be lacking. In such a situation the concerned teacher can utilize the teacher's edition of the text and other resources such as this textbook to build on the basic components that exist. The textbook with its suggested activities may provide good coverage of several worthwhile health units or topics, thus relieving teachers of much of the burden of program development. They can concentrate on the development of supplementary content to provide for topics of high interest or obvious need. In this situation individual teachers can strengthen the program by ordering free and inexpensive materials for their personal use and recommending the purchase of needed health-related materials to their local instructional materials director and/or librarian.

A GRASSROOTS EFFORT.   At this writing an unprecedented number of new health education programs are being developed in schools throughout the nation. It is to be hoped that elementary teachers who realize how important a good program of health education is to a child's general well-being, and how much satisfaction is gained in providing this education, will be ready to lend their support to any such legitimate effort that develops within their school system. These undertakings first require the general endorsement of the teaching staff if they are to be effective and next the participation of volunteers, who are often difficult to obtain even when properly compensated, in the arduous task of curriculum development. Some school districts underwrite this work by providing extra pay or release time for the participants.

Although the initiation of new programs is not for everyone, the elementary teacher who joins a school district with a weak or nonexistent health education program may gain considerable satisfaction in being the instigator of the needed program. Often only a small catalytic effort is needed to get something started. Most statements of educational goals and policies pay lip service to the need for health instruction and most school administrators are aware that their school or district should be meeting its health education responsibilities; often they have just procrastinated or they may feel that no one has noticed the neglect of this basic need. Also, it is not unusual to find that state laws requiring health instruction are already on the books and that the district is currently violating the law in its failure to provide this program. In these cases things often happen fast once this simple fact is brought to light.

Generally, however, the task of initiating a new program is far more difficult than simply pointing out a legal or philosophical responsibility. It is seldom appropriate for a beginning teacher to agitate for major changes in the curriculum. During the first year or two the teacher who would like to promote a health education program can accomplish useful groundwork by developing one or two high-priority health units within his or her own classroom. The successful implementation of health instruction on this small scale can provide concrete evidence of the need for a full K–12 program. One of the better approaches to curriculum development is based upon the assembling of field-tested pilot units into a well-articulated framework.

REFERENCES

AUBREY, ROGER F. "Health Education: Neglected Child of the Schools," *Journal of School Health,* Vol. 42, No. 5 (May 1972), pp. 285–288.

BYLER, RUTH, GERTRUDE LEWIS, and RUTH TOTMAN. *Teach Us What We Want to Know.* New York: Mental Health Materials Center, Inc., 1969.

FENTON, FLOSS. "The Helping Teacher," *The School Health Review,* Vol. 4, No. 1 (January-February 1973), pp. 24–25.

JACKSON, SHIRLEY A. "The Curriculum Council: New Hope, New Promise," *Educational Leadership,* Vol. 29, No. 8 (May 1972), pp. 690–694.

NASSTROM, ROY R. "Teacher Authority Over the Curriculum?" *Educational Leadership,* Vol. 31, No. 8 (May 1974), pp. 713–715.

NEWMAN, IAN M., and CYRUS MAYSHARK. "Health Education Planning and Community Perceptions of Local Health Problems," *The Journal of School Health,* Vol. 43, No. 7 (September 1973), pp. 458–463.

SLIEPCEVICH, ELENA M. *School Health Education Study: A Summary Report.* Washington, D.C.: School Health Education Study, 1964.

TABA, HILDA. *Curriculum Development: Theory and Practice.* New York: Harcourt Brace Jovanovich, Inc., 1962.

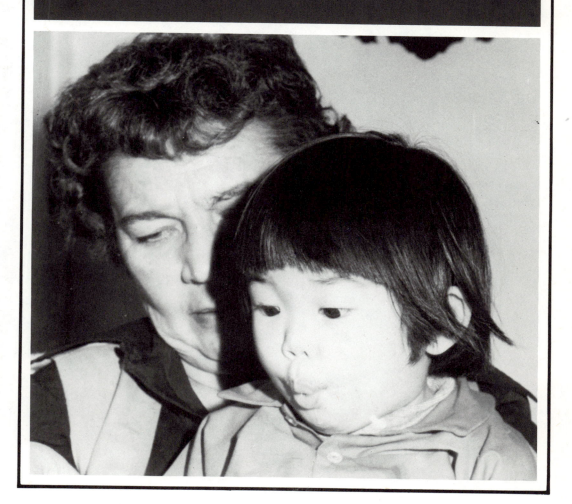

part 5

The Process

16

Teaching Strategies

Human beings are unified entities with inseparable qualities, but to study them effectively it is often convenient to direct attention to one aspect at a time, such as the physical or the emotional. In a similar fashion, the educational process has been somewhat artificially divided into separate processes for the purpose of analysis and discussion. It is useful to consider the selection of *teaching techniques,* which occurs in response to the question "How do we teach something?" as a process distinct from the selection of content, which presumably identifies what the something is that curriculum planners decide should be taught. In the study of health, as in most other subjects, these two processes are not interrelated, they often overlap and thus represent another instance where the medium becomes the message.

THE SELECTION PROCESS

Consider, for example, three fifth grade teachers preparing to teach a portion of a unit based on the objective "The pupil will demonstrate an awareness of the food situation in the underdeveloped countries of the world." Interestingly enough, this specific objective might be found in a unit on nutrition or community health or in a social studies unit focused on such countries, which illustrates the interrelatedness of various curricular areas. One teacher might ask the children to plan and construct a series of graphs to depict such things as per capita meat consumption in the underdeveloped as compared to the developed countries, the price of various food items in representative countries in comparison with the average daily income, estimated number of deaths due to malnutrition, and so forth. A second teacher might search out a good film combining such data with some emotionally charged scenes of hungry people. And a third teacher might bring up the matter in a general class discussion, which leads to a decision by the children to fast for a day and report their reactions to this experience.

347

CRITERIA

Any one of these three learning activities might prepare the children to demonstrate the type of awareness called for by the objective; however, the nature of this awareness would probably vary considerably in each classroom group. Each of the three teachers consciously or unconsciously considered the same general criteria in making their selection. Typically, these criteria are (1) the objectives of the lesson or unit of study, (2) the characteristics of the classroom group, (3) the individual style of the teacher, and (4) situational factors such as the availability of resources, the limitation of school policies, and the sensitivities of the community. A brief consideration of how each of these exerted their influence may lead to a fuller understanding of this process.

OBJECTIVE. The specific objective in this case was actually not so specific. Its behavioral component, "demonstrate an awareness," lends itself to a variety of interpretations because the particular mode of demonstration was not prescribed. Also, the content component, the "food situation in underdeveloped countries," likewise could lead to a variety of interpretations such as an emphasis on the economic, the agricultural, or the health aspects of the food situation. But vague as this objective is, it is probably as specific as one is likely to find in most curriculum guides, and in many districts curriculum guides for health education simply do not exist.

CLASSROOM GROUP. The teacher who used the graph construction activity had probably found that the children were capable of becoming enthused about this rather demanding activity; this would require a somewhat advanced group that is also perhaps "cooler" emotionally than the average group of fifth grade children. The teacher who used class discussion to choose a specific learning activity probably knew that this group had responded favorably to such oportunities in the past. The teacher who used the film as the main learning activity might have presented something more active as a follow-up, or he or she might be burdened with a group that does not respond to much beyond films or seatwork.

TEACHING STYLE. The personal style or preference of the teacher is a factor that often operates unconsciously. Teachers often do not think of their decision as resulting from their personal preferences or are perhaps reluctant to admit to these motives; instead, they tend to emphasize the external factors as logically supporting their particular selection of learning activities. The first teacher in our example might have a general preference for working with facts and figures as opposed to the more emotionalized or value-laden aspects of a topic, whereas the third teacher's tendencies might take the opposite direction. Although there is virtue in developing flexibility and versatility in one's teaching approach, there is also something to be said for

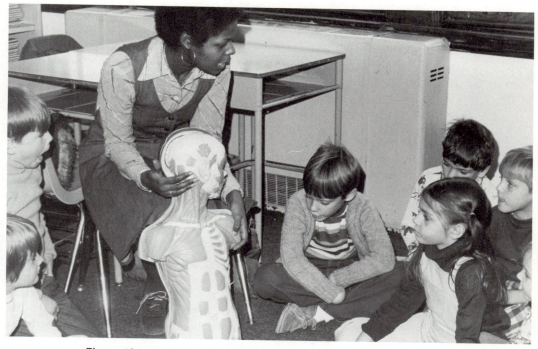

Figure 16.1. Individual Teaching Style, the Characteristics of the Classroom Group, and the Availability of Resources Interact in Each Teaching Situation. (Carol Ashton)

capitalizing on one's strengths on the assumption that if each teacher does what he or she can do best, the individual differences will tend to complement one another and provide a balanced program for each child's overall school career.

SITUATIONAL FACTORS. The term situational factors covers a multitude of "sins" and a multitude of opportunities. Schools vary greatly in the pattern of resources and obstacles they present to teachers. The second teacher may have been blessed with a well-stocked and well-managed district film library or a generous budget for film rentals. In another situation a teacher might have to rely entirely on free loans from various health-related trade organizations and voluntary health organizations for health films. The fasting experience adopted by the third teacher's class was voluntary; however, in some communities the parents would object to even the suggestion of such an activity, whereas in other locales the teacher would receive accolades as an innovative humanitarian. Many situational opportunities and constraints also arise out of school policies with respect to the time allotments for various curricular areas and the degree of freedom provided the teacher in terms of scheduling and selection of materials and learning activities.

DIMENSIONS of LEARNING ACTIVITIES

Most teachers seek to base their selection of learning activities on the educational needs of their children rather than on external considerations. The teaching situations presented herein can also serve to illustrate some of the common dimensions of these activities that merit attention during the selection process. This type of analysis will reveal each activity as possessing a unique pattern of strengths and limitations.

ABSTRACT VERSUS CONCRETE. The charts and graphs used by the first teacher are quite far removed from the realities of hunger; they are instead composed of abstract symbols. The fasting children of teacher three obviously had a much more concrete learning experience and the film viewers of the second teacher had a learning experience somewhere in between the other two in terms of realism. Edgar Dale provides an almost classic organizational pattern with his cone-of-experience concept.[1] As shown in Figure 16.2, he ranks verbal symbols as the most abstract, television and films in a middle range, and dramatic participation (playlets, role playing, etc.) and contrived experiences such as the fasting example as the closest activities to the real-life living experience represented by the base of his cone. Although the more concrete learning experiences are generally regarded as being more valuable in comparison to the abstract ones, they are also generally more costly in terms of time and resources. A field trip, for example, is more concrete than most classroom experiences but may consume an entire school day and cause added expenses. The same number of hours devoted to reading, discussion, films, role playing, and other classroom activities could normally provide a more comprehensive although less realistic coverage of any given topic.

COGNITIVE VERSUS AFFECTIVE. Some techniques are generally more useful in achieving cognitive objectives whereas others are more appropriate for classroom sessions directed toward affective objectives. The charts and graphs completed by the first group lead basically to cognitive outcomes; the children have the opportunity to develop a very precise view of the adequacy or inadequacy of diets among the people of underdeveloped countries, current trends toward improvement or deterioration of the situation, and perhaps priority needs in terms of money, loans, or technological assistance for the alleviation of the problem. The fasting experience obviously should carry more emotional impact and perhaps would be more effective in stimulating the desire to take action; however, by itself it provides little insight as to what the nature of this action should be. We have, in effect, "light without heat" in the first instance and "heat without light" in the

[1] Edgar Dale, *Audio-Visual Methods in Teaching* (New York: Holt, Rinehart and Winston, Inc., 1969).

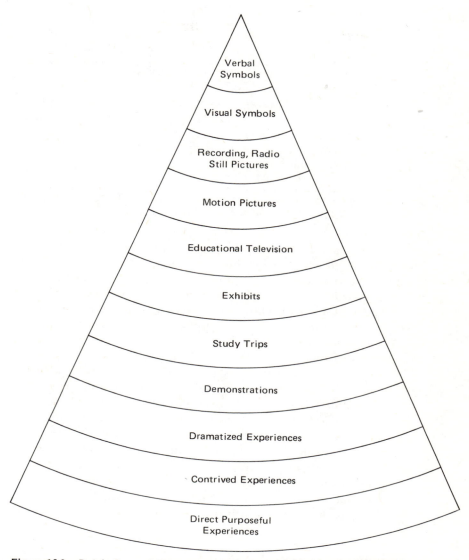

Figure 16.2. Dale's Cone of Experience. From **Audio-Visual Methods in Teaching,** Copyright © 1969, by Holt, Rinehart and Winston, Inc. Reprinted by permission of the Dryden Press.

second. Once again, the film experience probably falls midway between these extremes. The chart shown in Table 16.1 provides a classification of learning activities in terms of the cognitive–affective dimension.

TEACHER- VERSUS STUDENT-CENTERED.   The learning activities in the example obviously varied in the degree to which decisions within the activity

TABLE 16.1

COGNITIVE-AFFECTIVE CLASSIFICATION
OF TEACHING TECHNIQUES *

Cognitive	Affective	Composite
Reading assignments	Role playing	Films
Lecture-discussion	Playlets	Slide-tapes
Oral reports	Affective discussions	Field trips
Resource speakers	Values clarification	Demonstrations
Overhead projector	techniques	
Charts and graphs		
Programmed instruction		

* From Jenne, Frank H., and Greene, Walter H.: **Turner's School Health and Health Education, ed. 7** (St. Louis: The C. V. Mosby Co., 1976), p. 91.

were made by the teacher as opposed to the pupils; they also varied in the degree to which the children had active as opposed to passive roles in the learning process. Any degree of student activity or student decision making may exist in any single learning activity. For example, in the traditional lecture format the children generally have little voice in deciding what will be emphasized in the lesson and they have a very passive role in its implementation. In many laboratory activities such as dissecting frogs and completing experiments they are quite active but make few decisions concerning their actions. In other instances the children, with proper guidance, may plan and carry out an entire unit of study involving many activities in which the children both make the key decisions and play active roles in the activity itself. Generally, these latter activities are viewed as resulting in more meaningful learning, particularly when there is an important need to exert an impact on the attitudes or behavior of the children. However, teacher-dominated activities, when presented with enthusiasm and geared to the appropriate interests for the grade level involved, typically offer the advantage of covering more content per unit of time while making full use of the maturity and insights the teacher can bring to the topic of study.

HUMANISTIC EMPHASIS

The reader may have noticed that the information concerning teaching techniques thus far in this chapter applies to the instructional process in a generic sense, not merely to the teaching of health education. There are really no distinct methods for the teaching of health education; this should not be surprising when one considers the very broad scope of the subject matter normally found in a modern health curriculum. The basic knowledge incorporated in such curricula are taken on a nearly equal basis from the "hard" sciences such as anatomy, physiology, and epidemiology and the behavioral sciences such as psychology, sociology, and anthropology. Consequently, the teaching methods used for health education in the elementary school represent a composite of those normally used for science and for social studies.

FAVORABLE LEARNING CLIMATE

Another characteristic that the study of health shares with other curricular areas is the need for a favorable learning climate in the classroom. Although the subject matter of health education is extremely broad, all of it is focused on a single theme, namely, people—their nature, their concerns, their well-being. Furthermore, the concentration on this focal point is expected to yield results not only in knowledge gain but also in improved health behavior. It is not enough to know the facts related to nutrition; the child must improve his or her eating habits.

If learning experiences are to be translated into actual changes in everyday behavior, the child must fully accept or internalize the content. This internalization process seems to take place most readily when children learn in a positive rather than a negative motivational climate. A hard-driving taskmaster utilizing various threats could force the average class of sixth grade children to memorize the minimum daily requirements for the essential food elements, together with the composition of many common foods. Even though scores on the unit test might be impressive, the odds are that the main outcomes in overt behavior would be limited to attempts to avoid any future study of nutrition. However, if the teacher were to rely instead on interesting activities and material, together with a reasonable amount of pupil participation in the planning process, there might be a reduction in knowledge gain, but this would be more than offset by a favorable attitude toward nutrition information, better retention of knowledge, and a reasonable chance that behavior would be improved. For some strange reason, school programs of mathematics and language arts that yield high test scores are deemed successful even when the children involved still cannot manage their allowance money; however, few parents or administrators are impressed with a health education program that raises knowledge levels without producing a corresponding improvement in real-life behavior.

HUMAN RESOURCES

The development of a positive learning climate in the classroom offers obvious advantages in terms of the social and emotional growth of the children. Furthermore, from an academic standpoint, it provides the teacher access to the most valuable learning resource for the study of health, the children themselves, who constitute not only the prime subject of study but also one of the best sources of data currently available If the topic is nutrition, ask the children to keep a 5-day food diary and start with this information; if the human body is being studied, start with the height and weight data for the class; if the topic is family living, ask the children to share their family experiences if they are willing; and when studying mental health, which is essentially the study of human personalities, there is little need to rely on outside resources when the classroom is already filled with the real thing.

The suggestion to use the classroom group as a learning resource is not presented as a panacea. Many conventional resources and learning activities exist that are very useful to the teaching of health education. In this regard, the planning process does not differ greatly from that of any other subject; however, the teacher is well advised to first look to the characteristics and experiences of his or her children as a logical starting point. This material is valid, current, readily available, and possesses built-in relevance. As Clark Moustakas states in a more general yet appropriate context, "In an atmosphere of freedom and trust . . . the group becomes its own best resource and serves as the primary basis for emerging insight." [2]

AN INVENTORY of TECHNIQUES

The teaching techniques needed for the teaching of health education content do not differ substantially from those used for other subjects in the elementary school curriculum, particularly social studies and science. Thus it would be redundant to present detailed descriptions of these devices, which are commonly discussed in considerable detail in standard works and standard courses on teaching methodology. The elementary teacher need only apply these standard techniques to the task of health instruction. In an effort to assist this process, specific learning activities that many school health supervisors and health education consultants have found useful are defined and discussed in terms of their most useful applications. Cross-references are also provided for the examples of many of these techniques that have been described in the chapters related to specific content areas.

DISCUSSION TECHNIQUES

Class discussion in its various forms is one of the most widely used techniques in health education because of its simplicity and it effectiveness in tapping the human resources available in any classroom. It is quite useful in dealing with cognitive material, as through debates and panel discussions, which

[2] Clark Moustakas, *Teaching as Learning* (New York: Ballantine Books, 1972), p. 33.

are appropriate for the intermediate grades; however, it is essential to the accomplishment of many objectives related to the feeling and valuing aspects of the affective domain. The "magic circle" technique provides a highly successful example; here, "eight to twelve students gather daily in a circle for 20 to 30 minutes to discuss their thoughts, feelings, and behaviors." [3] It is based on the establishment of a "safe" discussion environment in which children are protected from verbal attack and never forced to contribute. Charlotte Epstein in her book *Affective Subjects in the Classroom* describes a similar technique and lists the sharing of differential feelings, the reduction of isolation, the elimination of secrecy, and the linking up of affect and cognition as the useful outcome of affective discussion. [4]

The establishment of a favorable emotional environment based on freedom and trust is also emphasized throughout Epstein's text as the most important prerequisite to any successful discussion. Also stressed is the teacher's ability to tolerate periods of silence. Teachers tend to fear "dead air," which they are generally too quick to fill with some extraneous remark; when they learn to remain quiet and relaxed they often find that useful comments begin to flow. Another useful procedure is to provide some stimulating experience immediately prior to the discussion, such as a film, a story, or some role-playing activity. There is a tendency to place discussion in a secondary role as a mere supplement to films, reading assignments, and other activities that often dominate the programs. Actually, these roles should frequently be reversed; a good discussion provides children with the opportunity to "sort things out," to reflect on the meaning and importance of the near-overwhelming flood of information to which they are commonly exposed.

NARRATIVES

The appeal of a good story to a child is well known, as is its potential for developing insights and stimulating thought and discussion. Perhaps the most important new development in this learning resource is the increasing tendency for children's literature to contain content related to many of the more sensitive and controversial health topics. David Sadker and associates note that death is a fact of life in children's books and provides several examples of such titles for all grade levels. [5] In her article on techniques for the study of love, Sylvia Jackson provides a bibliography listing 17 chil-

[3] Uvaldo H. Palomares, "Magic Circle: Key to Understanding Self and Others," *Educational Leadership*, Vol. 32, No. 1 (October 1974), p. 20.

[4] Charlotte Epstein, *Affective Subjects in the Classroom* (Scranton, Pa.: Intext Educational Publishers, 1972).

[5] David Sadker, Myra Sadker, and Carol Crockett, "Death—A Fact of Life in Children's Literature," *Instructor*, Vol. 75, No. 7 (March 1976), pp. 75–84.

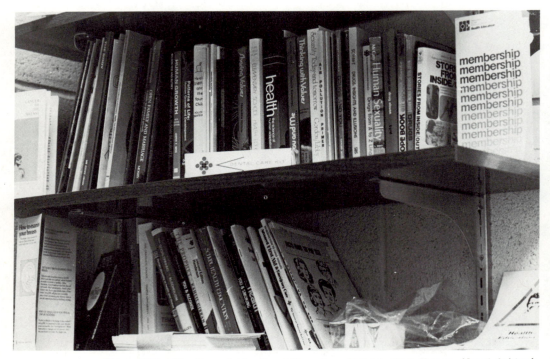

Figure 16.3.   The Appeal of a Good Story to a Child is Well Known. (Carol Ashton)

dren's books that include material on this sensitive but highly important topic. Lorna Flynn observes that "The Hardy Boys Didn't Have Wet Dreams," but lists several examples of more recent books for children which deal quite frankly with sexual topics.[6] Those who study children's literature are aware that the better stories and novels are well regarded because of their validity in terms of real-life situations. Very often they represent a far more valuable learning resource than many nonfiction books.

There are a great variety of uses of narratives in the teaching of health. Younger children enjoy listening to stories on health topics and they benefit both from the information the stories provide and from the discussion they stimulate. The familiar open-ended story in which the children devise their own endings is a useful variation for getting students actively involved.

[6] Lorna B. Flynn, "The Hardy Boys Didn't Have Wet Dreams," *SIECUS Report* (Sex Information and Education Council of the U.S.), Vol. 1, No. 2 (November 1972), pp. 1–2, 10.

In other instances they may be asked to create entire stories on assigned topics. Many teachers also find it worthwhile to write their own open-ended or completed stories to use as teaching resources; this is a good method for ensuring that the story will relate well to both the individual teacher's style and the needs of his or her classroom situation.

DRAMATIZATIONS

Children are natural practitioners of the art of make-believe. Betty Caldwell and Robert Yowell aptly describe the learning potential of this activity when they state:

> Young children engage in dramatic play not because of any inherent love of drama as an art form but because it is a fundamental way of learning how to behave in ways that are appropriate for their age and culture.[7]

They feel that no one is "more capable of 'role-playing' than a group of kindergarten children" and maintain that "fifth-graders can enact a simulated city council meeting every bit as heated as one actually held in City Hall." They thus support the appropriateness of this technique for use at all grade levels of the elementary school.

Dramatizations may be divided into two basic categories: those with prepared scripts, and those in which roles are assigned, a situation is described, and the actors are asked to improvise their responses. It is this latter category, termed role playing, that is most commonly used in health teaching. Within family living and mental health units this device can provide a safe exposure to anger, disappointment, elation, and many other such feelings that can then be discussed and more fully understood. Decision-making situations are another common category of health-related applications. The aforementioned town council, for example, could have been discussing the restrictions of automobile use in the business district to control air pollution. Personal decisions such as whether to sniff glue or begin experimenting with cigarettes also provide good themes for role-playing situations. Here, children can become aware of the function of social pressure in such situations and thus become better prepared to cope with it.

The conventional playlet with its prewritten script may be used to cover the same topics in a more systematic although less spontaneous manner. Generally, these dramatizations are written by the children themselves often after considerable study and investigation of the health issue involved. The children thus benefit from the creation, the presentation, and the viewing of the performance. In the growing number of schools that possess

[7] Betty Caldwell and Robert Yowell, "Action Dramatics," *Instructor*, Vol. 86, No. 5 (January 1977), pp. 118–124.

closed-circuit television systems, the plays and playlets written by various classroom groups can be viewed by the entire school. The prospects of this exposure provides an obvious stimulus for the children's work.

COMMUNITY RESOURCES

The teacher who seeks to utilize the usually substantial resources of the community has at least three basic alternatives from which to choose: the conventional whole-class field trip, the small-group field trip, and the resource speaker. Of these, the conventional field trip is clearly the most popular choice among the children if not among the teachers and administrative staff of the school. Fire stations, dairy farms, supermarkets, and other food-producing or -processing facilities rank high on the list of popular health-related sites. Other possibilities include nursing homes and hospitals when special arrangements can be made. Also, in urban areas, some medical schools, hospitals, or scientific institutes maintain health museums complete with guided tours.

The small-group field trip offers many of the same advantages of the large-group trip without its considerable logistical problems and expense. It can be school sponsored as when a volunteer parent, with suitable administrative clearance, takes three or four children to an appropriate visitation site for all or a portion of the school day. The children take photographs if possible, collect brochures, samples of the product involved, and similar items, and then report to the full classroom group. A step lower on the organizational scale is the independent visit where one or two children, with parental supervision, visit a facility as an optional assignment terminating in a class report.

An extremely thorough and useful planning aid for field trips of all types has been devised by the Group for Environmental Education and published as the *Yellow Pages of Learning Resources*.[8] This source provides a detailed analysis in the form of guiding questions for almost any conceivable visitation site; examples of the sections include "What Can You Learn at a Restaurant?" "What Can You Learn from a Taxicab Driver?" and "What Can You Learn at a Cemetery?"

Field trips are used to bring the children to the community; however, it is always less cumbersome and often more effective from an instructional standpoint to bring the community to the classroom in the form of a resource speaker. To be effective with elementary schoolchildren, such speakers must have adequate training or experience, for a favorable response usually requires the use of educational media in the form of films, puppets, or some similar activity designed to produce the active involvement of the children. Most city fire and police departments make regular presentations

[8] Group for Environmental Education, Inc., *Yellow Pages of Learning Resources* (Cambridge, Mass.: MIT Press, 1972).

on safety topics. Other possibilities include the local chapter of the American Cancer Society for cigarette smoking, and the American Heart Association on hypertension and other topics dealing with the circulatory system.

FILMS and TELEVISION

Educational movie films, filmstrips, and colored slides combined with cassette tapes (slide-tapes) dealing with a wide variety of health topics are currently available. Most of these materials are designed to serve objectives in the cognitive domain such as those related to acquiring information and developing concepts. Recently, however, there has been a number of efforts to develop material suitable for such affective outcomes as experiencing different emotional states and exploring self-concepts. Some of the more promising examples take the form of 5- or 10-minute modules depicting personal incidents involving anger, grief, or shyness; these are specifically designed to provide a concrete starting point for the discussion of these somewhat nebulous topics. Another interesting possibility involves showing a rapid series of colored slides selected to produce emotional involvement with a specific topic. A series showing children enjoying a variety of recreational sports could stimulate a discussion on exercise preferences, for example, or a series showing individuals and groups suffering from hunger and famine could be used to introduce the study of world food problems. Such slides can be produced by the relatively simple process of copying them from magazines, books, posters, and other such sources; suitable background music provided by a cassette is desirable but not essential. The process of finding and obtaining suitable slides and films from outside sources will be discussed in a following section.

Television in its various applications can provide support to health instruction ranging from the relatively passive viewing of health-related "specials" on commercial television to the active production of health programs for use on closed-circuit systems. Also, professionally prepared video-tapes on health topics such as the *Inside Out Series*[9] on mental health are becoming increasingly available. In suitably equipped classrooms these can be used much like conventional sound films. One of the simplest methods of using television is to review one or more of the popular weekly guides, or perhaps other sources of reviews such as the TV section of *Instructor* magazine, for programs related to the topic currently under study. Although the educational channels are usually the most fruitful, good programs periodically appear on the commercial networks. One or more children can then be asked to watch the program on a voluntary or extra credit basis and report to the class. Another possibility is the taping of programs "off the air" for later viewing in the class. Permission must be obtained from the

[9] *Inside Out Series* (Bloomington, Ind.: Agency for Instructional Television).

stations; however, this is routinely granted by most educational television stations.

PHOTOGRAPHY

Because of growing popularity of cameras using either self-developing films or cassette film cartridges, photography is being used to an increasing degree by elementary schoolchildren in the completion of projects and assignments. Also, the teacher with an interest in photography should consider the possible use of this hobby as a source of teacher-made teaching materials. A 35-millimeter camera, together with a relatively inexpensive electronic flash attachment and a close-up lens, can be used to record everything from mountain landscapes to magazine pictures on 2×2 slides for classroom projection. The audiovisual centers of many school systems provide both the equipment and the technical assistance needed to add synchronized narration and background music capable of transforming these personal collections into professional-quality slide-tape modules.

GAMES

An increasing number of attractive educational games are coming on the market including a few with health-related topics as their main theme. *Rules of the Road,*[10] a prominent example in this category, simulates traffic situations for pedestrians, bicyclists, and motorists, and requires correct answers and proper decisions to safely reach the finish line. Also, some companies and industrial groups, particularly those in the food industry, make classroom games available at a relatively low cost.

The construction of games to meet special education needs can bring considerable personal satisfaction as well as improved teaching effectiveness to the creative teacher. Although it requires a significant amount of time and effort, these costs can be recovered many times over in the several years of service a good classroom game normally provides. Often the basic format can be borrowed from a commercial board game with the new content and situation based on the unit at hand. Lorraine Strom describes her use of games as a fourth grade teacher and provides assurance that "it isn't that hard to be creative, and after the children's interests are sparked, they will be begging to do the art work, the cutting, the pasting—all the time-consuming details—and eventually they will beg to do it all."[11] She also found

[10]As developed by L. M. and F. D. Wiseman and distributed by Rules of the Road, P.O. Box 338, Campbell, Calif. 95008.
[11] Lorraine Strom, "Formulas for Fun," *School Health Review*, Vol. 4, No. 1 (January-February 1973), pp. 10–12. [*School Health Review* is now named *Health Education*.]

that once she developed the basic pattern or formula for a game, such as a thinking game, a classifying game, a card game, she could use it for the creation of a number of new games. She offers one final hint: use sturdy materials.

ARTS and CRAFTS

As with so many curricular areas, activities commonly found under the heading of arts and crafts provide a great many possibilities for the teaching of health content. Projects centered on posters and cartoons are very appropriate because of health education's traditional concern with behavioral change. Wall-sized murals, with the various components prepared by separate children or working groups, lend themselves to many health themes. Another ever-popular activity in this general category is the full-body "cutout," where each child lies on a large piece of "butcher paper" while a partner traces his or her body outline. This is then cut out and embellished with details reflecting the owner's self-concept. One class of fourth grade pupils at Horace Mann School in Clinton, Iowa, devised an interesting variation of this device in which cutouts of the internal organ systems were constructed and pasted on their body replicas. The enthusiasm of the children for this project is clearly expressed in this report provided by their teacher:

> Their motto has been "No Extra Entrails". . . . [They] wanted to have their bodies in living color. The brain and spinal cord were canary yellow, the lungs were sky blue, the eyes were white, the ears were lime green. . . . [They] labeled the body parts, attached them in proper position on their own body replicas, then hung them in "The Morgue." [12]

With the addition of one more dimension, cutout figures become models and thus open up another realm of possibilities. The various commercial kits of the whole body or large models of individual segments or organs can provide both a good construction experience and a permanent schoolroom aid if the money can be found for their purchase. Model towns planned with due consideration for the water supply, sewage treatment, pollution control, traffic safety, and so forth offer the advantage of integrating the study of health and social studies or even a core project for the total curriculum. Puppets in their various forms represent another extremely versatile medium for health teaching, with the construction, the play writing, and the presentation providing useful learning experiences.

[12] Marcia Martensen, "Body Building," *Instructor*, Vol. 85, No. 6 (February 1976), pp. 62–63.

LABORATORY ACTIVITIES

For teachers who can tolerate the "messiness" involved in the classroom, dissection and examination of kidneys, brains, and intestines (the famous "chitterlings" of the South) will always capture the interest of upper elementary schoolchildren. Living things are more appealing to most teachers and probably to most children, even if they only are bacteria cultured in glass jars containing peeled and cooked potatoes.[13] More engaging are such classroom pets as gerbils, hamsters, white rats, and guinea pigs, which among other virtues, provide interesting learning experiences in sex and reproduction.

The two more common formats for laboratory-type activities are the "demonstration," with the teacher, resource person, or student presenter carrying out the dissection or some similar activity for the class to view, and the "experiment," which is conducted by the children over a period of time as with the bacteria culturing already mentioned. Of these, the experiment tends to be favored because of the more active involvement of the children and the more comprehensive experience it provides in terms of planning, execution, reporting, and the many other skills related to an orderly investigation.

ACTIVITY CARDS

Teaching, of course, does not consist of one continuous sequence of exotic activities leading to new skills or insights. Children usually need considerable practice, reinforcement, and enrichment added to their educational diets. The activity card provides an effective device for meeting these needs with a minimal drain on teacher time or energy. As defined by Dorothy M. Lloyd,

> . . . the term *activity card* means any card which defines a task that takes the form of directions or questions, or a combination of the two. This task may be done by one student or by two or more students together. Such a card may be any size, shape or color.[14]

For example, one card for the study of nutrition reads as follows:

HOW'S YOUR NUTRITION?
1. List what you ate and how much you ate for breakfast today.
2. After lunch, list what you ate and how much you ate for lunch.
3. Tomorrow list what you eat and how much you eat for dinner tonight.
4. Look at the nutrition chart and divide the list of things you ate for the day into the four food groups: Meats, Milk Products, Vegetables and Fruits, Bread and Cereals.

[13] See Leslie W. Irwin et al., *Health in Elementary Schools* (St. Louis, Mo.: C. V. Mosby Company, 1966), p. 273, for detailed instructions of this activity.
[14] Dorothy M. Lloyd, *Classroom Activity Cards* (Danville, N.Y.: The Instructor Publications, Inc.), 1975.

5. Did you eat something from all groups? If not, which did you leave out?

6. Did you eat the amount for each group that is required? If not, which do you need to eat more of?

One of the principal advantages of activity cards is that children can generally use them on an independent basis, either individually or in a small group, without close supervision. For this reason they lend themselves readily to the "learning center" concept in which children who have finished their routine assignments may move to a designated table located at the back of the room, select a card, and complete the assignment, perhaps utilizing resources that were placed there beforehand. Instruction for the cards or general ideas for their creation may be found in various publications or with only moderate effort they may be completely produced by the teacher.

VALUES CLARIFICATION

During the past 10 years there has been an increasing emphasis placed on the development of techniques and approaches for the accomplishment of objectives in the affective domain. Although teachers, administrators, and other school personnel have always recognized the importance of how children "feel" about various issues or phenomena as compared with what they "know" about them, they have always been at somewhat of a loss as to how to treat this sensitive realm of human behavior. The basic problem is that, although important, feelings to a large extent are one's own business; outsiders cannot tell anyone what feelings are "correct" in any given situation in the same manner that "facts" can be established as "correct." Any effort to dictate how children should feel about very many things would, in most of our typically heterogeneous communities, soon run afoul of all manner of ethical and legal obstacles.

This basic problem is still not solved to everyone's satisfaction but a promising approach has been devised by Raths, Harmin, Simon [15] and others under the general heading of values clarification. The basic assumption on which this approach is based is that many personal values remain implicit, non-verbalized—perhaps subconscious—and thus not open to personal review and modification. This view provides the basis for literally dozens of classroom techniques designed to help children identify their values in explicit terms and thus make favorable changes or perhaps bring their behavior more in concert with these now "clarified" values.[16] For example, one sixth grade teacher posed this situation to the class

[15] L. Raths, M. Harmin, and S. Simon, *Values and Teaching* (Columbus, Ohio: Charles E. Merrill Publishing Co.), 1966.
[16] See Sidney B. Simon, Leland W. Howe, and Howard Kirschenbaum, *Values Clarification* (New York: Hart Publishing Company, Inc., 1977), for detailed descriptions of many of these techniques.

You have a new T-shirt. You want a slogan written across the chest that shows what you think of yourself—something that really shows "you." What would you write? [17]

Once the children have completed this task, the teacher asks them such "clarifying" questions as

- What makes you think so?
- What do you think is the reason for that?
- What makes you feel that way? [18]

Perhaps the most well known of the values clarification techniques is the values continuum in which two extreme positions are formulated and then placed at opposite ends of a line drawn across the chalkboard as in the following example:

Courageous Connie
Any problem can be
solved if you act
with enough courage

Careful Cal
Always choose the
safest way; nothing
is worth taking risks

Each child who wishes to participate is then asked to choose a point on the line that represents his or her view. This generally leads to a discussion of what each position means in terms of real-life situations. As the discussion progresses, individual children may become more firm in their position or perhaps change it in light of new insights. Although some question the long-term benefits of this general approach, it does serve to involve children in a systematic way with many heretofore neglected topics.[19]

FINDING and SELECTING MATERIALS

Although the quality may often be criticized, the quantity of health-related teaching resources currently available is virtually overwhelming. Health content tends to overlap directly with both science and social studies in many areas such as anatomy and physiology and community health problems. Also, health situations are a common theme in texts, work sheets, and other materials for language arts. Consequently, much of the vast quantities of commercially produced instructional materials for these curriculum areas

[17] Joyce W. Hopp, "VC for Sixth Graders," *School Health Review,* Vol. 5, No. 7 (January-February 1974), pp. 34–35.

[18] Ibid., p. 35.

[19] For a critical review of this approach, see Dennis Loggins, "Clarifying What and How Well?" *Health Education,* Vol. 7, No. 2 (March-April 1976), pp. 2–5.

often apply directly to health topics. Many multimillion-dollar industries are health related and make teaching materials available as part of their advertising program; examples in this category include drug and toothpaste manufacturers and life insurance companies. The voluntary health agencies such as the American Cancer Society and the health professional organizations such as the American Medical Association are two other sources that distribute health education teaching materials. Finally, there are a great multitude of governmental agencies that make materials available, often with no charge; these range from the local public health department to the more remote federal agencies. It must be noted, however, that careful selection is needed regardless of the source. Some of these items contain too much advertising material or other self-serving propaganda; however, many others are educationally valid and very effective.

TEACHER PRODUCTION

One unique solution to the formidable problem of finding and selecting good teaching media is to simply forego the entire task and create one's own materials. As has been emphasized throughout this chapter, this practice often results in better materials because of their tailor-made design with

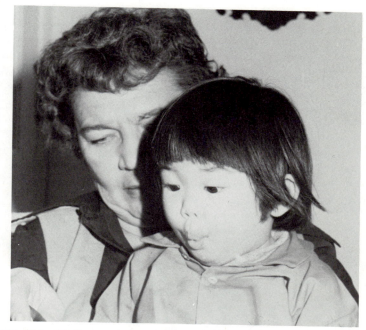

Figure 16.4. Finding and Selecting Appropriate Materials. (Carol Ashton)

not too much more effort. One further advantage is the opportunity this practice provides for professional growth; teachers who create their own materials invariably become more personally involved with the subject matter, the subtleties of the learning process, and the characteristics of children. This type of experience in time helps transform mere "clock-punching" technicians into fully committed professionals who know their craft "from the ground up."

Those with reasonable tolerance for occasional failure and who like to "tinker" with things often develop into good producers of materials with little or no outside help. A more systematic approach is followed by those who search out the many fine "how-to-do-it" sources that are available in this field.[20] Local personnel from the school's instructional media center and/or the district's audiovisual department are another source of aid, often providing materials, equipment, and advice. Finally, teachers with real enthusiasm for this activity often take summer or evening school courses from the educational media departments of local colleges and universities to both sharpen their skills and meet the inevitable requirements for maintaining one's teaching certification.

THE SEARCH

Despite the many virtues of teacher production, commercial organizations can do a better job in some areas because of their obviously larger resources. For this and a variety of other reasons most teachers find it necessary to enter the somewhat hectic marketplace for commercially prepared teaching media. One of the first stops in this search is often the school instructional materials center (IMC). To an increasing degree school libraries are evolving into facilities that emphasize both nonprint and print materials; whether the people in charge are termed librarians or IMC directors, they usually provide teachers with this type of assistance as part of their responsibility.

The local IMC or the local college or university library usually provides access to a few of the many indexes that list newly developed materials. Among the most popular of these are *NICEM Media Indexes* as prepared by the National Information Center for Educational Media.[21] Separate NICEM guides are published for each type of media such as 16-mm films, overhead transparencies, and film strips. Whereas these national guides are useful in long-term planning geared toward purchases for local collections in identifying sources of free and inexpensive materials, the catalogues and indexes for the local building or school district collection can alert one to items that are available through standard loan procedures.

[20] One of the most highly regarded of these is Jerrold E. Kemp, *Planning and Producing Audiovisual Materials* (New York: Thomas Y. Crowell Co., Inc., 1975).
[21] Available from the National Information Center for Educational Media (NICEM), R. R. Bowker Company, 1180 Avenue of the Americas, New York, N.Y. 10036.

The teacher's independent search for teaching media must logically begin with the various sections of such professional journals as *Instructor* and *Grade Teacher* that routinely review and identify sources of free and inexpensive materials. Within the specific field of health education, the *Journal of School Health* and *Health Education* both provide such information. From here, one could go to the "yellow pages" under the heading "Health Agencies" to identify the local offices of the American Heart Association, the American Cancer Society, the Lung Association, and other such organizations, most of which provide educational materials related to their specialty. The local public health department also falls into this general category. Although it is usually best to contact local offices first, they are sometimes not available. In this case requests mailed to national offices of health-related organizations will often yield good results.

SELECTION

Once a material has been obtained, a decision must be made as to whether it is acceptable in terms of the educational purposes for which it was selected. This is a difficult task, for virtually all items of media have limitations or negative points such as dated information, amateurish acting in the case of films, amateurish illustrations in the case of printed materials, or unwanted bias in the case of materials prepared by industrial groups or trade organizations. Often the teacher can offset these features by such tactics as warning the children against propaganda or correcting inaccuracies. There are no hard and fast rules on the selection of particular materials; however, Carlton Erickson and David Curl [22] provide 12 criteria that can help guide the review process:

1. Is the content useful and important to the learner?
2. Will it be interesting to students?
3. Is there a direct relationship to a specific objecive or problem-solving activity?
4. How will the format and presentation treatment affect the organization and sequence of learner activities?
5. Is the material authentic, typical, and up-to-date?
6. Have facts and concepts been checked for accuracy? Are the producers expert in the subject matter, or have they employed competent consultants?
7. Do the content and presentation meet contemporary standards of good taste?
8. If [the subject is] controversial, are both sides given equal emphasis? Should they be?

[22] Carlton W. H. Erickson and David H. Curl, *Fundamentals of Teaching with Audiovisual Technology* (New York: Macmillan Publishing Co., Inc., 1972).

9. Is bias or propaganda evident? If so, how should students deal with it?
10. Is technical quality satisfactory? Are images clear? Narration or dialog intelligible? Color, motion, and special effects used authentically and creatively?
11. Do content and structure reveal careful planning by the producer?
12. Has the material actually been *validated*, or tested with learners? If so, who performed the evaluation? Under what conditions? What were the characteristics of the students? How successful were the results?

REFERENCES

BROWN, JAMES W., RICHARD B. LEWIS, and FRED F. HARCLEROAD. *AV Instruction: Media and Methods.* New York: McGraw-Hill Book Company, 1973.

CALDWELL, BETTY, and ROBERT YOWELL. "Action Dramatics," *Instructor,* Vol. 86, No. 5 (January 1977), p. 118.

CORNACCHIA, HAROLD J., and WESLEY M. STATON. *Health in Elementary Schools.* St. Louis: C. V. Mosby Company, 1974.

DALE, EDGAR, *Audio-Visual Methods in Teaching.* New York: The Dryden Press, 1969.

EPSTEIN, CHARLOTTE. *Affective Subjects in the Classroom.* Scranton, Pa.: Intext Educational Publishers, 1972.

ERICKSON, CARLTON W. H., and DAVID H. CURL. *Fundamentals of Teaching with Audiovisual Technology.* New York: Macmillan Publishing, Co., Inc., 1972.

FRAENKEL, JACK R. *Helping Students Think and Value.* Englewood Cliffs, N.J.: Prentice-Hall, Inc., 1973.

Group for Environmental Education, Inc. *Yellow Pages of Learning Resources.* Cambridge, Mass.: MIT Press, 1972.

HOPP, JOYCE W. "VC for Sixth Graders," *School Health Review,* Vol. 5, No. 7 (January-February 1974), p. 34.

KEMP, JERROLD E. *Planning and Producing Audiovisual Materials.* New York: Thomas Y. Crowell Company, Inc., 1975.

LLOYD, DOROTHY M. *Classroom Activity Cards.* Dansville, N.Y.: The Instructor Publications, Inc., 1975.

LOGGINS, DENNIS. "Clarifying What and How Well?" *Health Education,* Vol. 7, No. 2 (March-April 1976), p. 2.

MARTENSEN, MARCIA. "Body Building," *Instructor,* Vol. 85, No. 6 (February 1976), p. 62.

MOUSTAKAS, CLARK. *Teaching as Learning.* New York: Ballantine Books, 1972.

PALOMARES, UVALDO H. "Magic Circle: Key to Understanding Self and Others," *Educational Leadership,* Vol. 32, No. 1 (October 1974), p. 19.

RATHS, L., M. HARMIN, and S. SIMON. *Values and Teaching.* Columbus, Ohio: Charles E. Merrill Publishing Company, 1966.

READ, DONALD A., and WALTER H. GREENE. *Creative Teaching in Health.* Macmillan Publishing Co., Inc., 1975.

SIMON, SIDNEY B., LELAND W. HOWE, and HOWARD KIRSCHENBAUM. *Values Clarification.* New York: Hart Publishing Company, Inc. 1977.

STROM, LORRAINE. "Formulas for Fun," *School Health Review,* Vol. 4, No. 1 (January-February 1973), p. 10.

Evaluation

In its most basic sense evaluation is an integral part of normal human behavior. As people go about their daily lives they are continually observing a wide variety of phenomena including the actions of other persons, the consequences of their own actions, and the effectiveness of various products—then judging the relative desirability of these things as they affect their own personal needs. Following this judgmental process one normally modifies his or her actions to avoid the "bad" and seek out the "good" people, behavior patterns, or services. Sometimes this process takes a very deliberate form as when a young couple selects an apartment after visiting and systematically gathering information on several that were available for rent. In others it takes place in an almost instinctive fashion as when one takes a new job just because "the 'vibes' were good when I talked to the people there." But regardless of how casual or formalized the process of evaluation may be, two vital elements will be present: (1) observations or data gathering, and (2) judgment of what is observed against some preconceived goal or standard that is, in effect, an evaluative criterion. These two basic steps should normally be followed by (3) modification or reaffirmation of some course of action as the results of the evaluative process are put to use.

APPLICATIONS to HEALTH EDUCATION

It seems clear that judgmental or evaluative behavior occurs as a natural part of any field of endeavor. And where educational activities are involved, those managing the program have an inherent obligation to conduct evaluative functions in the most effective possible way. If a subject such as health education is worth studying, pupils need to know whether they are learning anything of value from this study; if parents have a responsibility to help and support their children as they acquire an education, they must be informed as to the child's progress; if teachers are to continually improve

370

their teaching effectiveness, they must determine what techniques and what materials are producing the desired results; and, finally, those responsible for the total program with its curriculum, time allotments, supervisory assistance, and other teaching supports must decide if the program is on course and making worthwhile use of the time and money allocated to it. These needs are universally recognized; to deny them is to condemn people to a life of stumbling around in the dark. However, once one moves beyond this basic acceptance into the specific mechanics of evaluation a whole host of controversies soon arise.

BARRIERS to EVALUATION

Controversies related to evaluation are common in almost any teaching field; however, they are particularly troublesome as applied to health education with its traditional emphasis on producing changes in everyday behavior as opposed to mere improvement of classroom performance. A consideration of the formidable barriers to effective evaluation in health education may well discourage one from making the attempt; but in a more positive sense the realization of the real difficulties involved may help one tolerate the inevitable frustration that seems to be part of every evaluative task. These barriers tend to form three specific categories:

1. *Philosophical.* There are many disagreements as to the validity of various criteria used for evaluation. It is relatively easy to measure a child's degree of mastery of specific information, for example; however, the question of deciding whether or not the information was worth learning in the first place is essentially a matter of subjective judgment. Beyond this lies the whole issue of the relative value of knowledge gain versus attitudinal or behavioral change.

2. *Technological.* There are serious limitations to the instruments or techniques available for observing or measuring the various qualities related to the various criteria. One may conclude that it is highly desirable for pupils to develop a positive self-concept or to feel comfortable with their own health values, but how does one measure these degrees of positiveness or comfort with anything approaching precision or objectivity?

3. *Emotional.* The people involved in most evaluative processes generally have a vested interest in the outcome which interferes with the accuracy and validity of their judgments. The desire of pupils to obtain good grades or to simply preserve some cherished image of themselves as outstanding scholars may prevent their acceptance or use of this evidence provided by evaluation techniques; likewise, teachers and administrators may be more interested in justifying their current modes

of operating than identifying and correcting any weaknesses or short-comings.

If these barriers are to be overcome or minimized, it is necessary to approach any evaluative task with the presupposition that the people involved are worthwhile human beings with many good qualities, and that any shortcomings that may be revealed represent opportunities for further growth and improvement. One of the main emotional barriers to evaluation is personal feelings of insecurity; insecure persons tend to resist even the most fair programs of evaluation because of the unreasonable fear that they will reveal some terrible weakness about themselves. The secure person, however, feels that any weak points that may be found can be corrected or adjusted; therefore, schools that can foster this healthy atmosphere of acceptance and security will find much of the sting removed and the constructive aspects restored to their evaluation tasks.

The second most essential need in any program of evaluation is for the evaluators to keep their attention constantly focused on the underlying qualities they are assessing and avoid becoming unduly fascinated with any single indicator of these qualities. A pupil's knowledge of nutrition may be worth fostering and evaluating; his or her score on a nutrition knowledge test might or might not be a useful indicator of this quality depending on a variety of factors including the pupil's reading ability, his or her general attitude toward tests, and the basic reliability and validity of the instrument itself. High test scores have no intrinsic value; however, relevant knowledge presumably does. Because the relationship between these two is seldom perfect and often widely disparate, one is seldom justified in attaching undue significance to any single measure or indicator. In the case of nutrition knowledge, then, oral responses in class and work on assignments and projects should normally receive proper consideration. This necessity to develop a broad basis for one's evaluation is perhaps most important when one seeks to assess pupil status in relation to attitudes, values, or behavior; here, the objective techniques of measurement are even more limited in their effectiveness.

EVALUATION of PUPIL RESPONSE

The basic reason for providing pupils with instruction in health is to exert some favorable impact on the health behavior they manifest in their everyday lives. In an ideal sense the progress of individual pupils in their study of health could be determined by evaluating this behavior. This approach might be justified if one were able to devise some omniscient device that would monitor this behavior on a 24 hour a day basis over a period of years; however, it is obvious that no such instrument exists.

HEALTH BEHAVIOR as CRITERION

Although it is true that a number of less ideal but useful techniques are available for the assessment of practical everyday health behavior, their limitations preclude their use as the primary measure of pupil progress. Some health behavior may be observed directly by the teacher, as when pupils cover their mouths and noses when coughing or sneezing or when they make a special effort to be friendly to a new pupil, but these incidental observations cover only a small portion of daily health behavior. Another approach is the pencil-and-paper behavior inventory in which pupils are systematically questioned as to their out-of-class behavior; however, pupils are not always accurate or truthful in the way they respond to such instruments. Also, an unfavorable answer doesn't always indicate an educational lack; a child may not have had fruit or juice for breakfast, for example, simply because none was available. An even more serious problem with this general approach to evaluation is the fact that a pupil often may acquire the potential to apply good health behavior but not have any occasion to use it during the period of observation. A pupil might acquire an effective understanding and appreciation of the miraculous functioning of the human respiratory system with its delicate alveoli and microscopic cilia in the fifth grade and have no occasion to act on this learning experience until he or she resists the temptation to begin cigarette smoking 2 years later in junior high school.

INDIRECT CRITERIA

The many problems inherent in the assessment of health behavior have prompted most health educators to fall back on the evaluation of demonstrable knowledge and attitudes as the main criteria for determining pupil performance. Although it is often difficult to demonstrate a direct relationship between knowledge gain and immediate behavioral change, as when the frequency of cigarette smoking is polled after instruction on this topic, most health educators believe that a long-term acquisition of meaningful health knowledge will eventually manifest itself in improved health behavior. The relationship between general educational levels and good health behavior has been quite clearly established, and it seems logical that specific knowledge gain in health should augment this established trend.

The case for the relationship between favorable health attitudes and overt health behavior is even more clearly established and has fewer detractors than does health knowledge. This added support for attitudes as a valid criterion is somewhat moderated by a generally lower level of confidence in current methods of attitude assessment. Attitude assessment may also be questioned by some as an unwarranted invasion of a student's right to privacy. But both factors carry the great advantage of assessability and, to a large extent, accountability. Teachers can establish rather specific knowledge and attitudinal objectives as classroom goals and then determine whether or not individual pupils attained these objectives with reasonable precision. The link between these factors and the ultimate criterion of health behavior must then be defended by logic; however, this is generally true for any subject in the curriculum.

SPECIFIC TECHNIQUES

If one accepts the proposition that evaluative activities are an integral part of human behavior and thus an integral part of the education process, then it becomes quite logical to accept a wide variety of specific techniques as useful to the completion of this task. This approach is also compatible with the modern trend away from excess reliance on single examinations, surveys, or opinionnaires as the basis for judging the performance of any student, teacher, or program. Health goals are complex and the instruments that measure progress toward these goals are imperfect; therefore, several specific factors should be observed.

CLASSROOM FEEDBACK. Pupil manifestation of high interest is not always a sure sign of effective learning, but its lack casts grave doubts as whether anything worthwhile is taking place. Classroom discussions provide a prime opportunity to observe both individual and general class interest in a particular health topic. The willingness of particular children to voluntarily contribute specific remarks is an obvious indicator of interest in most cases; however, the behavior of the nonspeaking pupils is even more significant. Their eye contact with the teacher or the classmate speaking, their facial expressions, their spontaneous laughter or sighs, and the physical posture they display all provide evidence of interest and participation that do not require formal training in body language for a reasonably accurate assessment of their significance. In addition to formal discussion, there are a host of behaviors that merit attention. As applied to a particular topic such as health, these include getting assignments in on time; exceeding the requirements of the assignments; bringing in newspaper clippings, magazine articles, and other outside materials; checking a health-related book out of the library for free reading; and other such indicators.[1]

Thus far these "feedback" behaviors have been discussed as indicators of interest; however, they also have obvious value in the assessment of knowledge gain. Although they do not provide the systematic and comprehensive evaluation of a pupil's knowledge on a particular health topic that a well-

---

[1] Adapted for the elementary school level from the general concept described by Robert F. Mager, *Developing Attitudes Towards Learning* (Palo Alto, Calif.: Fearon Publishers, 1968), pp. 21–30.

constructed knowledge test does, these spontaneous behaviors often provide a more valid indicator that the child has internalized a particular health fact or principle and is willing to apply it to real-life situations.

CLASSROOM ASSIGNMENTS.   Just as a good test has auxiliary value as a learning device, many teaching–learning activities also contain built-in evaluative features. Written assignments such as essays and workbooks are obvious examples, but many others should be added to this category. Poster construction and art projects provide pupils with the opportunity to show that they can identify the main points of a nutrition unit, for example. The construction of simple dioramas depicting pollution and soil erosion or models of water treatment or waste water treatment plants are within the ability of many fifth or sixth grade pupils and can provide tangible evidence of their knowledge of these important subtopics. Within the realm of mental health, pupils can demonstrate their knowledge of basic behavioral dynamics such as the concealing of emotions or the need for support and encouragement in role-playing activities or pupil-devised playlets related to these concepts.

TEACHER-CONSTRUCTED INSTRUMENTS.   However useful the teacher's random observations may be, they must normally be supplemented from time to time with the systematic sampling of the behavior of every pupil that a well-constructed evaluative instrument can provide. Such devices can be used to determine (1) current health habits and practices, (2) health attitudes, and (3) health knowledge. The construction of such instruments can be infinitely complicated and time consuming if one has the time, energy, and expertise to apply the sophisticated technology of formal test construction to the task. Those designed to test behavior and attitudes must be constructed with sensitivity as to students' home environments and their right to hold attitudes consistent with their families' political and religious beliefs. In contrast to these idealized procedures, many other teachers routinely use instruments that they devised in total ignorance of the basic principles of test construction. In most cases the practical course lies somewhere between these extremes where the sound principles are applied but the process stops short of the often impractical application of statistical refinements characteristic of standardized tests. Although teacher-constructed instruments are seldom as refined as standard tests, they offer the major advantage of being constructed for a specific class and a specific evaluative need.

STANDARDIZED TESTS.   Although they have come under increasing public criticism in recent years, standardized tests offer many advantages if they are properly selected and applied. Generally, they are designed for use in all parts of the country; this broad market makes it commercially feasible to hire expert consultants both for subject matter consideration and to oversee the technical aspects of the construction and refinement process. A particular test may begin with a pool of 300 carefully formulated test items designed to thoroughly cover a subject. These may be reduced to a more practical size of 50 items by statistical techniques, yet still yield scores related to what the child would have received on the original 300. Another advantage is the broad-based norms that are generally developed for such instruments; these are a compilation of scores achieved by pupils from a wide geographic area, which are organized into some readily understandable form such as percentiles. These permit school-to-school comparisons and provide an external measure of at least one aspect of a program's effectiveness.

Standardized tests can provide a useful supplement to a total program of evaluation if they are properly used. Their usual pattern of organization into subtests on specific areas such as nutrition and mental health makes them useful as diagnostic devices to determine either individual or general class needs. Also, their generally high levels of reliability permit relatively accurate measurement of knowledge gain when used on a test–retest basis before and after a particular unit of study. This is useful in specific situations as when a new unit of study or a new teaching approach is being added to the curriculum for the first time. Finally, when administered annually to the same school population, such instruments can provide one useful indication of overall program effectiveness.

Unfortunately, many people, including teachers, administrators, pupils, and parents, often feel unduly threatened by the results of standardized tests. Because of the frequent abuse of test scores, these fears are often well founded. In defense of these instruments, it should be noted that the abuses are seldom built into the test by the test developers. The injustices occur when teachers, administrators, and special interest groups exaggerate the importance or distort the meaning of the results, either because of lack of understanding or occasionally in an overt effort to lobby for some cherished cause. These abuses can be controlled only by making all parties aware of the strengths and limitations of any instrument used. Most tests measure some relatively narrowly defined area; even health exams that include all major health topics generally only measure one type of behavior such as knowledge, attitudes, or actual practices; typically, a health education program is concerned with all three. A single test score should seldom be the sole criterion for any evaluative process; it is more properly used as simply one more useful piece of evidence.

GRADING. The process of reporting the quality of a pupil's performance to the parents and to the pupil in the form of a letter grade, a single number, or some similar scheme provides a focal point for much of the criticism of the public schools. School systems that rely on more broad and constructive forms of reporting such as anecdotal reports and various combinations of parent–teacher, pupil–teacher conferences receive heavy criticism as being "wishy-washy" and diffuse; we hear the lament "I don't know where my child stands." On the other hand, school systems that retain the conventional letter system are accused of being arbitrary, unfair, and needlessly cruel.[2]

One of the somewhat "backhanded" advantages of health education's public image as one of the auxiliary subjects of the curriculum is that parents tend to be less concerned about health grades. The unwholesome attitudes and inflamed emotions that sometime surround reading and mathematics grades, for example, occur much less frequently. However, if one views learning to care for one's health as equally vital to the child's welfare as learning to read, despite the public tendency to downgrade health education, then it seems clear that the task of grading pupils in health education is similar or identical to the task of grading any other subject. There are two essential criteria that any grading or progress reporting system must meet: (1) pupils and parents must be effectively informed as to how thoroughly essential competencies or skills are being acquired, and (2) the system must not produce damaging side effects in the form of negative attitudes, distortion of teaching emphasis, poor teacher–pupil or parent–pupil rapport, and so forth.

As implied earlier, many schools seek to satisfy these sometimes conflicting criteria by placing emphasis on conferences, anecdotal reports, and self-evaluation activities. The inherently practical and humanistic nature of a good program of health education lends itself well to this type of approach. Although specific scores, assignments, texts, and standardized examinations may contribute to the reporting process, these are interpreted in the context of the total task and do not dominate the process. Although these broad-based reports are essential, many schools feel it necessary to supplement them with periodic report cards that represent the traditional single-symbol grade in forms of A–F; O, S, U; 1–5; or some similar scheme. Where such is the case, it is important that it be fairly determined and not allowed to assume undue importance among pupils or parents. At its best, a grade merely represents how well one performed in a relatively narrow area of concern, classroom activities in a particular subject, over a relatively short period of time; it is not a reflection of one's overall worth and value as a person, nor is it often an accurate reflection of how effectively one might apply these competencies, insights, or skills outside the classroom.

CONSTRUCTION of EVALUATIVE INSTRUMENTS

Even after discounting the common tendency to exaggerate the importance of test scores, it is difficult to deny their usefulness in the general evaluative process. Although standardized tests are highly useful for specific purposes, the large majority of tests are teacher constructed.

[2] For a critical evaluation of grading practices presented in narrative form, see Howard Kirschenbaum et al., *Wad-ja-get?* (New York, N.Y.: Hart Publishing Co., Inc., 1971).

KNOWLEDGE TESTS

Most teachers can develop reasonably good knowledge tests if they will give proper consideration to (1) *scope* and *balance,* which are associated with test validity, and (2) *comprehensiveness* and *clarity,* which are related to reliability. If the scope of an unit on communicable disease included material on causes, prevention, and treatment, then a test designed to determine the knowledge gain in this should have a similar scope of causes, prevention, and treatment. Also, the number of test items for each of these three categories should reflect the proportion of time devoted to them during the course of the unit if the test is to have proper balance. This principle can also be applied to other dimensions of the subject matter presented; for example, if approximately 50 per cent of the emphasis was placed on building a factual background and 50 per cent on understanding practical applications of the knowledge, the test items should reflect this balance. A useful device for planning for balance and scope is a simple "table of organization" as shown in Table 17.1.

Although it may not be necessary to actually devise such a table, its basic principles must be kept in mind to avoid the common error of unduly loading the test with questions from one aspect of the unit, such as disease terminology, simply because it was easy to devise these types of questions.

As used here, comprehensiveness refers to the principle that the more questions that are included on a particular topic, the more likely a pupil's score will reflect his or her knowledge of a subject. For example, if a unit on dental health included 20 basic facts related to the structure of teeth and yet the test included only one question on this particular subtopic, a pupil who was inattentive or perhaps absent during the unit might by chance give the correct answer whereas a pupil who learned a great deal might miss it. This would be far less likely to occur if five questions were involved. Clarity is based on many factors, including the pupil's reading ability; it is seldom wise to try to assess both health knowledge and reading ability in the same test even though both are important. Generally, it is a good idea to design

TABLE 17.1
An example of a table of organization for planning
a short test on communicable diseases.

		Facts and Principles 50%	Applications 50%	(Total)
Causes	25%	4	4	8
Prevention	50%	8	8	16
Treatment	25%	4	4	8
(Total Questions)		16	16	32

health tests for the poorer readers in the class so that all may have an equal chance to demonstrate their health knowledge. The clarity of a test question depends also on the logic or semantics involved in its structure. A good test often includes some difficult and challenging questions; however, deceptive questions are seldom justified. Consider for example, the following true–false question:

> T F The food poisoning caused by putting food in the refrigerator before it has cooled should be treated right away.

The teacher in this case wanted to determine if the children realized that food poisoning does not result from putting warm food in the refrigerator, but has chosen rather deceptive wording. A more straightforward form would be

> T F Food poisoning is often caused by putting warm food in the refrigerator.

True–false items are relatively easy to construct and do offer the advantage of testing several facts in a short period of time as children can answer them relatively quickly. However, they also lend themselves to ambiguities, spurious guessing, and undue emphasis on factual knowlege as opposed to application or analysis. These problems can be minimized by use of the multiple-choice item which is regarded as the best form for most purposes. For example, the same item of information used in the example above could be tested in the following form:

Food poisoning is often caused by:
   a. putting warm food in the refrigerator.
   b. letting leftover food sit outside the refrigerator.
   c. storing food in the refrigerator in open cans.
   d. refreezing frozen food that was thawed by accident.

Perhaps the most challenging task for the elementary school is the assessment of knowledge levels among kindergarten-primary level children. The simplest solution is to rely completely upon classroom observation of general performance and foresake the use of instruments. This policy works well in most situations; however, there are times when it is useful to systematically test each pupil to obtain data that only a well developed test can provide. Many second and third grade children can handle simple matching and identification items if the wording is kept simple and if the children have made reasonable progress in reading ability. Perhaps the simplest form is

CIRCLE THE FOOD THAT IS BEST FOR YOU

CANDY   SODA POP
APPLE   GUM

A bit more challenging are matching items such as this example

GREEN	STREET
CHILDREN	SIDEWALK
RED	GO
CAR	STOP

For the younger children either one of these basic formats can be presented in picture form. For example

CIRCLE THE FOOD THAT IS BEST FOR YOU

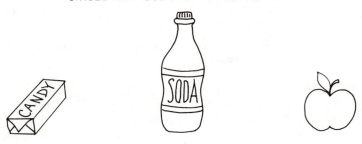

When a "test" composed of such items is presented to kindergarten children, for example, it becomes more a game than an examination and provides many opportunities for learning as well as evaluation.

ATTITUDE ASSESSMENT

The definition of the term "attitude" varies considerably among psychologists and this disparity of opinion exists to an even greater degree among educators who tend to give less attention to fine distinctions. In a very general sense attitude tends to be regarded as a somewhat emotionalized tendency to act or react in a consistent way towards particular phenomena or situations. As such it is usually regarded as an affective factor somewhat less intensive than a value but one that nonetheless exerts a significant effect on behavior patterns. There is a tendency among teachers to profess a serious concern for the development of positive health attitudes yet to evaluate and defend their teaching purely on the grounds of knowledge gain. This apparent inconsistency is partially a result of professed philosophy and partially a result of the difficulty of assessing attitudes in any systematic way.

Because of these measurement problems there is considerable justification in the common practice of assessing attitudes purely on an observational feedback type basis provided that this informality does not lead to an ignoring of the basic importance of attitudes. Actually it is difficult to construct a pencil and paper instrument that will do better than this subjective evaluation of informal pupil comments and actions that appear related to underlying attitudes; however, one very definite advantage of the development of an attitude test is that it can be used to survey a wide variety of attitudes covering a number of health areas in a relatively short period of time. The format for attitude items is basically simple consisting in its more common form of a statement together with a scale upon which the pupil may indicate his or her degree of agreement. For example:

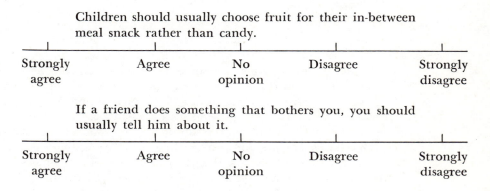

These items, in effect, represent a pencil and paper version of values voting which was described in Chapter 16 as a teaching device. Therefore, the oral form can be used as an attitude evaluation device among the younger pupils who are not yet reading. In this case the statement is read to the class and each child is asked to raise his or her hand if they agree, fold their arms if they "don't care" and give the "thumbs down" sign if they disagree. It is usually unnecessary to tell them to wave their hands or thumbs for "strongly agree" or "strongly disagree." Kindergarten-primary children will usually display any strong feeling they may have without special encouragement.

BEHAVIOR ASSESSMENT

A considerable amount of useful information about the health behavior of children can be gathered simply by asking them. And among children with reading ability such questions can often be presented more quickly and effectively by use of a written "behavior inventory." This approach also elicits more honest response than oral questions because of the obvious privacy that is provided. The format for these types of items are similar to those for attitude except for some obvious changes in wording. For example

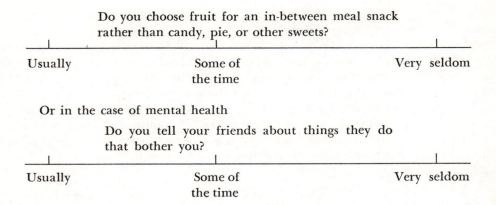

Do you choose fruit for an in-between meal snack
rather than candy, pie, or other sweets?

Usually	Some of the time	Very seldom

Or in the case of mental health

Do you tell your friends about things they do
that bother you?

Usually	Some of the time	Very seldom

The tasks of selecting the areas of behavior about which to question and formulating the questions are somewhat burdensome to the teacher but no more so than constructing an equal amount of knowledge items. A review of the unit material in the forms of chapters assigned, films viewed, and other such resources will provide the reasonably creative teacher with ideas for the development of appropriate items for a good inventory.

One important precaution regarding behavior inventories merits special emphasis. Both children and their parents sometimes object to questions regarding certain sensitive areas. Undue criticism or trouble is almost always avoided when the teacher (1) restricts the scope of the questions to behavior related to topics that have been approved for the curriculum, (2) clears the questions with an appropriate administrator such as the building principal and (3) allows children the option of passing on questions that concern behavior they do not wish to reveal. Also if the inventory contains particularly sensitive items it is sometimes useful to let the children remain anonymous by not putting their names on their papers; this provides the added benefit of increasing the truthfulness (validity) of many of the responses. An obvious disadvantage of this practice is the loss of the ability to use the results for individual guidance; however, they still may be used to guide curriculum or unit emphasis and to help determine if instruction is having any effect on the behavior of the class as a group.

INTEREST ASSESSMENT

Health interests are ordinarily not measured as a planned objective or outcome of instruction. They are more appropriately assessed before a particular unit of instruction as a clue to pupil needs; quite often, although not invariably, pupil interest in a particular item or sub-topics closely parallels a genuine educational need to understand it. The assessment effort may be very simple in scope as before a single unit of study or very broad and sweeping as might be the case if a school district wanted student input for a major curriculum effort.

Health interests may be assessed by use of an inventory type of approach using items similar in format to the attitude and behavior items described above. However, this approach tends to structure the thinking of the respondents and sometimes inhibits the spontaneous expression of interests that didn't happen to be included in the instrument. Many curriculum workers consider the more open-ended approach as used by Byler and her associates in their recent study to be more productive. As they describe

> A brief list of leading questions such as, "What do you wish to know about your body?" "What do we mean by being healthy?" were offered as sample discussion topics. The interviewers were encouraged to develop their own discussion leads which might be more closely related to their students . . . . The possibility of using a structured check-list or questionnaire was rejected from the very beginning of the study by all concerned, on the basis that these devices would suggest to students what they ought to be interested in, and could easily inhibit the creative responses the study was seeking.[3]

EVALUATION of the HEALTH EDUCATION PROGRAM

Regardless of whether one's attention is focused on health education, language arts, social studies, or any other component of the total school program, the task of determining its general effectiveness is becoming increasingly important. During an era in which expectations of a long and satisfying life are high, we find the pathway to this goal cluttered with such obstacles as alcoholism, premature heart disease, mental illness, and divorce; these and similar modern problems provide evidence of serious and pressing educational needs. Many of the same factors in modern society that are exacerbating these health problems are also contributing to unemployment, mismanagement of personal finances, political unrest, and other problems more closely related to social studies, mathematics, and other teaching fields; thus we find the curriculum crowded and time in short supply. Finally, this whole array of modern problems demands an increasing amount of money, whether for attacking these problems as they exist in society at large or studying about them within the school; therefore, we find that funds are always limited. These factors put every area of the curriculum under increasing pressure to use the evaluative process to guide its growth and justify its existence.

[3] Ruth Byler, Gertrude Lewis, and Ruth Totman, *Teach Us What We Want to Know*. New York: Mental Health Materials Center, Inc., 1969, p. xiii–xiv.

MECHANICS of EVALUATION

The evaluation of the health instruction that takes place in a particular school or school district is commonly based on two basic categories or sources of information. These are (1) the reactions of people involved in the program such as knowledge on the part of the pupils, enthusiasm on the part of the teachers, and so forth, and (2) the external features of the program in terms of such factors as time allotments, availability of resources, and the training level of personnel. Because evaluation is an imperfect process at best, both categories must be fully utilized if optimum results are to be obtained.

HUMAN REACTIONS. The fundamental goal of health education is the improvement of health behavior; therefore, evidence of such change becomes the most logical evaluative criterion. But as related earlier in this chapter, the many practical limitations to its assessment may easily lead to invalid conclusions if it is relied upon too heavily. In addition to the obvious problems in determining behavior that takes place out of the classroom and that may take place in the future, it is usually impossible to determine what relationship, if any, health instruction had with behavioral change. A well-taught unit on first aid and safety, for example, might raise the accident rate in a particular school as pupils bring more minor cuts and bumped heads to the attention of the school nurse that otherwise might have been unreported and untreated. This is but one of several possible examples where better behavior leads to "poorer" statistics. It also illustrates an extremely pertinent point: numbers such as test scores or frequency of accidents are helpful in evaluation, but of far greater importance is the human judgment involved in the proper interpretation of these numbers.

Although still far from perfect, the technology that has been developed for the measurement of knowledge is further advanced than is the case for perhaps any other human attribute involved in education. Those promoting health education should not discount the value of demonstrable knowledge gains as evidence of a good program; however, the fact that this factor typically appears as "hard data" in the form of numbers often leads teachers and administrators to exaggerate its importance.

The subjective opinion of teachers and pupils is another potent evaluative factor that requires careful interpretation. Enthusiasm and interest on the part of the children are usually an indication that valuable learning is taking place, and the same can be said in regard to teacher enthusiasm. Occasionally the satisfaction of pupil and/or teachers is based upon the entertainment value of the subject matter rather than its intrinsic worth; however, such positive reactions when coupled with other external evidence that the content is indeed relevant provide strong evidence of a good program.

EXTERNAL FEATURES.   Although less direct, the external features of a health education program are equally as important as are indications of pupil response because of the greater assessibility. These features were discussed in Chapter 15 under the general headings of the availability of (1) a health supervisor or resource person, (2) a well-planned health curriculum, (3) adequate instructional resources, (4) sufficient time allotments, and (5) specific professional training in health on the part of the teacher. The presence of these features in a particular program provides evidence that the teachers have a good opportunity to teach and that the children have an opportunity to learn about health.

Generally, where such conditions prevail one will find that effective learning is taking place and that improvement is taking place in the health practices of the children involved. But like the person with no apparent physical abnormalities who nonetheless does not function well, school programs sometime fail to produce good results even when all the visible components of the program seem to be strong. The health supervisor may be well trained but possess an abrasive personality that prevents him or her from working effectively with the teacher; the curriculum may have a beautiful design and an impressive array of concepts and behavioral objectives, yet be inappropriate to the particular needs of the pupils. These and other flaws in a program that "looks good on paper" may not be revealed until one systematically polls the opinion of the teachers, test scores of the pupils, and other more direct indicators. In this manner human reactions and external features serve to cross-validate one another.

THE CRUCIAL COMPONENT

Despite all the recent improvements in the design of school curricula and the effectiveness of teaching materials and media, the teacher remains unchallenged as the single most important factor determining the quality of any educational program. Although teachers can find some compensation in this importance, it does make them the target of considerable scrutiny and criticism. One authority described health progress as the "periodic redefining of the unacceptable" to illustrate the open-ended quality of that particular endeavor. It seems clear that this definition can be applied to progress in education as well; if teachers are to gain enduring satisfaction from their jobs, they must, among other things, learn to thrive in an atmosphere of criticism.

The solution to this general problem appears to be bound up with the general concept of professionalism. The true professionals, although recognizing appropriate authority, are above all working for themselves in their own unique way. They have internalized the goals of their profession; they see intrinsic value in their work. They tend to be more critical of their own performance than outside evaluators, and their own self-evaluation tends to be more important than any formal plan that the school district might implement. At its best, self-evaluation leads to the real satisfaction of continuous professional growth, reduced anxiety concerning outside criticism, and, as a frequent fringe benefit, the recognition, promotions, salary advancement, and other advantages that often accompany good performance.

Good programs of teacher training tend to equip the new teacher with tools needed for self-evaluation even though they may not be explicitly taught. Generally, this process can be effectively carried out if one keeps in mind the same basic categories that outside evaluators might employ. These are as follows:

1. *Professional Training*. In regard to health teaching, the teacher might ask: Have I had at least one health course? Do I need more such training for specialized topics such as sex education or mental health? Am I reasonably prepared in both knowledge of subject matter and skill in the use of appropriate teaching techniques?

2. *Class Preparation*. In regard to any subject, the teacher might ask: Have I planned carefully in terms of both the overall unit of study and the individual presentations for each lesson? Did I review the subject matter? Search for interesting media or materials? Select teaching techniques appropriate to the intended learning experiences?

3. *Teaching Behavior*. Here the teacher might ask: Did my actions in the classroom serve to implement the lesson effectively? Did I display enthusiasm? Explain assignments clearly? Deal effectively with off-task behavior? Adjust to individual needs and situations?

4. *Pupil Response*. Did the children display interest in the assignment? Did they work effectively? Did they show evidence of knowledge gain? Attitudinal change? Behavioral change?

Although individual teachers can learn to become quite objective in regard to their own work, it is a good idea to recognize the vital role that others, particularly professional colleagues, can play in one's search for the truth. The sharing of the problems, frustrations, and satisfaction of one's job with other teachers provides one with the opportunity to bring strengths and weaknesses into sharper focus. Throughout this sharing process it is best kept in mind that the personal needs of other teachers often influence what they tell you of their own teaching experiences and how they respond to your reports. Some will be quite honest and sincere, but other more insecure types may be simply interested in sharing excuses for poor work or may talk as if they have all the answers and no problems in an effort to reassure themselves that they are competent.

Formal evaluative efforts in the form of classroom observations by principals, supervisors, or other such persons usually provide the opportunity to gain a truer picture of one's own effectiveness provided that one trusts the competence and constructive intentions of the visitor. Throughout the total process of self-evaluation, one needs to strike a balance between excessive emphasis on one's shortcomings and an equally irrational refusal to consider them.

REFERENCES

"Alternatives to Grading" (special series of ten articles). *Educational Leadership*, Vol. 32, No. 4 (January 1975), pp. 243–277.

ANASTASI, ANNE. *Psychological Testing*. New York: Macmillan Publishing Co., Inc., 1976.

COMBS, ARTHUR W. *Educational Accountability*. Washington, D.C.: Association for Curriculum Development, 1972.

CRONBACH, LEE J. *Essentials of Psychological Testing*. New York: Harper & Row, 1970.

GLASSER, WILLIAM. *Schools Without Failure*. New York: Harper & Row, 1969.

GRONLUND, NORMAN. *Measurement and Evaluation in Teaching*. New York: Macmillan Publishing Co., Inc., 1976.

GRONLUND, NORMAN. *Preparing for Criterion-Referenced Tests for Classroom Instruction*. New York: Macmillan Publishing Co., Inc., 1973.

HASTINGS, J. THOMAS. "Evaluation in Health Education," *The Journal of School Health*, Vol. XL, No. 10 (December 1970), pp. 519–522.

KIRSCHENBAUM, HOWARD, RODNEY NAPIER, and SIDNEY B. SIMON. *Wad-ja-get? The Grading Game in American Education*. New York: Hart Publishing Company, Inc., 1971.

MAGER, ROBERT F. *Developing Attitudes Towards Learning*. Palo Alto, Calif.: Fearon Publishers, 1968.

REMMERS, H. H., N. L. GAGE, and J. FRANCIS RUMMEL. *A Practical Introduction to Measurement and Evaluation*. New York: Harper & Row, 1965.

SOLLEDER, MARION K. "Evaluation in the Cognitive Domain," *The Journal of School Health*, Vol. 42, No. 1 (January 1972), pp. 16–20.

WILHELMS, FRED T. (editor). *Evaluation as Feedback and Guide*. Washington, D.C.: Association for Supervision and Curriculum Development, 1967.

Index